CLINICAL PROCEDURES
for the Canadian
MEDICAL OFFICE ASSISTANT

CLINICAL PROCEDURES

for the Canadian

MEDICAL OFFICE ASSISTANT

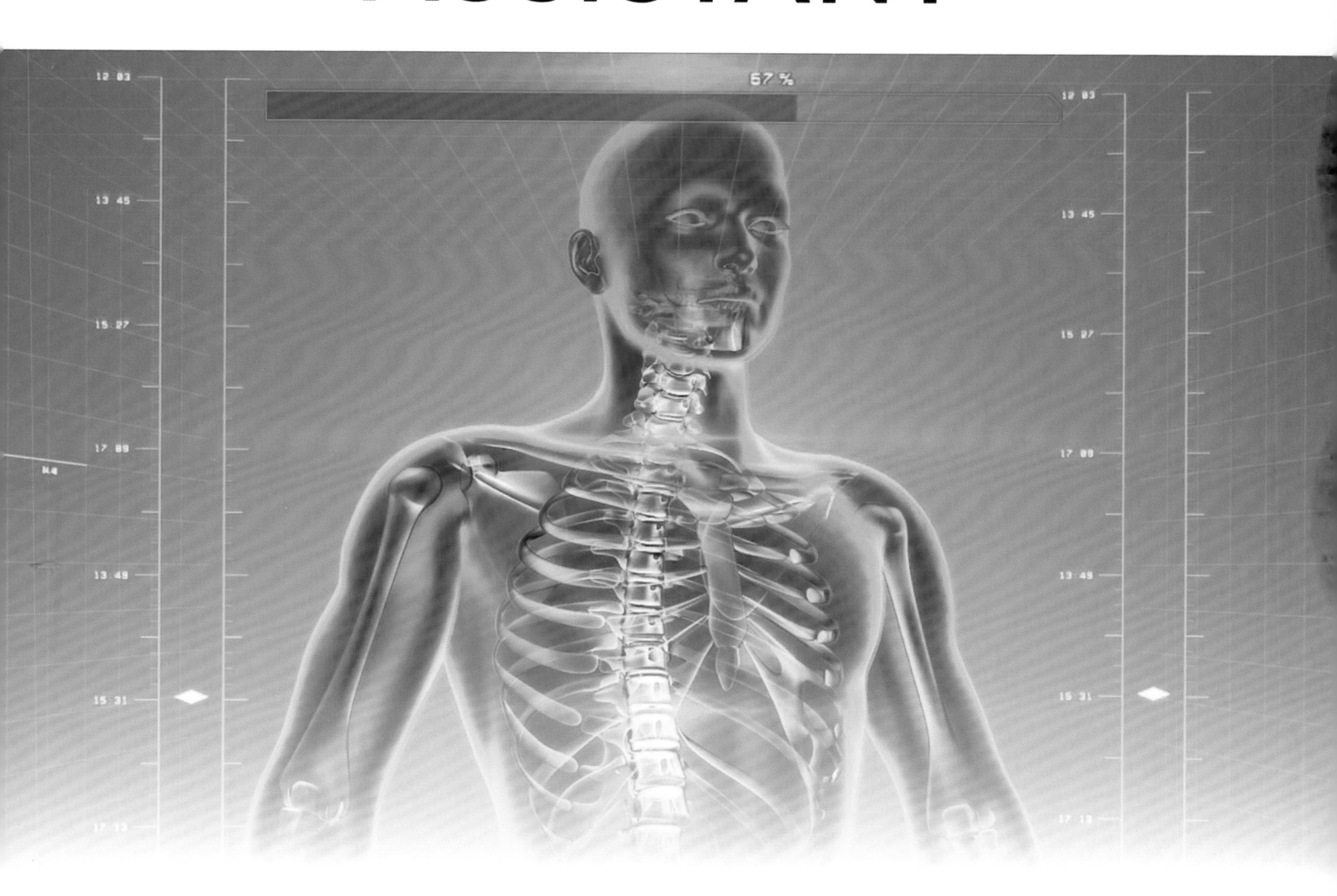

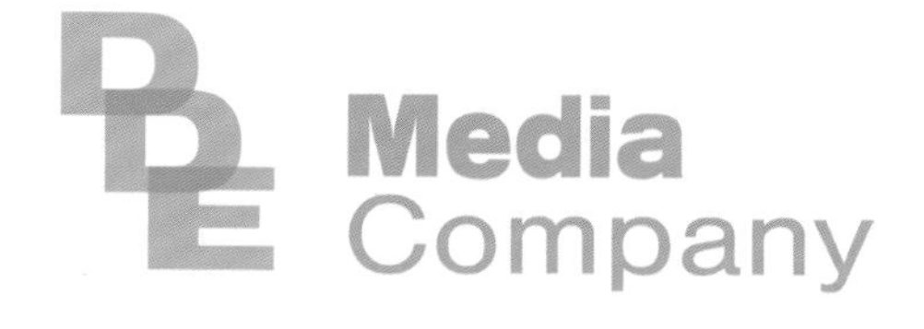

Clinical Procedures for the Canadian Medical Office Assistant

DDE Media Company

Guelph, ON

Printed in China.

1 2 3 4 11 10 9 8 7

Library and Archives Canada Cataloging in Publication

ISBN 978-0-9940225-9-2

Writers: Sandy Ho, Adrien Potvin, Lyle Shepherd

Editorial Director: Lyle Shepherd

Proofreaders: John Charles, Jessica Groom, and Jason Regular.

Layout Design & Illustrations: Cornelia Svela

Cover: Photo (upper left): “Selected by freepik”

Special thanks to Amy Pytolowany for her guidance and expertise and to Michele Brydges for her help with the photos in this textbook.

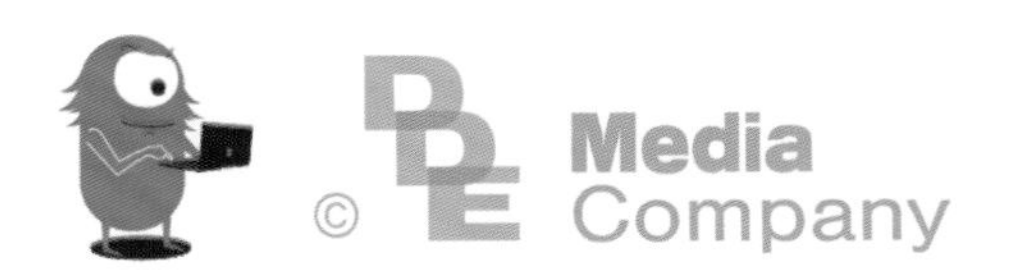

Contents

1 Clinical Infection Theory 1

2 Standard Procedures for Preventing the Spread of Infection 37

3 Standards and Safety 71

4 Drugs, Prescription, and Handling Patient Prescription Requests 91

5 Diagnostic Testing Theory 123

6 Types of Testing 131

7 Diagnostic Imaging 155

8 Assisting with Physical Examinations and Assessment Procedures 193

Chapter 1

Clinical Infection Theory

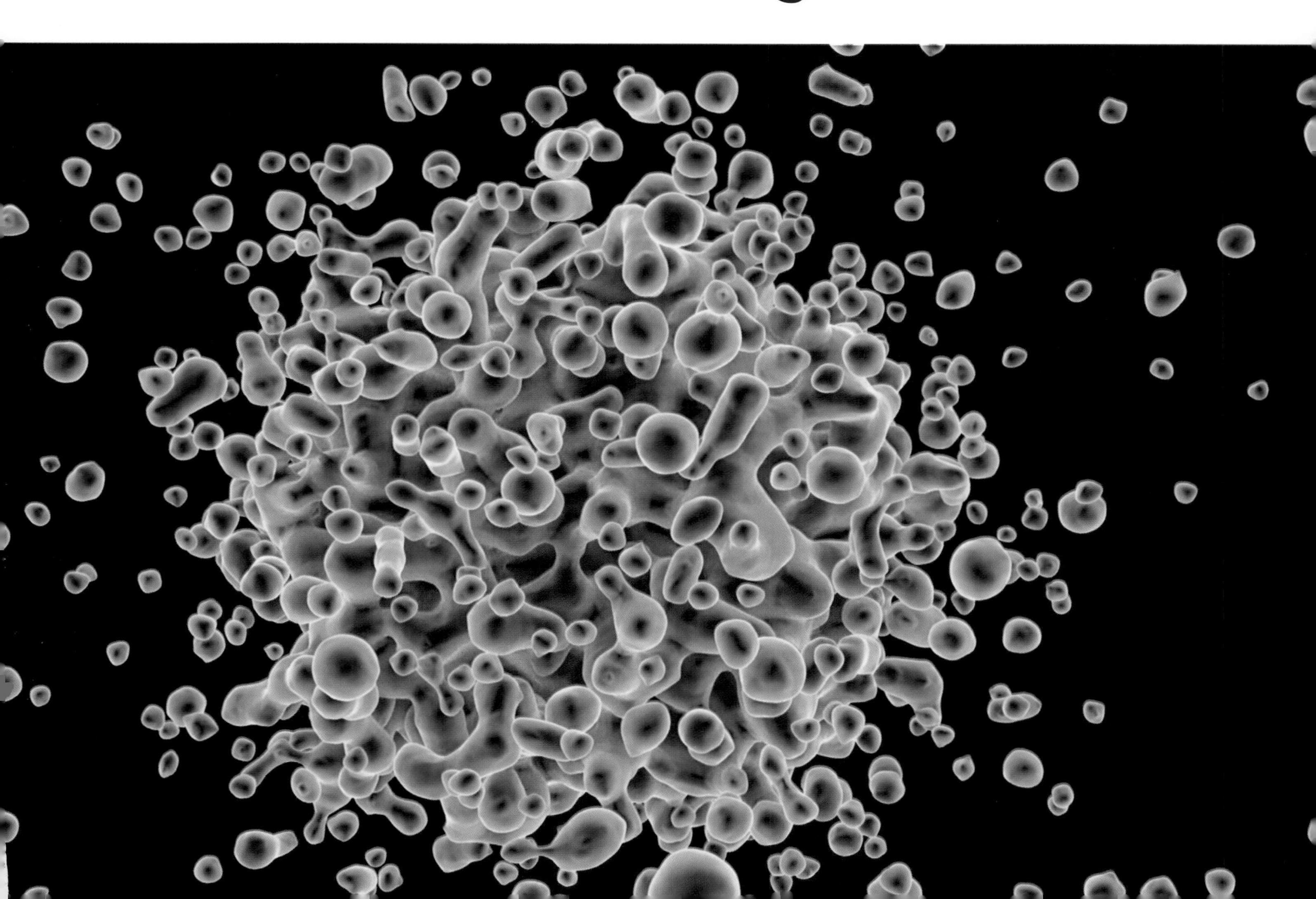

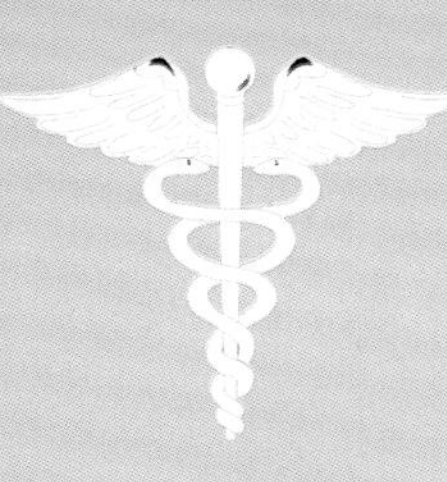

CHAPTER ONE LEARNING OBJECTIVES

After completing this chapter, you should be able to:

- ❑ Define the term infection
- ❑ Understand and explain the stages of infection
- ❑ Identify and define microorganisms
- ❑ Classify different types of bacteria
- ❑ Distinguish the difference between Gram-positive and Gram-negative bacteria through gram staining
- ❑ Describe viruses, fungi, and protozoa
- ❑ Understand and explain the patterns of infection
- ❑ Describe the chain of infection
- ❑ Recognize the different immune system defences
- ❑ Define and explain immunity, and the role that vaccines play
- ❑ Know the recommended immunizations and tests for health professionals

Infection

An infection is a disease process resulting from the entry and spread of microorganisms such as bacteria, viruses, and parasites that are not normally present in the body. Many common infectious diseases have human reservoirs, but may or may not show the effects of an illness. It is important for medical office assistants to recognize the signs and symptoms that indicate when an infection is present.

Infection: *A disease process that results from the entry and spread of a microorganism such as bacteria, viruses, and parasites not normally present in the body.*

Knowing these signs and symptoms will allow the medical office assistant to be mindful when scheduling a patient's appointment—if signs of an acute infection are present, it is a clear indication that the patient should be seen sooner rather than later.

Infection can be introduced whenever there is exposure to an unprotected or vulnerable area of the body. Broken skin, wounds, insect bites, ingestion, inhalation, or even direct contact can result in infection.

When an infection is a possibility, the medical office assistant must know how to prepare the patient for assessment. This includes taking the patient's temperature and asking the appropriate questions to obtain a medical history.

Body temperature is a good indicator of a potential infection. If a person has a fever, infection may be spreading (**sepsis**) throughout their body and they need to be seen by a physician right away. An infection may remain localized, or it may spread through the body via blood or lymphatic vessels. A medical office assistant should warn patients that when certain symptoms arise, they should seek medical attention as soon as possible.

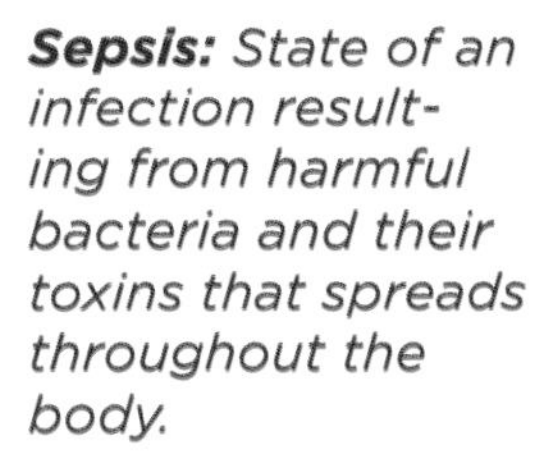

Sepsis: *State of an infection resulting from harmful bacteria and their toxins that spreads throughout the body.*

When a patient presents with a wound, symptoms of serious illness include:

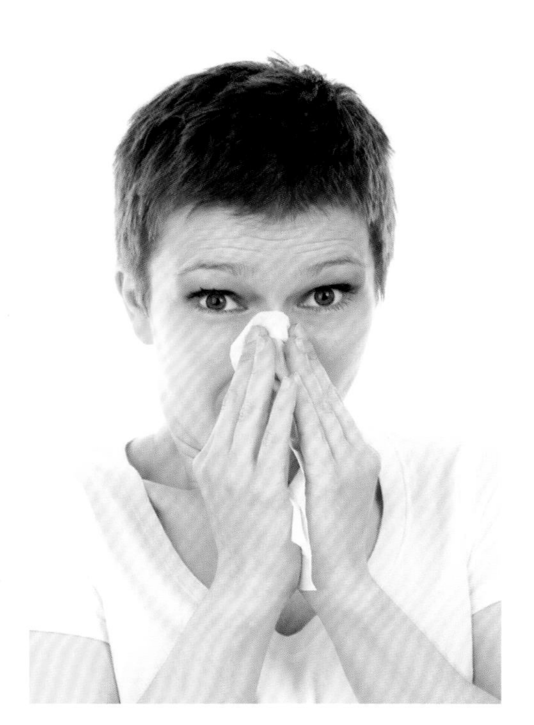

- Fever
- Persistent or increased pain, swelling, or draining of fluid from the wound
- Red streaks radiating away from the wound
- Increases in redness or warmth around the wound

Infected individuals should contact their physician to ensure early diagnosis and treatment before symptoms worsen. Catching an infection early increases the probability and speed of recovery.

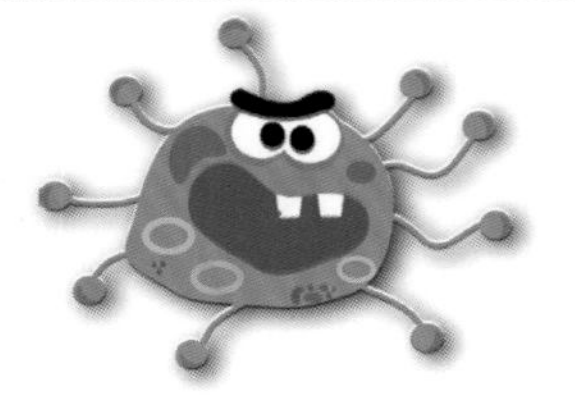

Stages of an Infectious Disease

Pathogen: *A microorganism or biological agent that can cause disease.*

Latent period: *The time from initial infection until the start of infectiousness.*

Incubation period: *The length of time it takes between the initial infection and the individual displaying the first symptoms of the disease*

Prodromal period: *The period where early symptoms, such as a headache, suggest the approach of the disease.*

Period of communicability: *The time during which an infectious agent can be transmitted directly or indirectly from an infected person to another person, from an infected animal to humans, or from an infected person to animals.*

Acute period: *When the disease and its symptoms are at their strongest.*

Pathogens, which are microorganisms or biological agents that can cause disease, are important to understand for anyone working in the medical field. A thorough understanding of when a worker is at risk will protect everyone in the medical office against infectious diseases.

There are five stages of disease occurring after a person is exposed to an infectious pathogen. These stages are: exposure, incubation, prodromal, acute, decline, and convalescent periods. When discussing contagiousness, there are two stages. There is also a latent stage and a period of communicability.

1. After a host is infected, there will be a period where they are not contagious and another in which they are shedding the contagion. These are known as the **latent period** and the **period of communicability**.

2. The **incubation period** is the first stage following infection before the individual will begin to display symptoms of the infectious disease. The length of the incubation period varies based on the type of disease. During incubation, the pathogens will continue to reproduce.

3. During the **prodromal period**, the **period of communicability** begins, during which the infected individual (human or animal) can transmit the infectious agent to another person or animal.

4. The infected individual enters the **acute period** when the infectious disease and its symptoms are at their strongest. Symptoms, such as fever, can present at their worst.

5. Symptoms of the disease begin to taper off during the **decline period**, marking the start of the recovery process.

6. The individual completes the recovery process and returns to good health in the **convalescent period**.

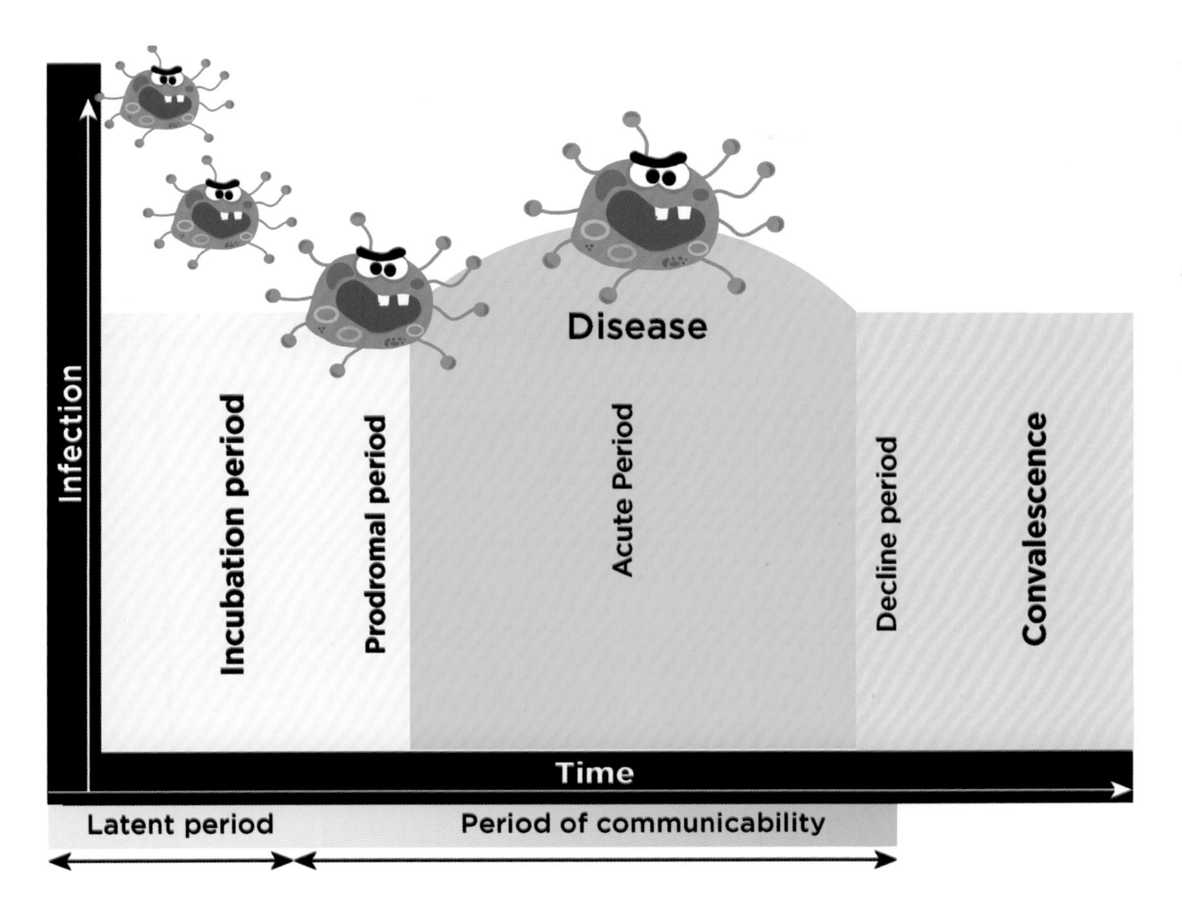

Decline period: *Time during which symptoms of the disease taper off.*

Convalescent period: *Stage in which the individual returns to good health.*

The pandemic outbreak of H1N1 virus in 2009 is a good example of the necessity of infection prevention and control measures. Originally referred to as "swine flu" as it also circulates in pigs, the contagious H1N1 flu virus caused a worldwide panic when it first surfaced, as many people started developing flu-like symptoms. The spread of this virus was rapid and made its way around the world, causing more serious complications such as pneumonia and respiratory failure

The H1N1 virus still continues to circulate, but without the same vigour as the first outbreak, thanks to the flu vaccine. The Centers for Disease Control and Prevention (CDC) have tracked seasonal flu activity, including H1N1. It's hard to tell the difference between seasonal flu and swine flu symptoms, but a lab test should clear up any questions.

The development of new products, medical equipment, techniques, and clinical procedures must change as new infections are identified. New standards, directives, and guidelines should be developed by provincial, national, and international organizations, followed by updated medical practices to keep patients and health care workers safe.

Practicing good medical asepsis techniques, living a healthy lifestyle, obtaining proper rest, and using good hygienic measures all play a part in helping to prevent and control the transmission of infectious diseases. Medical office assistants must aid in the education of patients about daily living practices that help to reduce the transmission of pathogens. Spreading accurate information helps in the control of infectious diseases.

Microorganisms: *Organisms that are tiny living plants or animals so small that they can only be seen under a microscope.*

Virulence: *The power of a microbe to produce disease in a particular host.*

Microorganisms

Microorganisms are tiny living organisms so small they can only be seen under a microscope. There are three different types of microorganisms that can either be harmful or helpful to us, such as viruses, bacteria, and fungi. As a medical office assistant, there are many opportunities to come into contact with potentially harmful microorganisms, so it is essential to practice good hygiene to avoid transmitting microorganisms between people, equipment, and surfaces.

The power of a pathogen to produce disease in a particular host is its **virulence**. Virulence is determined by both the potency of the strain of organism and the number of organisms present in the body. Let's look at the different types of microorganisms

Types of Microorganisms

Normal (Resident) Flora

Resident flora: *Non-pathogenic microbes that exist on all surfaces of the body that are exposed to the external environment.*

Naturally present in the human body, these life-long microbes are a part of the body's normal microbial community. **Resident flora** exists on all parts of the body exposed to the external environment, including the skin, urinary tract, respiratory tract, and gastrointestinal tract.

In their normal environment, they are non-pathogenic and often beneficial, as they feed on the cellular waste and dead cells of the host's body. Resident flora attaches to the deeper skin layers on your hands where basic hand washing does not typically reach. A problem arises when resident flora from one system invades another system. The invading flora is often pathogenic.

For example, E. coli exists normally in the lower gastrointestinal (GI) tract with no issues, but if it manages to make its way into the urinary tract, an infection occurs.

Another example of the benefit of resident flora is the breakdown of certain vitamins such as vitamins B and K. As it is difficult for your body to break these vitamins down, preventing other microorganisms from colonizing. This is a good thing!

Transient flora

Transient flora: *Microbes that grow and develop on superficial skin layers.*

Transient flora, which is often pathogenic and lives and develops on the superficial skin layers, can be thought of as tourists that are just passing through. This type of flora may attempt to colonize in some areas, but is unable to remain in the body for extended periods. The body has defence mechanisms to prevent transient flora from colonizing; including competition from established resident microbes, the body's own immune system, and physical or chemical changes within the body that discourage the growth of transient microbes.

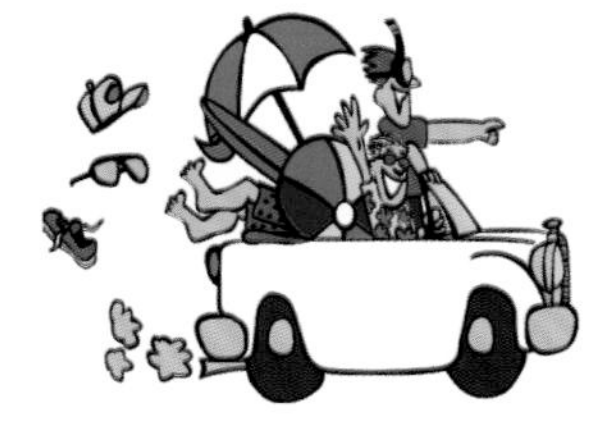

People often pick up transient flora on their hands during regular daily activities. In a medical office environment, a medical office assistant is at risk when interacting with infected patients, equipment, and contaminated surfaces. You can easily remove transient flora by engaging in the proper hand washing technique as it is only loosely attached to your skin.

Medical office assistants preparing for a well-baby exam, or working in the neonatal care department in the hospital, may find themselves exposed to higher levels of bacterial contamination. Routine neonatal care exposes medical assistants to bacterial contamination in a number of ways: respiratory secretions, diaper changes, and direct skin contact with patients.

The transmission between individuals depends on the species of microorganism present, the number of microorganisms on the surface, and skin moisture.

Bacteria

Bacteria are single-celled organisms that multiply by cell division and can be pathogenic or non-pathogenic. All bacteria need moisture, nutrients, warmth, and darkness to thrive. Some bacteria also need oxygen—these bacteria are known as **aerobes**. Bacteria that do not need oxygen are known as **anaerobes**.

Bacteria: *Single-celled organisms that multiply by cell division and can be pathogenic or non-pathogenic.*

Aerobes: *Bacteria that require oxygen to survive.*

Anaerobes: *Bacteria that do not require oxygen to survive.*

Microorganisms found on uncooked foods can be killed when the food is cooked properly at the required temperature. Food that is not fresh, or has not been cooked properly, may contain harmful microorganisms. In the medical office, designate a fridge for food to be consumed by people and a separate fridge for storing patient laboratory samples. Avoid contamination and the transfer of harmful microorganisms by posting signs to clarify the purpose of the fridges.

While bacteria are normally assumed to be pathogens, not all bacteria are harmful. There are useful microorganisms in the body and even in foods that we eat, such as yeast in bread (used to make dough rise), or the use of bacteria and fungi for cheese making. Yogourt is made by boiling milk with added bacteria to turn the milk's sugar into acid. The acid then thickens the milk and prevents any harmful bacteria from growing.

Classification of Bacteria

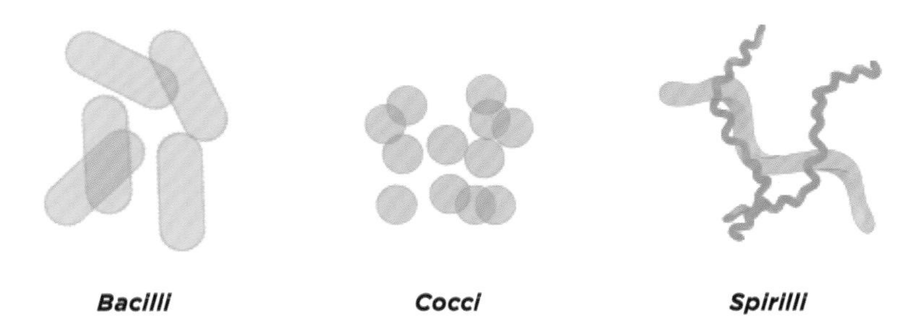

Bacteria are classified by their need for oxygen, response to stains, and their shape. When examining which type of bacteria is present under a microscope, there are distinctive ways to differentiate the bacteria that is on the slide. It is crucial to classify bacteria and not confuse them with viruses, as this can lead to misdiagnoses. This is especially important when it comes to prescribing antibiotics—antibiotics combat and control bacteria; they are not effective on viral infections.

Cocci

Cocci: *Bacteria that is spherical in shape.*

Cocci are spherical and fit into one of several groups. Grape-like clusters are known as *Staphylococci* and can be found in pus production, like abscesses and infected wounds. All Staphylococcus have a layer of slime that protects the bacteria from drying out on our salty skin and allows it to adhere to surfaces. This allows the Staphylococcus to take up space and resources making it hard for non-resident flora bacteria to grow.

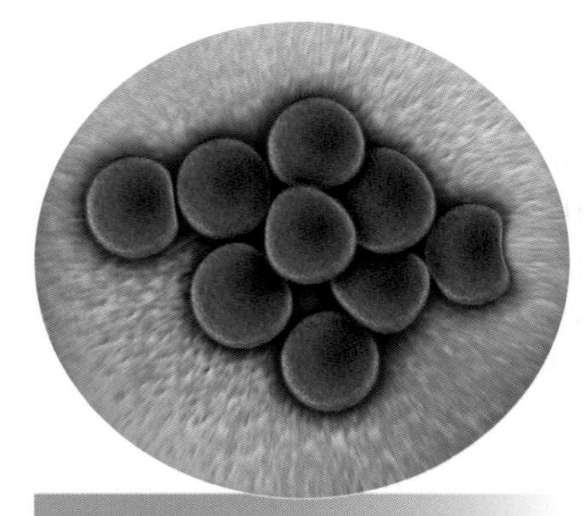

Staphylococci

The slimy layer acts like a biofilm, and this can be problematic when it begins to grow on internal medical devices such as catheters.

Streptococci are chains of bacteria, often found with strep throat and septicemia. When a patient displays symptoms of strep throat, the doctor must confirm this diagnosis by identifying the streptococci bacteria. The symptoms of strep throat can also be the result of a viral infection.

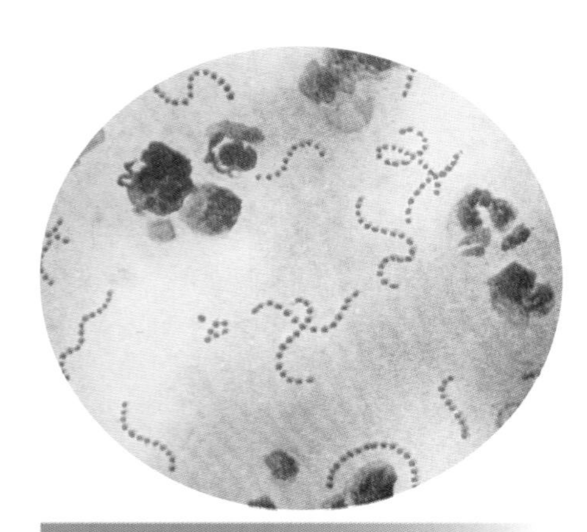

Streptococci

If antibiotics are prescribed for a sore throat that is the result of a viral infection, there will be no effect from the antibiotic. This might even do more harm than good as the misuse of antibiotics is linked to the growing problem of antibiotic resistance.

Streptococcal infections are communicable diseases that develop when bacteria normally found on the skin, intestines, mouth, nose, reproductive tract, or urinary tract invade other parts of the body and contaminate blood or tissues. Bacterial tests are invaluable, as some strep infections do not exhibit symptoms in patients but can still be fatal if the bacteria infect blood or tissues.

Diplococci can be distinguished under the microscope as round pairs (as a result of incomplete cell division), and are found as parasites or saprophytes. Diplococci are responsible for infectious diseases such as meningitis, pneumonia, and gonorrhea.

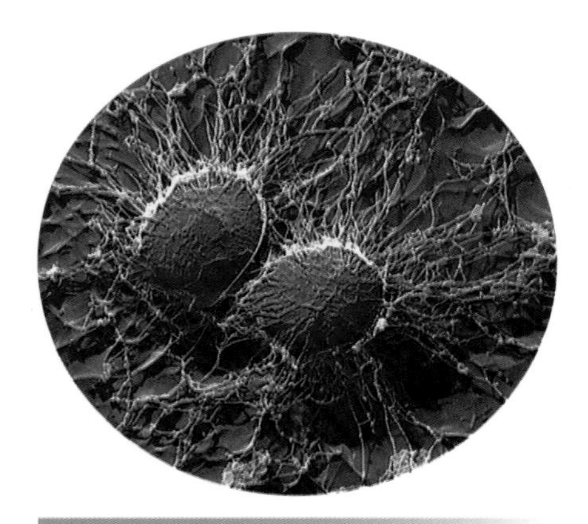

Diplococci

Bacilli

Bacilli are rod-shaped bacteria that can be found in patients with tuberculosis, tetanus, and diphtheria. Some bacilli are able to form spores, which provides them with the ability to resist adverse conditions such as disinfectants and heat. This bacterium is common in the body, but if it enters the urinary tract due to poor hygiene or lowered resistance, it may cause a urinary tract infection (UTI).

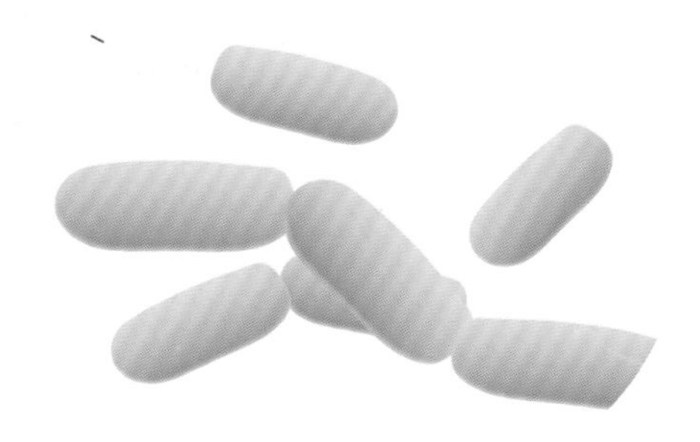

Bacilli

Bacilli: *rod-shaped bacteria.*

Clinical manifestations have been found in a wide range of infections, including abscesses, bacteremia/septicemia, wound and burn infections, ear infections, endocarditis, meningitis, ophthalmitis, osteomyelitis, peritonitis, and respiratory and urinary tract infections. Most of these infections are secondary or mixed infections, or they occur in immune-compromised individuals. This is the reason elderly and younger people are more susceptible to infections.

Spirilla

Spirilla are long and spiral shaped bacteria. The illnesses syphilis and cholera are a result of spirilla bacteria. Illnesses caused by spirilla can be detected using blood tests. Cholera results from a different strain of spirillum, Vibrio cholerae. To eliminate these bacteria, proper methods of sanitation and water purification are crucial.

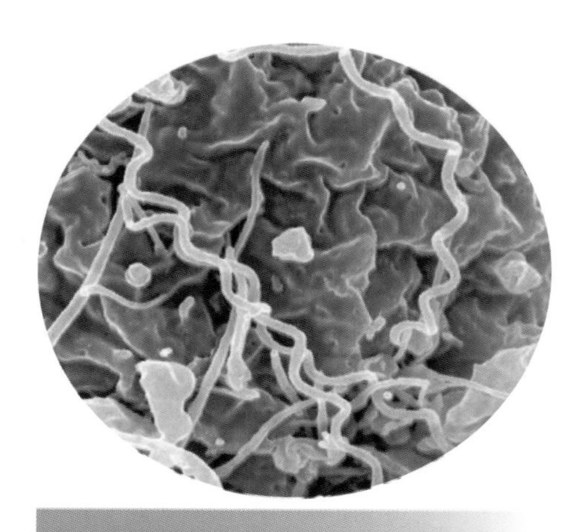

Spirilla

- Syphilis

Spirilla: *Spiral or curve-shaped bacteria.*

Bacteria and viruses are responsible for causing human diseases—for a physician to reach a proper diagnosis and prescribe the correct medication, the cause and type of infection must be identified. Further testing, such as staining, may be required to determine the type of bacteria present.

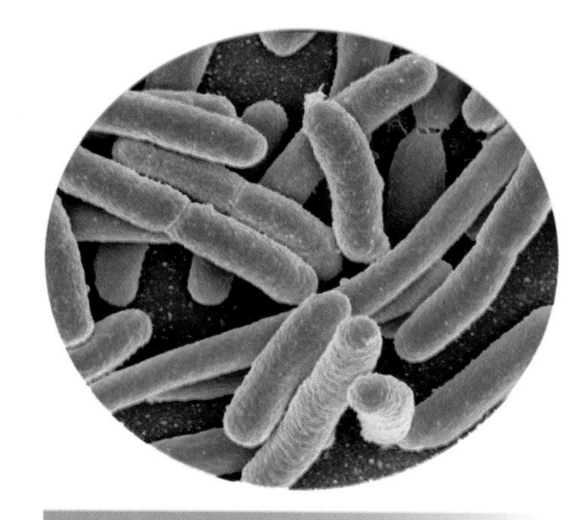

Spirilla

- Cholera

Activity

BACTERIAL CLASSIFICATION

Draw an example of the following bacterial shapes.

Cocci	Bacilli	Spirilla

Staining Gram-positive and Gram-negative Bacteria

The technique used to differentiate these two groups of bacteria is based on the differences in cell wall constituents, which are determined by coloring the cells either red or violet. Staining allows the observer to view the shape, size, and growth pattern of the bacteria. Classifying which bacteria are present helps a physician to reach an accurate diagnosis.

How Does Gram Staining Work?

Gram staining is a three-step process: staining with water-soluble dye called crystal violet, de-colorization, and counterstaining with another dye (usually safranin). The difference in thickness of a peptidoglycan layer in the cell membrane between Gram-positive and Gram-negative allows for the gram staining to work.

In order for this to be done properly, the cells must be stained with a crystal violet dye. Next, a Gram's iodine solution is added to form a complex between the crystal violet and iodine. Gram-positive bacteria will stain violet due to the presence of a thicker layer of peptidoglycan in their cell wall. The cell wall retains the crystal violet that has been stained.

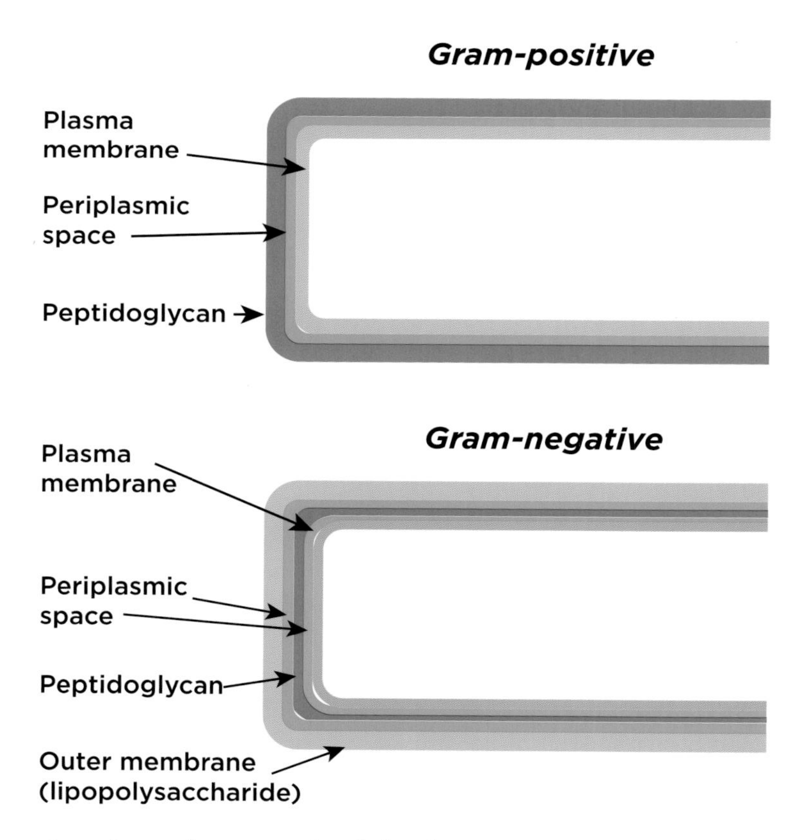

Gram-negative bacteria stains red as a result of the thinner peptidoglycan wall. It doesn't retain the crystal violet during the decolouring process, where it is stained by the safranin in the final staining process. This is explained in "How To: Staining Sample Slides" on the following page.

How to

STAINING SAMPLE SLIDES

Equipment/supplies needed:

- **Crystal violet (primary stain)**
- **Iodine solution/Gram's Iodine**
- **Decolourizer**
- **Safranin (secondary stain)**
- **Water (preferably in a squirt bottle)**
- **Slide forceps**
- **Sterile swab**
- **Microbiological specimen**
- **Clean glass slide**

1. Wash and sanitize your hands following the proper hand washing technique.

2. Wear appropriate laboratory clothing and apply gloves while handling the slide, especially during the staining process. Assemble all of the supplies needed.

3. Obtain a slide and label it with the patient's name and date of birth, as well as the date of sample collection.

4. Hold the slide between your thumb and index finger. Beginning at the right side of the slide, spread the material in a gentle, rolling motion over the slide, ensuring that you make it even. Cover one half to two thirds of the slide with the material. Avoid leaving clumps and rubbing the material over the slide with force. When finished, discard the contaminated swab into a biohazard waste container.

5. Before moving on with the staining process, air-dry the smear for a minimum of 30 minutes.

6. Fix the sample by applying heat to the slide to prevent the cells from rinsing off the slide during the staining process. Use the slide forceps to hold the slide. With caution, quickly pass the slide over a Bunsen burner flame two to three times.

Note: To avoid overheating the sample, make sure that the Bunsen burner flame is a small blue flame and not a tall orange one. If you overheat the sample, this could distort and damage the cells you have collected on your slide.

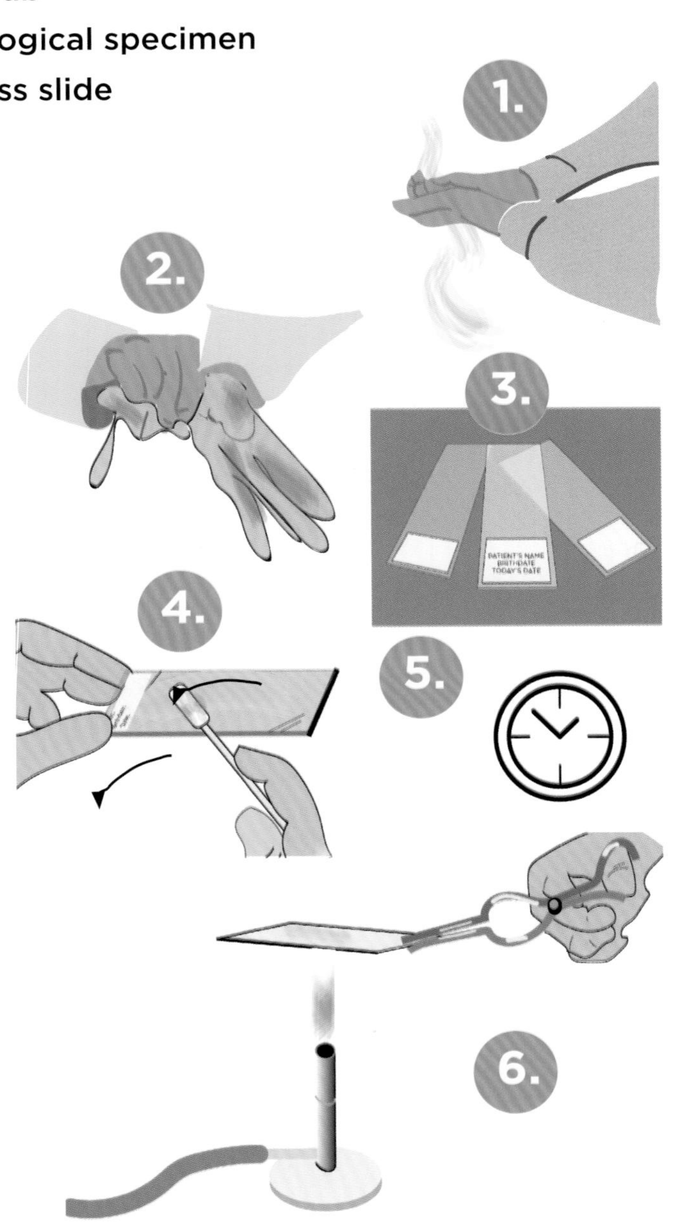

7. Add the primary stain—the crystal violet—to the sample slide, and let it sit for one minute. Rinse the slide with a gentle stream of water from your squirt bottle for a maximum of five seconds to remove any unbound crystal violet.

8. Add Gram's Iodine for one minute. This agent fixes the crystal violet to the bacterial cell wall.

9. Rinse the sample slide with acetone or alcohol for approximately three seconds and rinse with a gentle stream of water. The alcohol will decolourize the sample if it is Gram-negative, removing the crystal violet. However, if the alcohol remains on the sample for too long, you may also decolourize Gram-positive cells.

10. Add the second stain—the safranin—to the slide, and let it sit for approximately one minute. Wash the slide with a gentle stream of water for a maximum of five seconds.

11. Place the slide under the microscope and adjust the settings accordingly until a sharp clear image is formed.

12. If the bacteria cultured are Gram-positive, it will retain the primary stain and none of the second stain, resulting in a violet colour under the microscope. If the bacteria are Gram-negative, it will not retain the primary stain, but instead the secondary stain will hold, resulting in a red appearance under the microscope.

13. Relay the results to the physician and inform the physician that the slide is ready for examination.

14. The physician will record the results on the patient's chart and use the findings to reach a proper diagnosis.

Identifying the proper bacteria present in the specimen helps the physician to properly diagnose the problem. A Gram stain provides valuable information regarding the size, shape, type, and growth of bacteria. These procedures will give the medical office assistant the confidence to accurately distinguish between Gram-positive bacteria and Gram-negative bacteria. Who knew the thickness of the peptidoglycan of a cell wall could play such a crucial role in Gram staining?

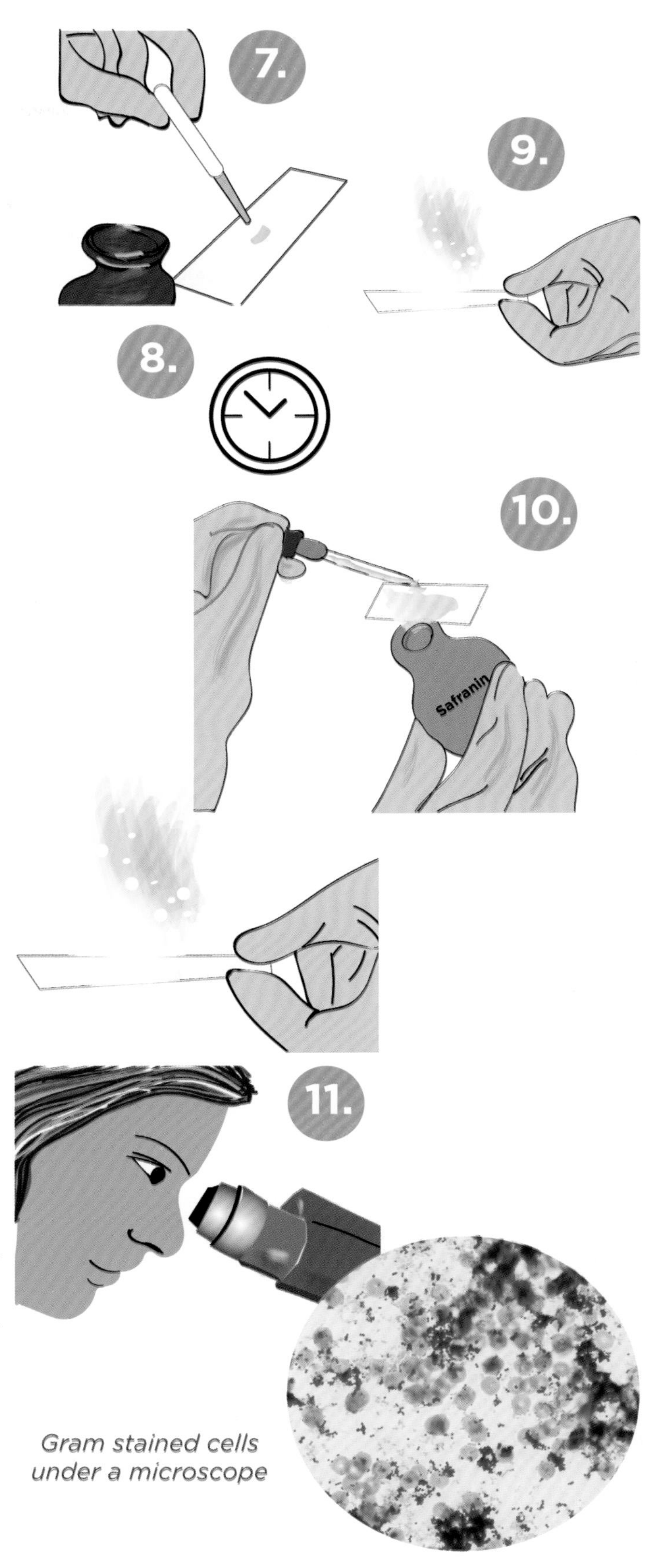

Gram stained cells under a microscope

Activity

GRAM-POSITIVE AND GRAM-NEGATIVE BACTERIA. WHAT'S THE DIFFERENCE?

Draw a diagram of Gram-positive and Gram-negative bacteria. Label the different structures and where the staining will occur after the staining process.

Gram-positive	Gram-negative

Viruses

Viruses are microscopic infectious agents that cannot be seen with a regular light microscope—they require the precision of an electron microscope to be viewed. Viruses cannot live or reproduce on their own, which means they need a host organism to allow metabolic and reproductive functioning. With the ability to infect plants, animals, and humans, viruses can easily spread from one host to another.

Viruses:

Microscopic infectious agents that can alter or damage living cells.

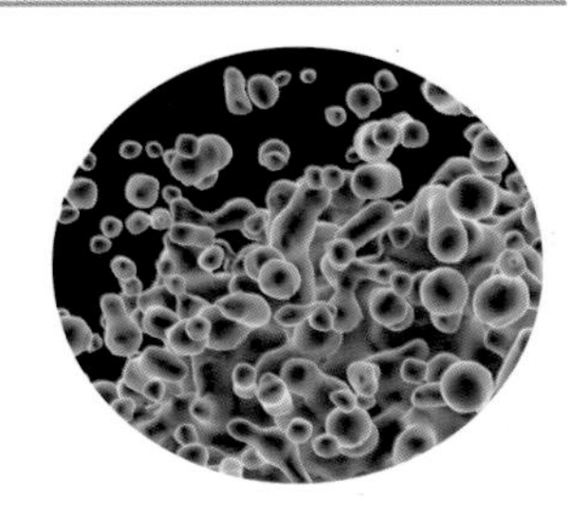

virus

Common viral infections causing infectious diseases include: influenza, chicken pox/shingles, measles, mumps, herpes simplex, hepatitis, and diseases of the upper respiratory tract (including the common cold). Illnesses caused by viruses do not respond to antibiotics—instead, there are antiviral medications that are used against certain viruses.

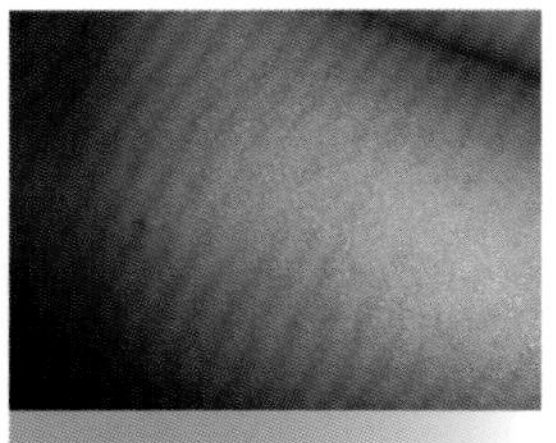

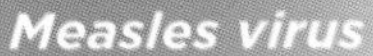

Measles virus

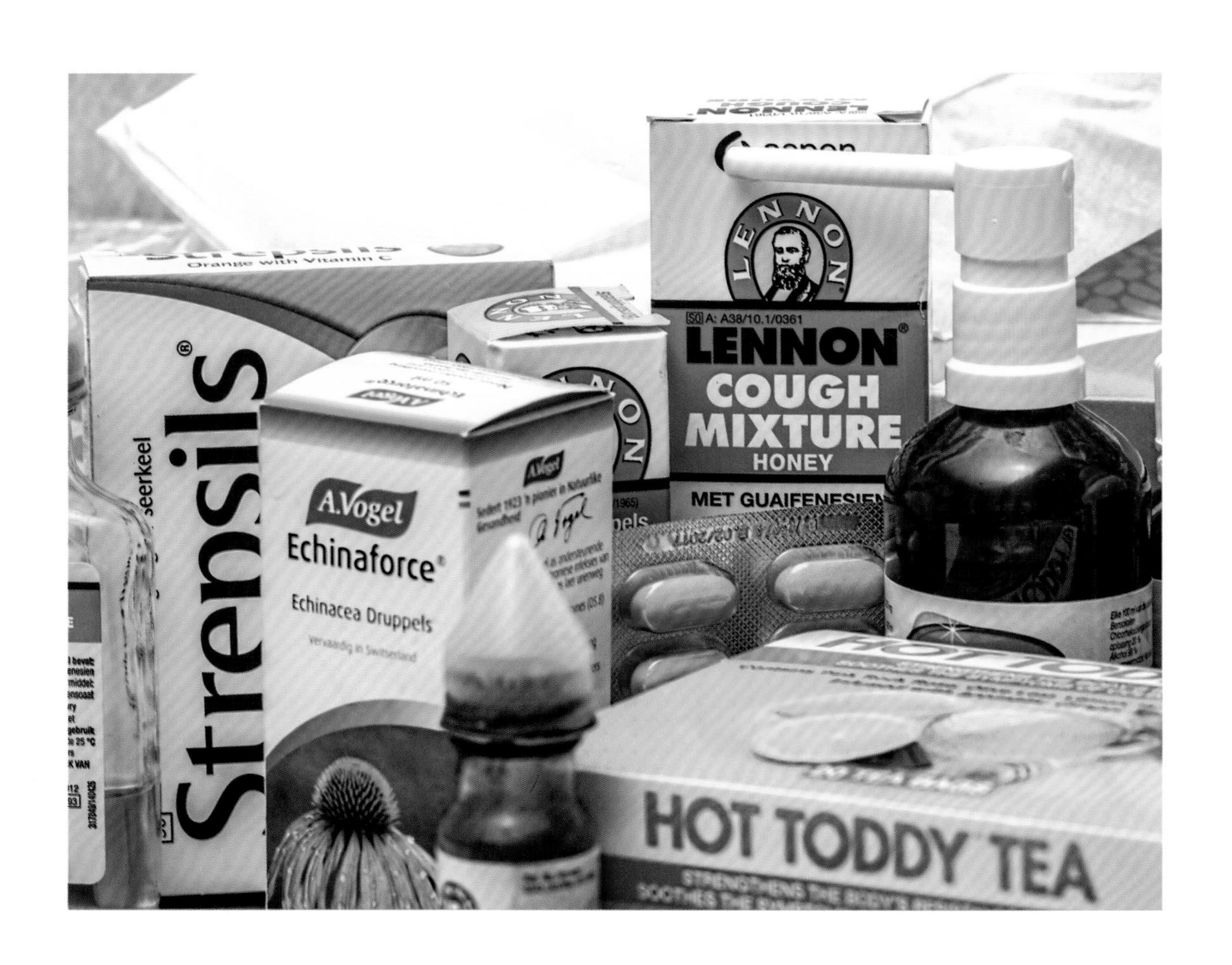

Fungi

***Fungi:** Living organisms that use spores to reproduce and rely on eating other organisms to survive.*

Organisms that use spores to reproduce, such as yeasts and molds, are classified as **fungi**. Fungi survive by metabolizing organic matter, and cannot synthesize their own food like plants can. Existing as single-celled living things such as yeast, and multicellular clusters such as molds or mushrooms, fungi come in a variety of shapes and sizes.

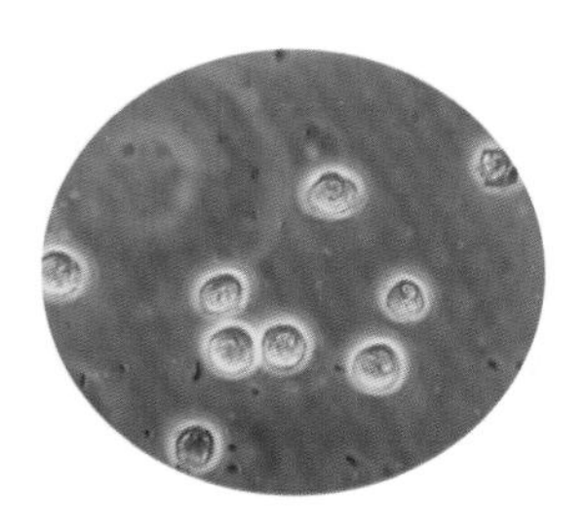

single-celled yeast

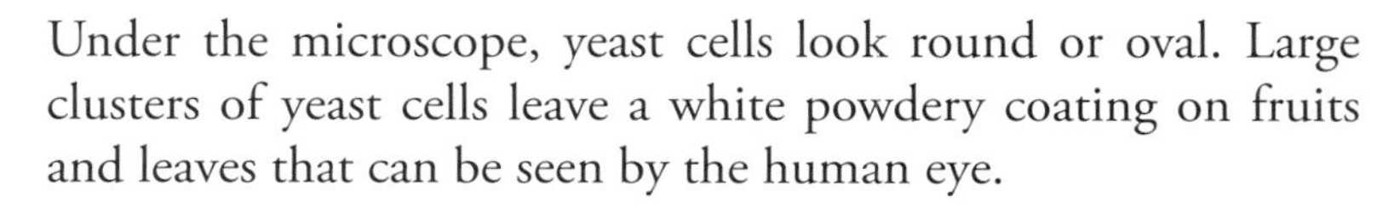

Under the microscope, yeast cells look round or oval. Large clusters of yeast cells leave a white powdery coating on fruits and leaves that can be seen by the human eye.

Molds can also be fuzzy in appearance—this is caused by hyphae, which form long, filament-like strands of cells.

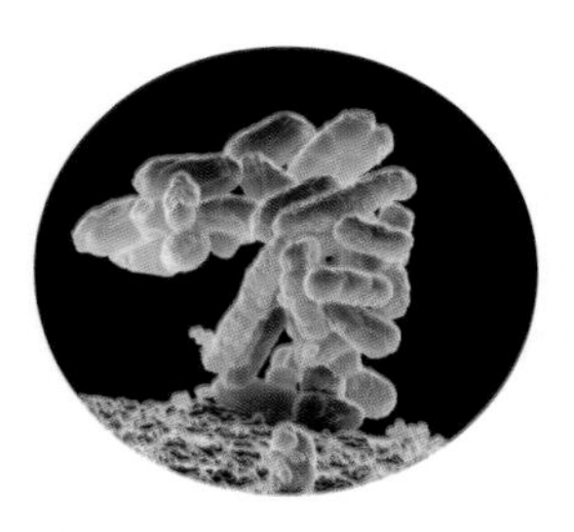

clustered yeast cells

Multicellular fungi have the ability to form fleshy bodies, such as that of a mushroom. It is strange to think that the mushrooms we eat began as tiny microbes!

Reproductive spores help fungi spread by extending their hyphae. In order to grow, fungi absorb nutrients from living or dead organic matter, such as sugars absorbed through cell walls. Special digestive enzymes are given off to help break down complex nutrients, freeing those nutrients for absorption by the fungi.

There are many advantages and disadvantages to fungi. Antibiotics are made from several kinds of fungi that can help fight bacterial infections due to the competitive nature of fungi. The fungi compete against the bacteria for nutrients and space, which results in an effective strategy for clearing up bacterial infections.

As mentioned, fungi are helpful for everyday uses. For example, baker's yeast is used to help bread rise, and plays a role in brewing beer. Very few fungi cause diseases in humans, but those that do can result in discomforts such as Athlete's Foot or yeast infections. Understanding the roles and functions of fungi can not only prevent detrimental fungal infections, but can also be beneficial for developing medicine.

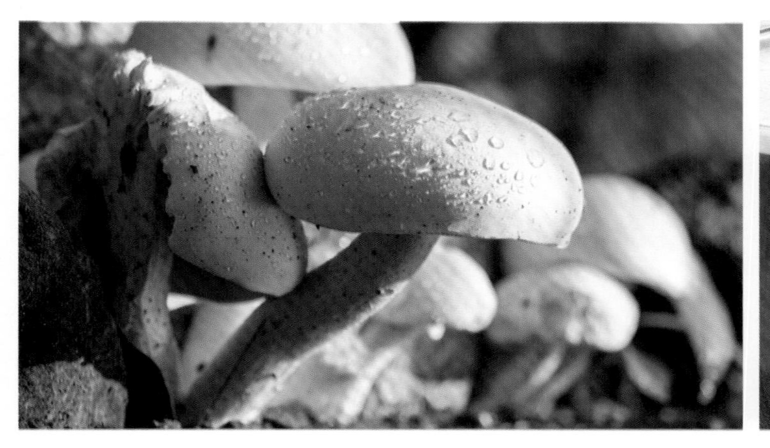

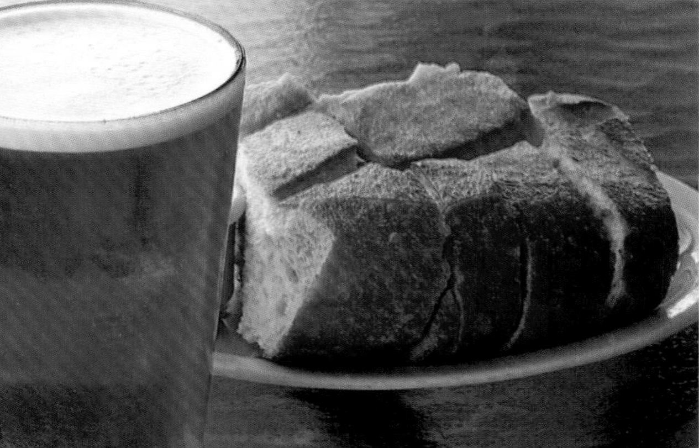

Protozoa

Protozoa are single-celled organisms found in almost every possible habitat. These organisms have a nuclei and organelles, which carry out a variety of functions such as digestion, excretion, respiration, and coordination. With these complex membranes and organelles, protozoa are able to survive harsh environmental conditions. As microscopic organisms, protozoa display essential life activities similar to those of higher metazoan eukaryotes, such as survival, feeding, and reproducing.

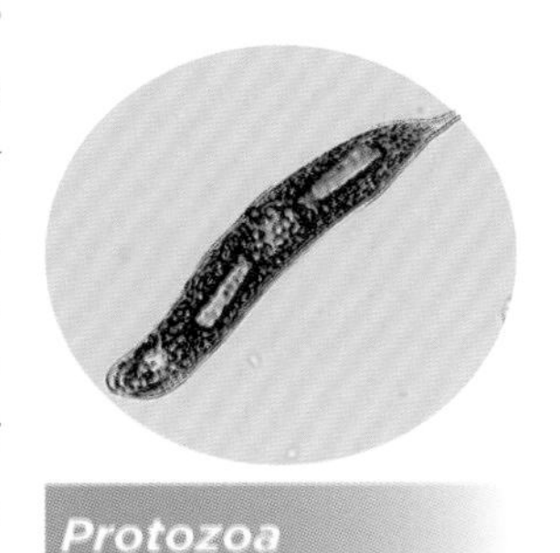
Protozoa

***Protozoa:** Single cell organisms with complex membranes and organelles. They can be harmful and are transmissible in several different ways.*

Harmful protozoa are seldom encountered thanks to water treatment protocols in place by the *Ontario Water Resources Act* and *Environmental Protection Act*. As a result, the water we drink is safe and clean. Illnesses from protozoa arise when water sources are contaminated, or individuals come into contact with untreated water or sewage. Sewage and untreated water sources are the leading causes of giardia and malaria, among other diseases. Infection from protozoa ranges from asymptomatic—showing no symptoms—to life threatening, depending on a few factors:

- the host's resistance;
- the strain of parasite present;
- the species of parasite.

There are many ways to transfer, infect, and transmit protozoa to a person. A person can become ill from giardia through the fecal-oral transmission route. In this case, another person ingests an environmentally-resistant cyst passed through the feces of the original host via food or water. For malaria, this protozoa is a vector-borne transmission where trophozoites (a growing stage in the life cycle of parasites in which they absorb nutrients from the host) are taken up by blood-sucking insects such as mosquitoes, and passed to a new host the next time the vector feeds.

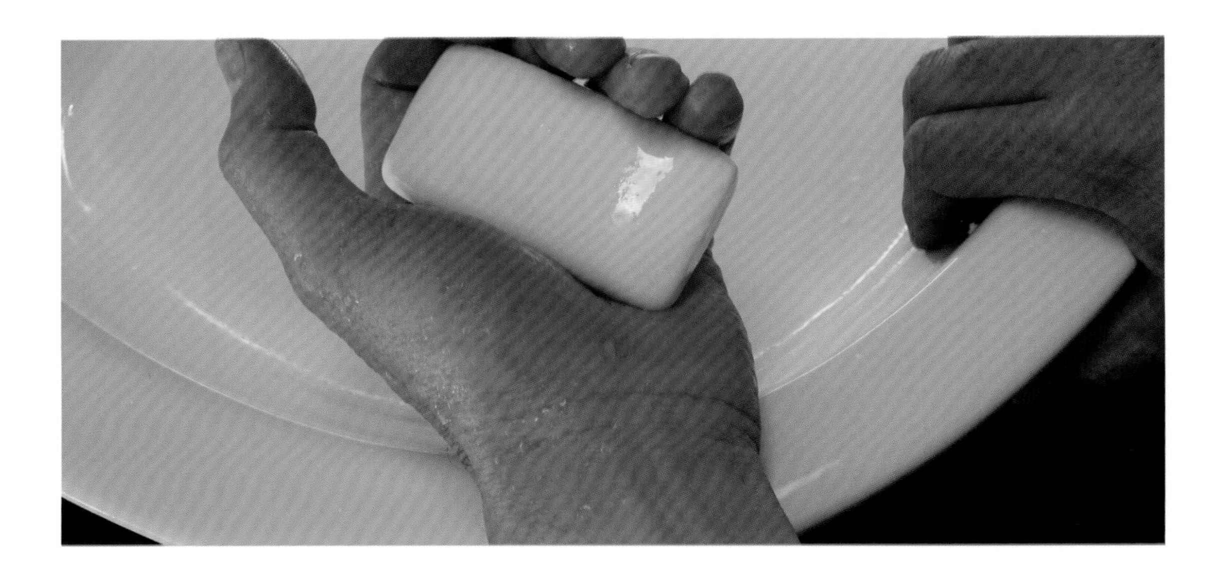

The last two routes of transmission are direct transmission through intimate body contact, such as sexual transmission and predator-prey transmission. The tissue of a prey animal is infected and eaten by a predator, which sheds the spores into the environment to be ingested by new prey animals. The cycle continues, allowing the reproduction cycle of the protozoa to be propagated by other hosts.

Avoiding the spread of harmful microorganisms in a medical office is crucial in protecting yourself, your coworkers, and patients that come into the practice. Knowing which steps to take in order to break the cycle of reproduction in microorganisms decreases the chances of transmission between individuals. Exercising hygiene, hand washing, and keeping a clean environment will deter harmful microorganisms from taking up residence in the medical office.

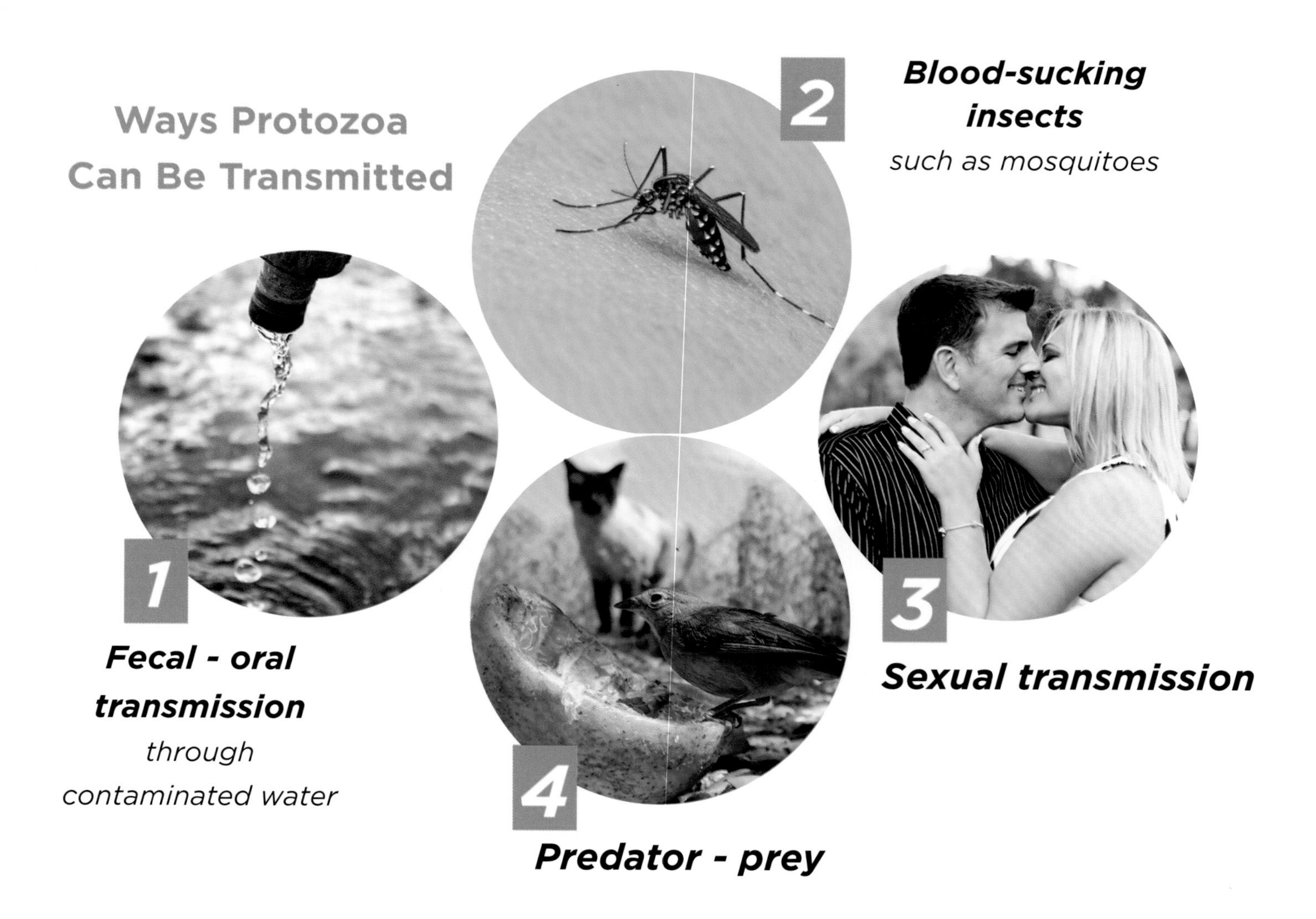

Activity

IDENTIFY THE TYPE OF MICROORGANISM AND THE DISEASE EACH CAN CAUSE.

Organism	Type	Disease
Epstein-Barr		
Giardia lamblia		
Stachybotrys		
Streptococcus pyogenes		
DENV 1		
Borrelia burgdorferi		
Trichophyton rubrum		
Trypanosoma brucei		
Varicella zoster		
Rickettsia rickettsii		
Aspergillus		
Toxoplasma gondii		
Bacillus anthracis		
Plasmodium		

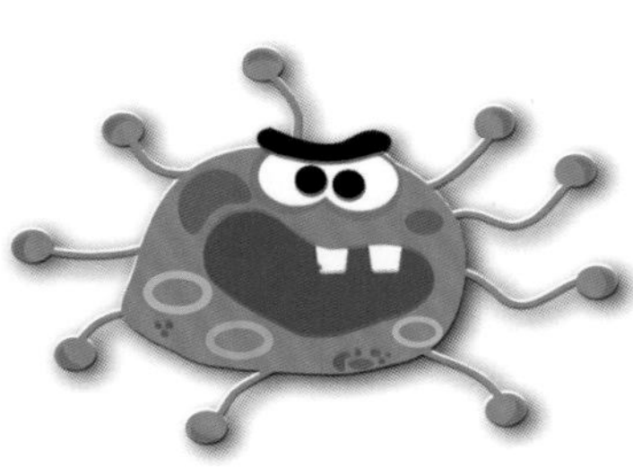

Infection by any microorganism can occur anywhere in the human body. There are six different patterns of infection that a person can encounter at any point in their lifetime. A medical office assistant should be aware of these patterns in order to identify how the infection may have occurred, and how to take the appropriate steps in breaking the chain of infection (to be discussed later in this chapter).

Local or Systemic

Infections can be local or systemic—**local infection** is confined to one location and is identified by redness, swelling, and increased warmth in the area. The body's own pre-existing antimicrobial mechanisms function as a barrier to cell surfaces, and these can quickly clear up any infection present in the body. The production of mucus or pus is the body's own defence mechanism to combat infection. If the symptoms cannot be controlled, managed, or maintained with over-the-counter medication, schedule the patient for an appointment with the physician.

Local infection: *An infection isolated to one location of the body. A local infection is often identified by redness, swelling, and increased warmth to the area.*

Systemic infections affect the whole body and are characterized by general fever, as well as an increased pulse and respiratory rate. When bacterial infection is severe enough that it overpowers the first lines of defence, the infection has the opportunity to spread through other areas of the body. A bacterial infection that progresses to systemic infection is known as septicemia, which is an infection present in the blood. In the event that an infection has become or will become systemic, it is crucial to seek medical help immediately. Schedule the patient to see the physician right away or direct them to go to an emergency room as soon as possible.

Systemic infections: *An infection of the whole body, characterized by general fever, as well as an increased pulse and respiratory rate.*

Acute or Chronic

Acute infection onset is rapid and severe, but its duration is usually short. Signs and symptoms of acute infections can take anywhere between a week to six months for the body to fight off the cause of infection. Once the body's immune system has killed off the cause of infection, the body then produces antibodies. Antibodies ensure that you will not be afflicted a second time with the same infection. Some acute infections can become serious and lead to long-term damage or death, such as a common cold turning into pneumonia.

Acute infection: *The onset of infection is rapid and severe, but the duration is usually short.*

Chronic infections often progress very slowly and will last for a longer period of time. These may last two weeks or longer. Some people may not be aware that they are infected and will transmit it to others. For example, those with hepatitis C—a chronic infection that affects the liver—may not know they are infected unless a blood test is done. A carrier of hepatitis C could be spreading infection without ever realizing it. Recovery from this chronic infection is rare, and the majority of people afflicted become carriers of this virus throughout their lifetime.

Chronic infections: *Infection that often progresses very slowly and will last for a longer period of time. These may last two weeks or longer.*

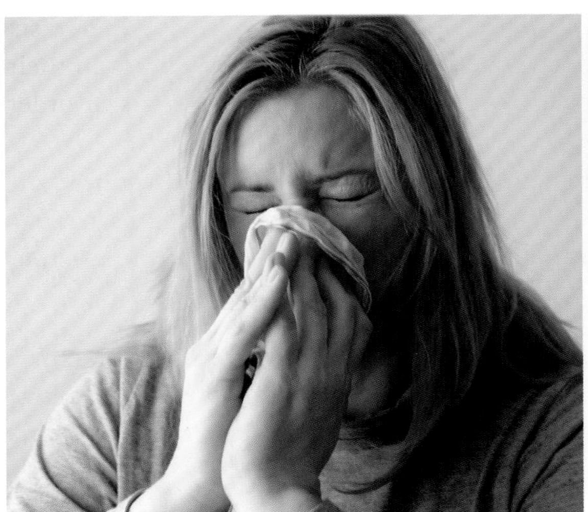 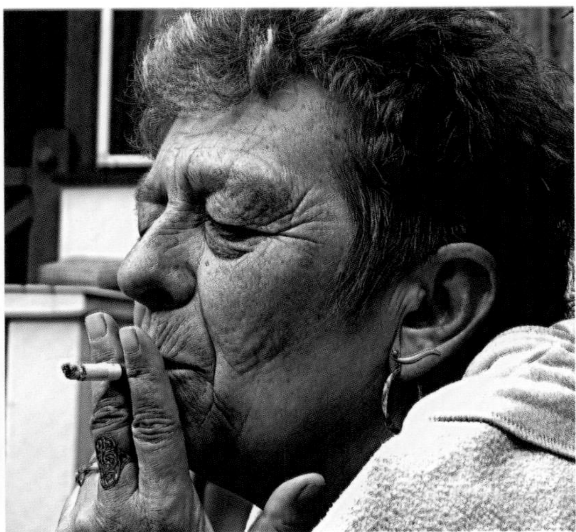

Fortunately, chronic infections can go into a cycle of asymptomatic periods called **remission** (also known as a latency period). At this point, the infection may become silent or hidden, with symptoms no longer present after the first acute episode. An example of remission is chicken pox—after the first episode, the virus goes into hiding in the body and potentially emerges as shingles in adults years later.

Remission: *Infection remains but symptoms are not present.*

Chronic infections may undergo cycles of symptomatic periods called **exacerbation** (also known as an active period). This is when latent microbes in the body suddenly wake up and become active in the body. Not all active microbes will always cause symptoms, but some may resurface off and on for months or years. During these flare ups, you can transmit these active microbes to other people. An example would be herpes simplex viruses (HSV), where the cells remain latent in nerve cells for a short or long period of time, but can still be transmitted to other people.

Exacerbation: *Chronic infections that may undergo cycles of symptomatic periods.*

Opportunistic

An **opportunistic** pattern of infection only occurs under special circumstances. Usually children and the elderly are most susceptible to infections of this variety. Under normal conditions, resident and transient microbes can live in balance with the body without causing any harm, but if the opportunity arises, some microbes can cause disease.

Opportunistic: *A pattern of infection that only occurs under special circumstances.*

Disease can occur when resident flora are traumatically introduced to an area of the body where it was not found originally, or does not naturally occur. Invasive medical procedures that use catheters or surgical wounds—procedures that allow microbes into areas of the body that are normally sterile—can cause infections.

These infections occur as a result of a number of different conditions, such as a compromised immune system, an imbalance in resident flora, or when resident flora is found outside of their particular body conditions. Resident flora can be disrupted and the unbalanced number of microbes present in the body can result in illness or infection. For example: AIDS patients can get very rare types of infections because they are already imunodeficient.

Primary or Secondary

__Primary infection:__ The original or initial infection a patient displays where the body has had no opportunity to build antibodies.

A **primary infection** is also known as the original or initial infection a patient displays—it is an infection with which the body has no opportunity to build antibodies.

__Secondary infection:__ An infection that follows or complicates a condition already present.

A **secondary infection** occurs when an infection follows or complicates a condition already present. It can be a completely new infection that comes along to infect a patient who is already sick, making them even more ill. The treatment for another pre-existing infection itself can cause a secondary infection due to changes in the immune system.

A secondary infection can also result from the first infection when progression of the first infection in the body travels elsewhere. For example, an untreated urinary tract infection, causing an infection in the kidneys, can travel into the blood and cause septicemia.

Recurrent

__Recurrent infection:__ The repetition of an infection after recovery.

Recurrent infection is the repetition of an infection after recovery. There are distinct episodes of recurrent infections, and they may be an indication that the first infection was not fully eradicated during the initial treatment. When the persistence of the same bacteria or virus is the cause of the infection, it is classified as a recurrent infection. An example of this is recurring respiratory infections in children who go through three episodes of the same infection within a six-month period.

my notes

Nosocomial

Nosocomial refers to any disease that has been acquired in a health care facility or originated in a hospital. It is also known as a hospital acquired disease, especially in reference to an infection. Patients are particularly sensitive in hospitals because they may be already in a weakened state.

Nosocomial:
A disease that has been acquired in a health care facility or originated in a hospital.

Hospitals host a greater variety of microorganisms, so there is a higher chance of acquiring a secondary infection in addition to the initial infection. Health care professionals can carry nosocomial infections, so the disruption of disease and pathogenic pathways is the first step in decreasing the number of hospital-acquired infections.

Medical office assistants work in an environment where they may be exposed to all six patterns of infection—to limit the risk of becoming infected, it is crucial to understand these patterns. There are many ways in which microorganisms can be destroyed when the routes of transmission are understood. Prevention and breaking the chain of infection are the key steps to avoiding infection.

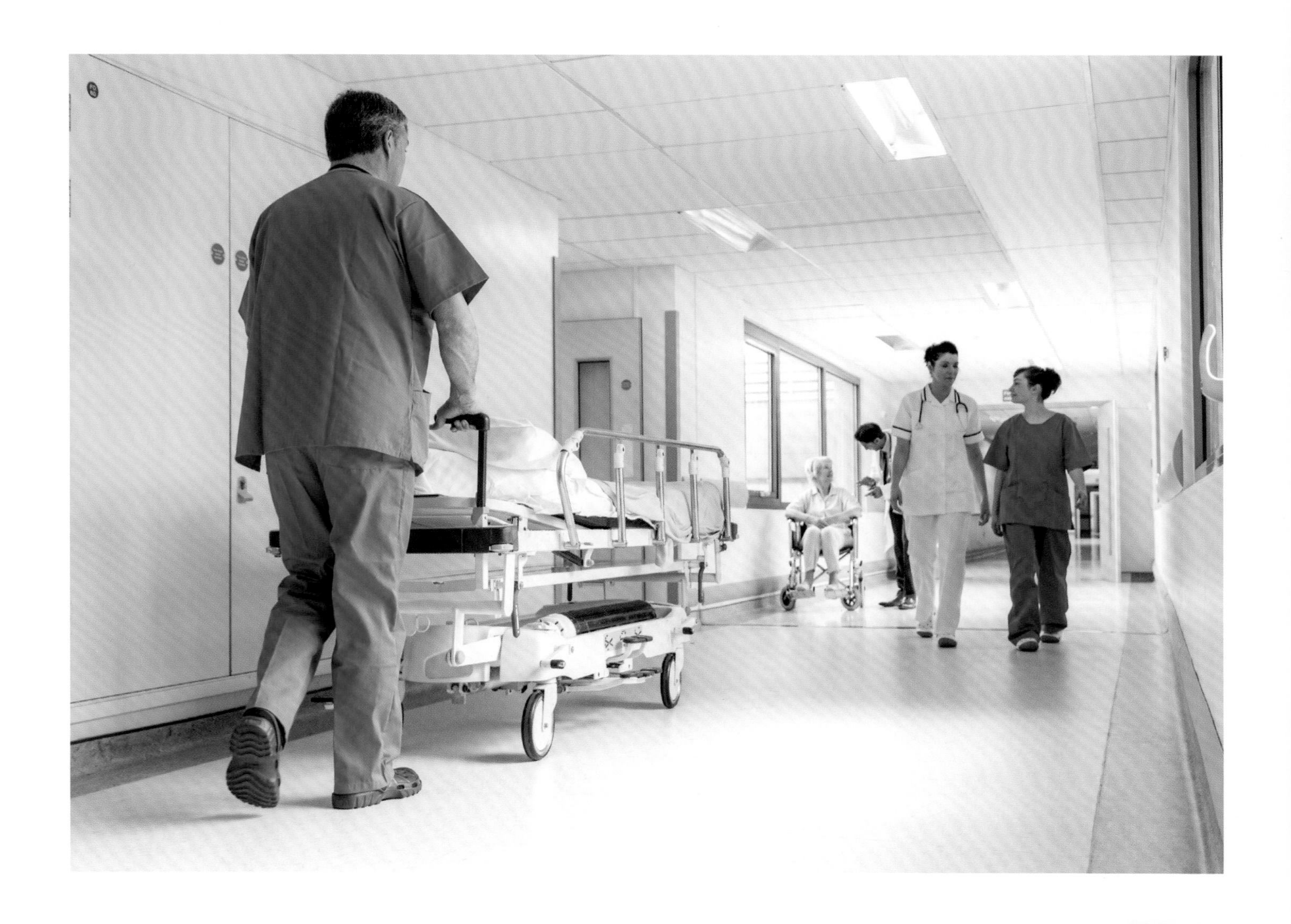

Chain of Infection

It is important to understand the progression from healthy state to infectious state, as a medical office assistant is exposed to many opportunities for infection to occur. Understanding the lifecycle of a pathogen and knowing how to break the chain of infection is crucial for preventing transmission.

The chain of infection has six elements, and all six elements must be present in order for an infection to occur. The pathogen will die without transmitting the infection to another individual if the cycle breaks at any point. Practicing good medical asepsis techniques is one way in which medical assistants can help to break the pathogen's chain of infection.

Activity

MODES OF TRANSMISSION

Find one example of infection for each of the modes of transmission:

Direct contact:	
Indirect contact:	
Droplet transmission:	
Vehicle:	
Airborne transmission:	
Vector:	

CHAIN OF INFECTION

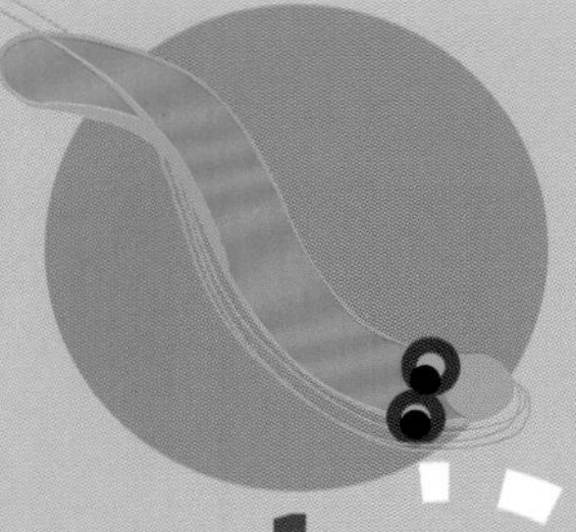

1. Causative Organism:

The pathogenic microorganism, such as bacteria, virus, or fungi.

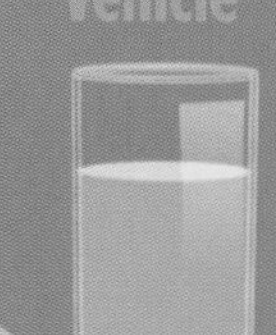

Droplet Transmission

Coughs or sneezes

Vehicle

food, water, blood, bodily fluids

Indirect Contact

Person to object to person

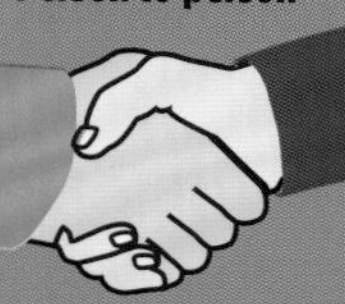

Direct Contact

Person to person

Airborne

dust and airborne particles of skin, etc.

Vector

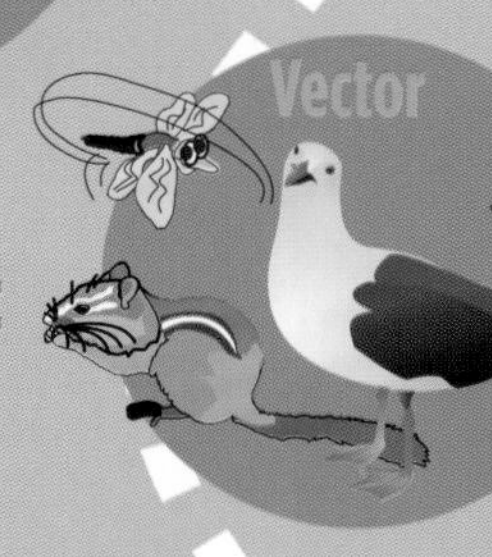

bird, animal, or insect carries the infectious agent

2. Reservoir Host:

The individual (person or animal) the pathogen infects. Depending on the pathogen, the reservoir host may also include water or soil. The host provides the nourishment the pathogen needs in order to develop and reproduce. It is where the pathogen is originally found.

4. Transmission Method:

How the pathogen moves from one host to another.

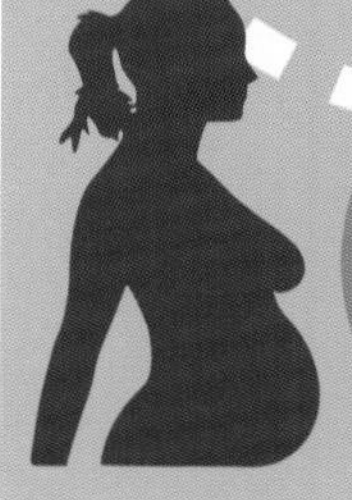

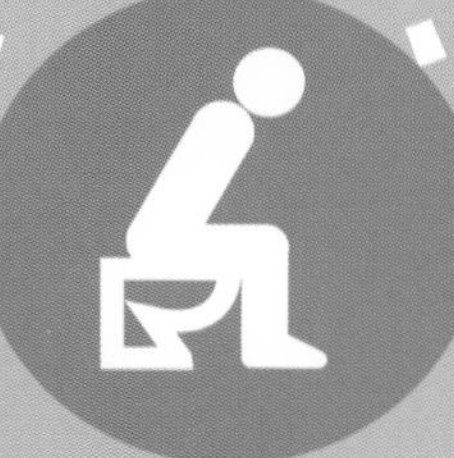

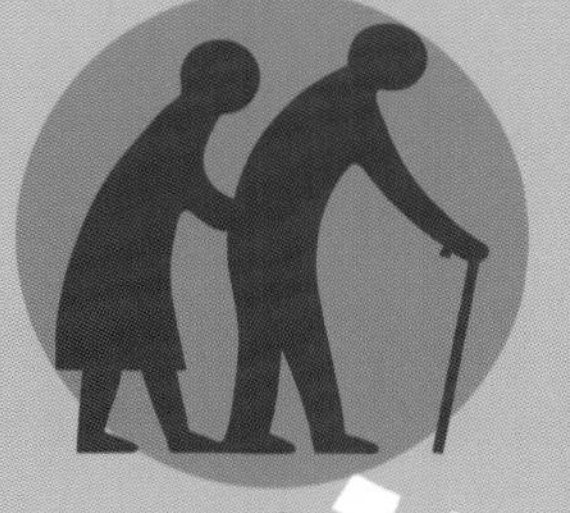

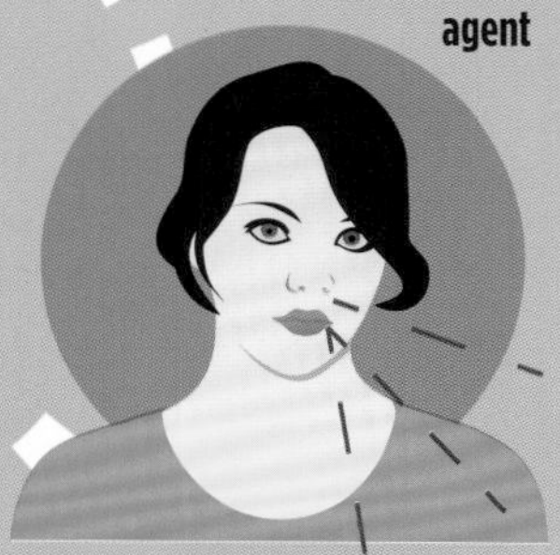

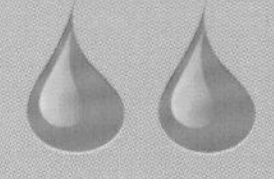

3. Portal of Exit:

The way in which the pathogen leaves the reservoir host. This includes through the nose, mouth, urinary tract, eyes, open wounds, reproductive trace, and ears. Another portal of exit can be the trans-placental route between the mother and her unborn child.

6. Susceptible Host:

Determined by the host's immune system and other defenses, this is the next individual the pathogen infects. Factors that may increase an individual's chances of being infected include a compromised immune system, poor nutrition, and stress.

5. Portal of Entry:

This is how the pathogen infects a new host. Similar to the portal of exit, this can include the mouth, throat, eyes, ears, nose, open wounds, and the reproductive tract.

Immune System and Defences

Our body's immune system is made up of defences to prevent the invasion of microorganisms. In order to survive, the human immune system protects us against potentially dangerous microorganisms that can lead to life-threatening infections. The medical assistant-patient interaction often occurs when the patient's immune system is under attack.

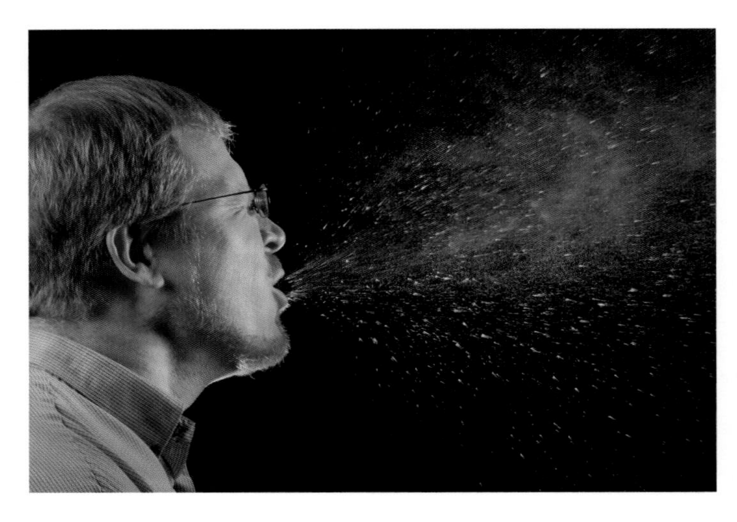

Mechanical Defences

The body is comprised of mechanical defences and is the primary level of defence against harmful microorganisms; these include barriers such as skin and mucous membranes. Cilia in the respiratory system, hairs, wax, secretions (such as tears, mucus, and sweat), and reflexes (such as coughing or sneezing) are also part of the body's defence system.

Immune System Responses

Antigen: *A foreign substance that enters the body and stimulates an immune response.*

Antibody: *Also known as immunoglobulin, it is a Y-shaped protein produced by plasma cells that is used by the immune system to identify and attack invading substances such as bacteria and viruses.*

Immunity: *The body's resistance to the effects of harmful agents, such as pathogenic microorganisms.*

Any foreign substance that enters the body and stimulates an immune response is an **antigen.**

An immune response includes phagocytosis (in which cells engulf microbes to destroy them) and **antibody** production. When antibodies are produced, they have a memory. If the antigen is again introduced into the body, the antibodies will immediately attack the invading substance. This response by the body is known as **immunity**.

Antibody and effector T cells

Initial Response | Protective Immunity | Memory

Weeks

Years

First exposure

Inapparent reinfection

Mild or inapparent reinfection

Immunity

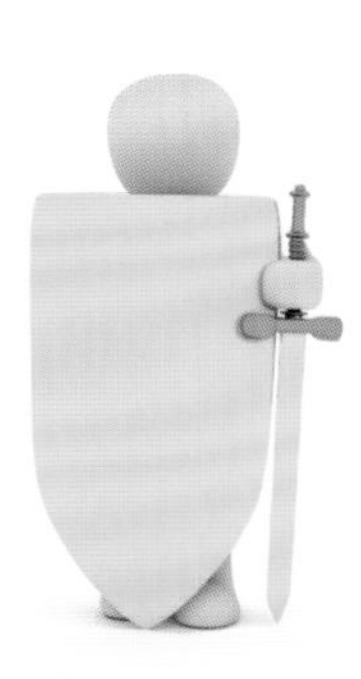

Immunity is the body's ability to resist the effects of pathogens and other harmful agents. The purpose of building immunity is to strengthen the body's defences and protect the individual from the attack of infectious diseases. There are four types of immunity that the body can produce on its own, in addition to making replicates of antibodies to resist diseases.

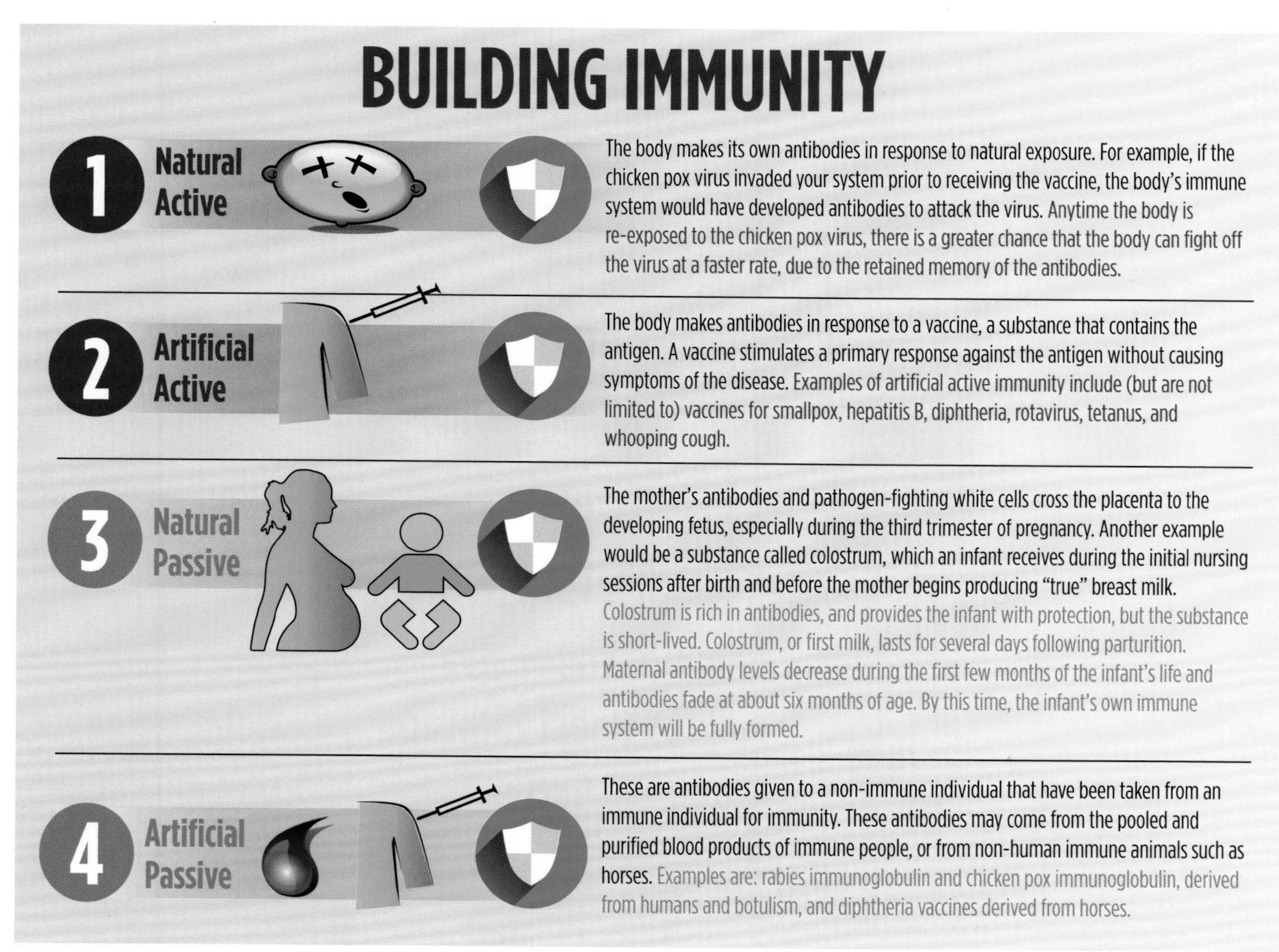

There are certain factors that can affect the immunity of a person. Some general considerations for a person's overall health are adequate rest, a balanced diet, adequate exercise, and stress management. As such, people have different baselines of how strong or weak their immune system is compared to others.

Diseases that target the immune system include—but are not limited to—AIDS, rheumatoid arthritis, lupus, multiple sclerosis, and scleroderma. There are ways to build up the immune system and prevent the invasion of germs that successfully attack your body. Keep in mind that your immune system is complex and is not made up of one single entity. In order for the immune system to function properly, balance and harmony is needed.

To enhance your immune system, adopting a healthy active lifestyle can be your first line of defence. Factors that need to be taken into consideration include diet, age, and psychological stress, as well as the base line factor on the immune response of the individual. Every part of the body functions better when your immune system is bolstered by healthy-living strategies such as:

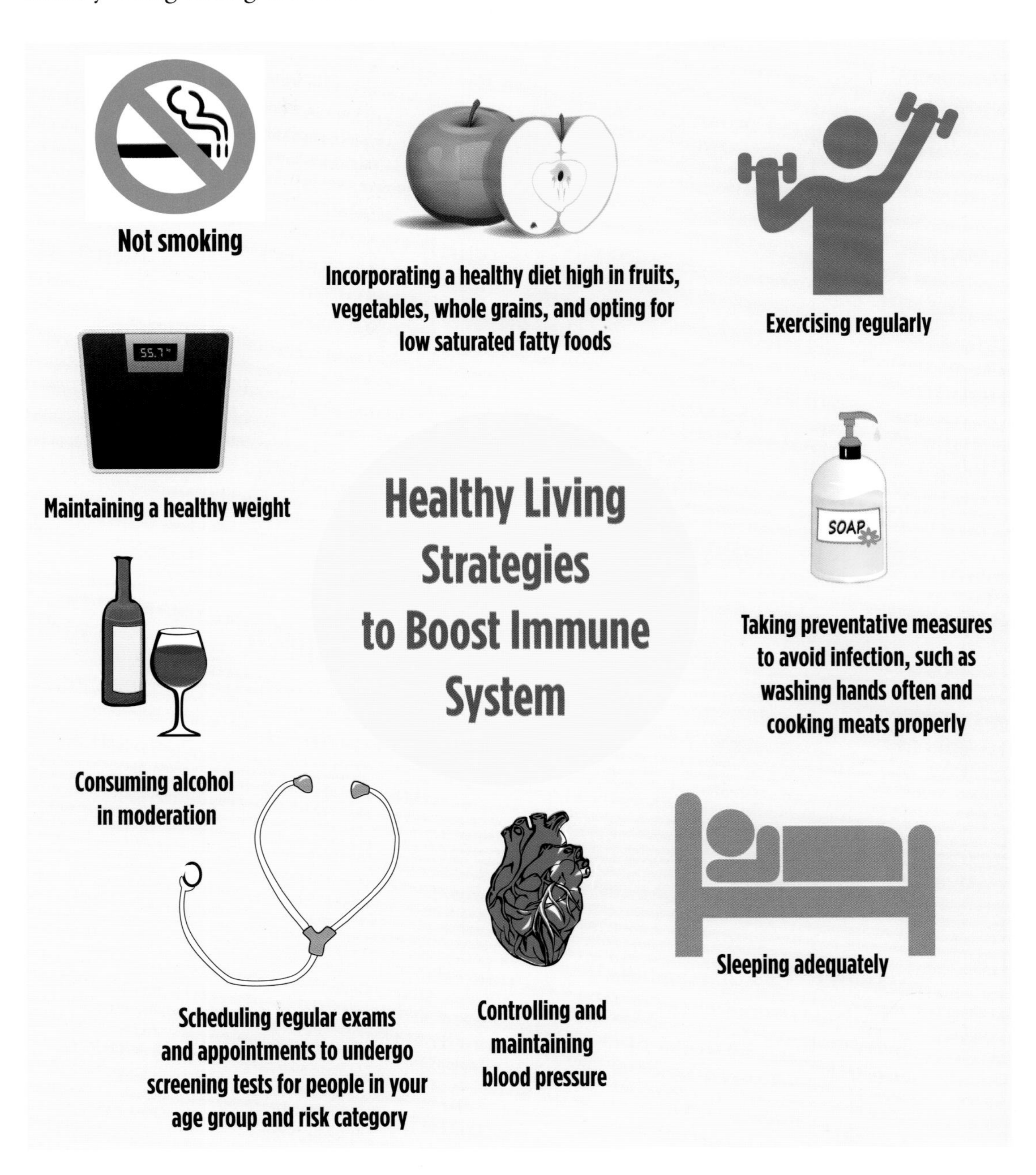

Vaccines

Vaccines are made of a serum prepared from a causative agent of a disease, its products, or a synthetic substitute. They are treated to act as an antigen without actually inducing the disease. It is introduced to stimulate an antibody response so that the body is prepared for any subsequent infection by that organism. Some patients will have adverse effects from the vaccine, but that number of patients is far fewer than those who would be harmed by the disease. The medical assistant should be familiar with every immunization that is given, including its use, common side effects, dosage, route of administration, and method of storage.

Vaccines: *A serum prepared from a causative agent of a disease, its products, or a synthetic substitute, treated to act as an antigen without inducing the disease.*

To ensure the efficacy of the vaccines given to patients, a medical office assistant should be familiar with the proper method of storing vaccines. Be aware of the medication and the vaccine manufacturers' storage and handling instructions. Keep vaccines refrigerated within the recommended temperature range and, whenever possible, store vaccines on the middle shelf. Never store vaccines on the door shelves, as the temperature may vary as the door is opened.

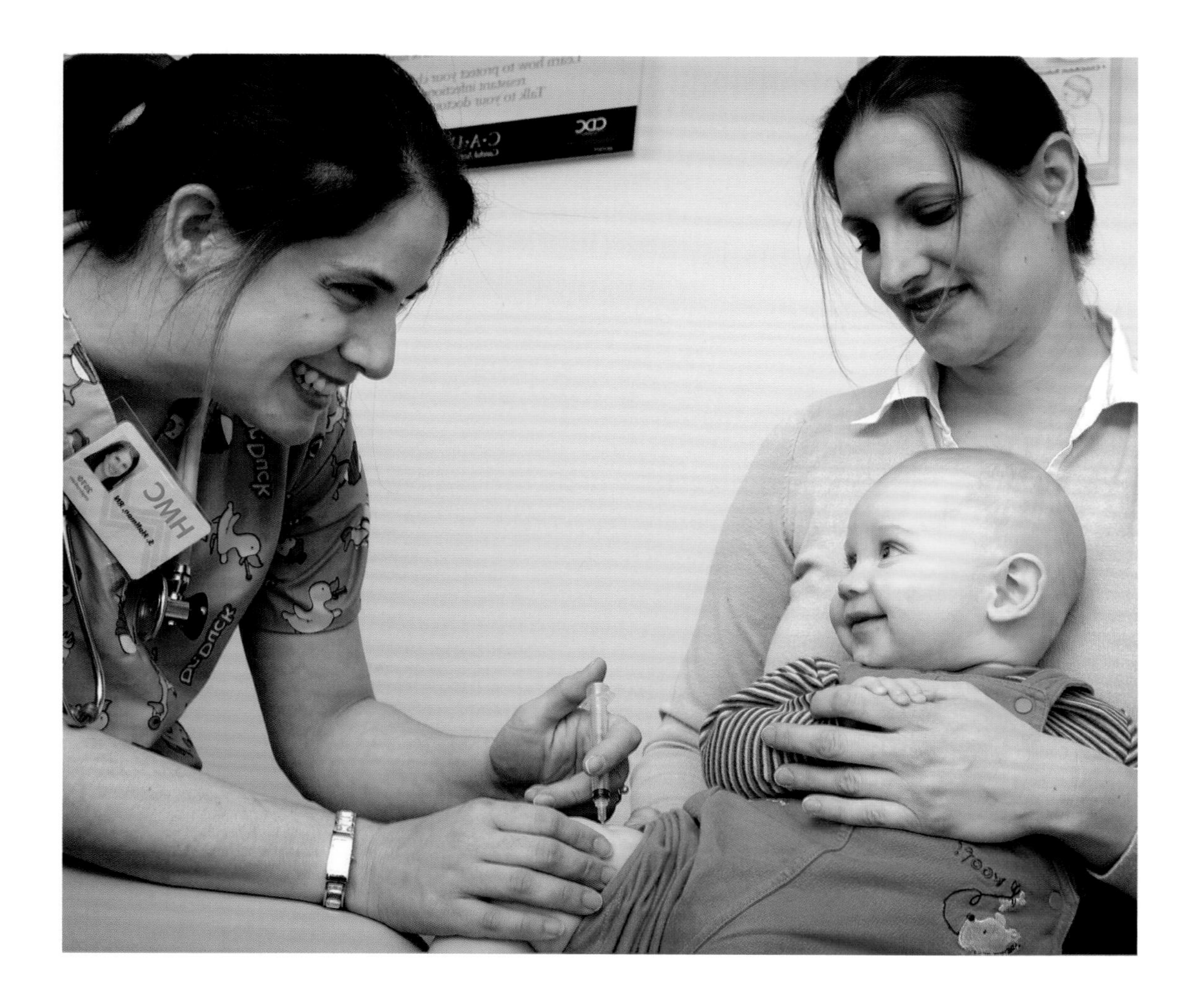

Vaccine check list

	Policies and procedures for the handling and storage of vaccines are listed somewhere accessible to everyone in the office.
	There is a dedicated medication or vaccine refrigerator.
	Food/specimens are not stored in the same refrigerator.
	There is a thermometer in the refrigerator.
	The refrigerator temperature is appropriate to store vaccines, the refrigerator is checked twice daily, and the results are recorded.
	There is an alarm on the vaccine refrigerator to warn when the temperature falls outside the recommended range.

Vaccines are:

	Kept refrigerated at a temperature between 2°C to 8°C.
	Protected from light (if required).
	Not stored in refrigerator doors, but on the middle interval shelves.
	Stored with space between the vaccine packages in the refrigerator to allow air to circulate.
	Diluents should be stored with vaccines and be kept within 2°C to 8°C.
	If refrigerator temperatures are less than 2°C or greater than 8°C, report immediately to the public health unit for assessment of vaccine potency.

Do not leave vaccines out of the refrigerator unless you are preparing the syringe for a patient, as this can compromise the efficacy of the vaccine. Never prepare vaccine doses in advance of seeing the patient by pre-filling the syringes, or leaving the syringes ready on the counter. Before preparing any vaccines, check the expiration date regularly and only have a one to three-month supply of vaccines on-hand at any given time.

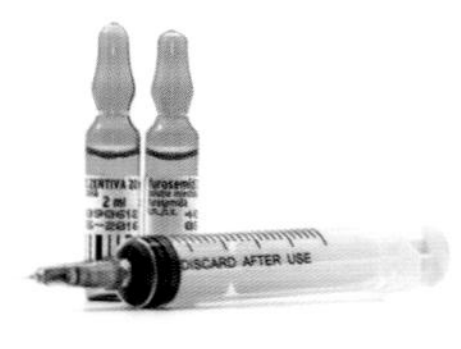

If vaccines have expired, discard them as recommended by your office's disposal protocol. The supplier of the vaccines will often accept returns and dispose of them appropriately. Never throw away expired vaccines in a normal waste receptacle, as vaccines contain dead or weakened infectious agents. In the case of power failures or malfunctions of the refrigerator, keep ice packs in the freezer or cooler bags in the office to prevent spoiling.

Activity

GROUP SCENARIO

Set up and prepare routine immunization trays for various ages. Discuss with the group the number of doses required for each vaccine, the age for the first dose, and when the booster dose is to be given.

- **Newborn**
- **Ages 2 months**
- **Ages 4 months**
- **Ages 6 months**
- **Ages 12 months**
- **Ages 15 months**
- **Ages 18 months**
- **Ages 4-6 years old**
- **Grade 7 students**
- **Grade 8 females**
- **14-16 years old (ten years after 4-6 year old booster)**
- **≥18 years old**
- **65 years old**
- **Every year**

As an immunization provider, medical office assistants play a key role in ensuring the safety and efficacy of vaccines. The time and space between administering vaccine doses are important when it comes to appropriate use of vaccines. Encourage patients to adhere to recommended schedules, maintain good record keeping, and organize patient vaccine histories to ensure vaccine efficacy.

Recommended Immunizations and Tests for Health Professionals

- Influenza
- Hepatitis A and B
- Boosters of MMR and Diphtheria/Tetanus/Pertussis
- Tuberculin Testing
- Poliomyelitis
- Rubella

Quiz

CHAPTER 1 QUIZ

1. What is the difference in cells that allows Gram staining to work? How do you differentiate between Gram-positive and Gram-negative bacteria?

____

____

____

____

____

____

2. Fill in the blank: The __________________ period is when the patient regains strength and can return to a good state of health.

3. When which of the following symptoms is present should you advise a patient to seek medical attention as soon as possible?

    a. Fever

    b. Appearance of green streaks

    c. Increased pain and swelling

    d. All of the above

4. True or false? Viruses cannot live or reproduce on their own—they need a host organism to provide metabolism and reproductive mechanisms.

5. When the symptoms of a disease begin to subside, this is known as the __________________.

6. Headaches and an overall feeling of illness are the first symptoms felt when disease is in the process of occurring. This is known as:

    a. Incubation period

    b. Prodromal period

    c. Acute period

    d. Decline period

    e. Convalescent period

7. What results from the entry of microorganisms not normally present in the body?

8. Fill in the blanks accordingly: The interval between the invasion by a __________________ microorganism and the appearance of the ______________________ from the disease is known as the incubation period.

9. Viruses, bacteria, and fungi are all different types of:

   a. Pathogen

   b. Microorganisms

   c. Flora

   d. Virus

10. What is transient flora and how can it be removed from equipment or contaminated surfaces?

____

____

____

____

____

____

11. True or false? Yeasts and molds are classified as protozoa.

12. Is normal (resident) flora harmful? How about when it is found outside of their normal environment? Give an example.

____

____

____

____

____

____

____

____

____

____

____

____

____

____

13. Bacteria that need oxygen are known as __________________ and bacteria that does not need oxygen is known as __________________.

a. Aerobes, anaerobes

b. Aerobes, aerobics

c. Anaerobes, aerobes

d. Anaerobes, aerobics

14. True or false? Chronic infection onset is rapid, severe, and lasts for a longer period of time.

15. What is the difference between local infections and systemic infections? Provide an example for each.

____

____

____

____

____

____

____

____

16. The original or initial infection a patient displays for which the body has had no opportunity to build antibodies is known as __________________.

17. What is nosocomial?

____

____

18. When a bacterial infection follows or complicates a condition already present or when a completely new infection comes along to infect a patient who is already sick and becomes even more ill, it is known as __________________.

19. An individual who is capable of being infected by a pathogen determined by the host's immune system and other defences is considered which part in the chain of infection?

a. Reservoir host

b. Portal of exit

c. Portal of entry

d. Susceptible host

20. Fill in the blank: ________________ is when the body makes antibodies in response to a vaccine.

21. The direct contact from one person to an infected person or discharge (since microorganisms cannot travel on their own) is part of which stage in the chain of infection?

    a. Reservoir host

    b. Portal of exit

    c. Mode of transmission

    d. Susceptible host

22. Fill in the blank: ________________ is when antibodies are passed from mother to child during pregnancy.

23. Fill in the blank: ________________ is when the body in response to natural exposure produces antibodies.

24. True or false? Vaccines are made of serum and contain live, robust antigens that prepare the body against harmful organisms.

25. True or false? The time and space between administering vaccine doses are important issues when it comes to appropriate use of vaccines.

my notes

my notes

Chapter 2

Standard Procedures for Preventing the Spread of Infection

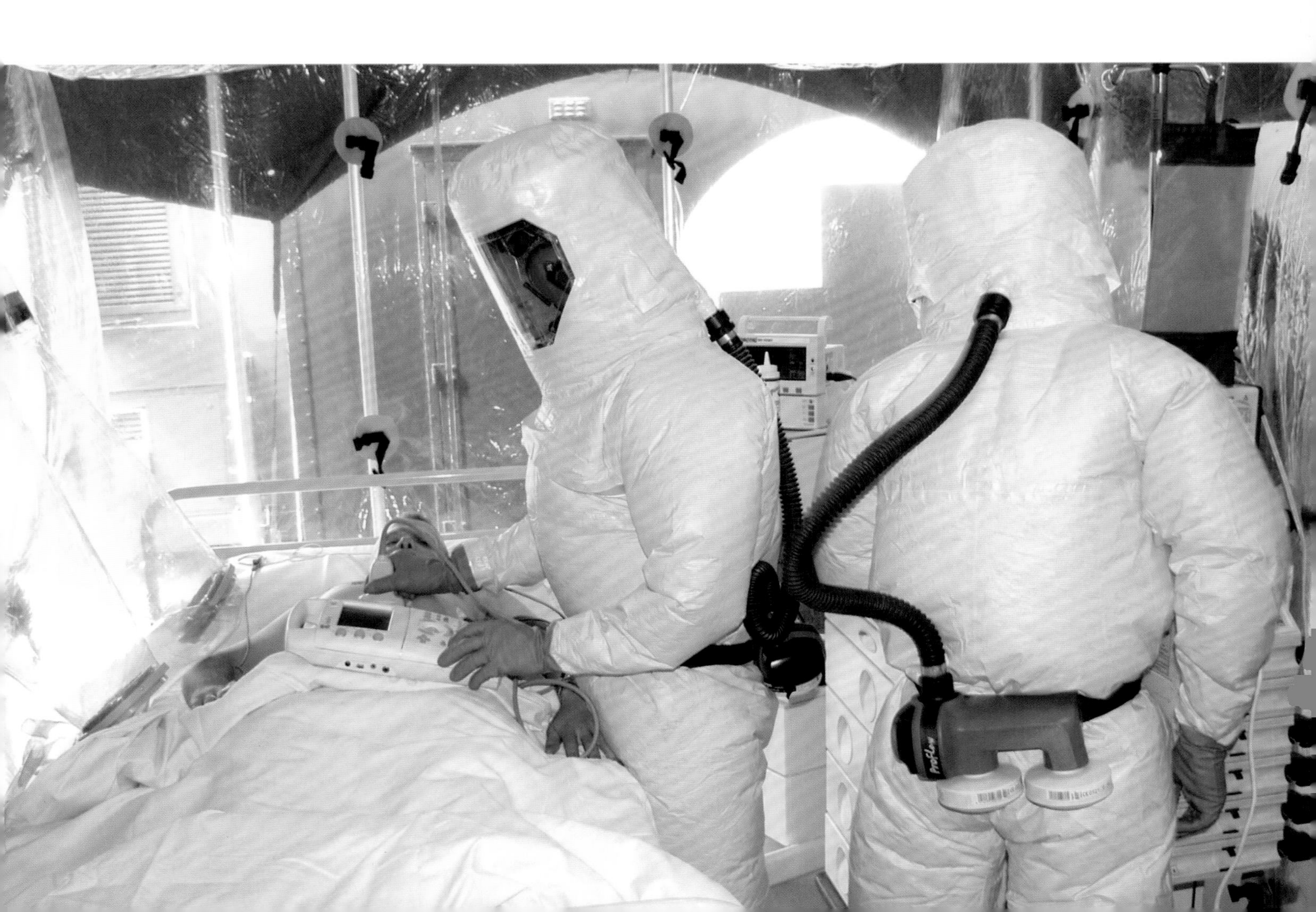

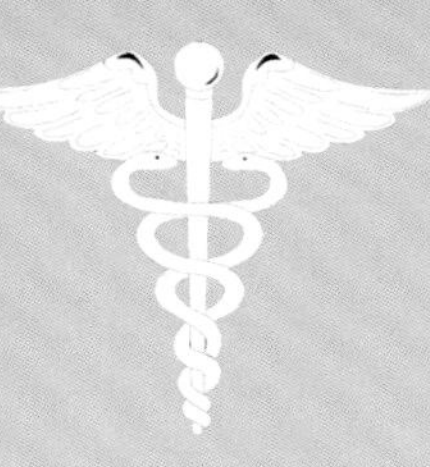

CHAPTER TWO LEARNING OBJECTIVES

After completing this chapter, you should be able to:

- ❑ Explain and define infection control
- ❑ Distinguish between medical asepsis and surgical asepsis
- ❑ Understand and apply proper hand washing technique
- ❑ Understand and apply proper gloving technique
- ❑ Identify and describe three levels of hygiene
- ❑ Understand and apply the technique of wrapping surgical packs
- ❑ Understand proper waste disposal

Infection Control

In order to break the chain of infection, the most effective method is to control the mode of transmission. It is crucial for a medical office assistant to know if a patient coming in for treatment is infectious—or potentially infectious—in order to implement the steps needed for quarantine.

Newborn infants, young children, elderly people, or immune-suppressed patients should not be in the office at the same time as someone with an infectious disease. Limit contact between the patient and office surfaces, as well as their interactions with other people. If microorganisms cannot transfer from the reservoir to the susceptible host, no infection will occur. Do not forget to wipe down any surfaces that the patient has come into contact—this lowers the chance of transmission via **fomites**.

Mode of transmission: *The movement of pathogens from a reservoir to a susceptible host. The transmission can be by direct or indirect contact. It can also be transmitted through the air.*

Fomites: *Any object, surface, or substance that can harbor an infectious organism.*

Asepsis

Practicing **asepsis** controls the modes of transmission: asepsis is *a state in which pathogens are absent or reduced*. Asepsis prevents contact with disease-causing organisms—this is why gloves should be worn at all times when handling samples, performing tests such as urine analysis, and while assisting the physician during examinations.

Asepsis: *A state in which pathogens are absent or reduced.*

There are two principal types of asepsis: medical asepsis and surgical asepsis. As a medical office assistant, it is crucial to know and practice both types to lower the presence of pathogens in the office. By controlling the pathogens present in the environment, the chain of infection can be broken, which prevents the transmission of microorganisms between people and fomites.

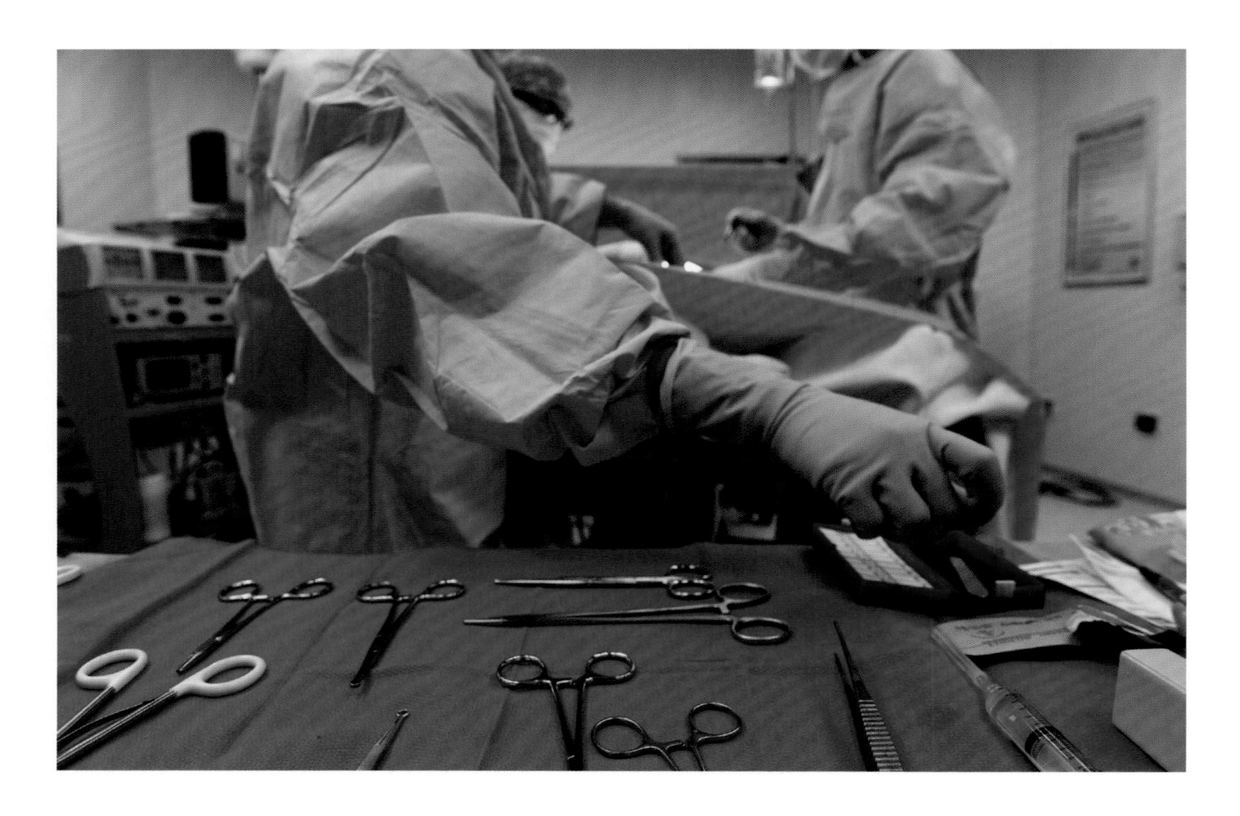

Environmental Cleaning Check List

	There are procedures for cleaning the office.
	Approved and appropriate disinfectant products are available for patient surfaces, equipment, and instruments.
	Approved hospital-grade cleaning and disinfecting agents are used for environmental cleaning.
	Clinic/examination areas and other high touch surfaces are to be cleaned and disinfected daily. Areas in direct contact with the patient are cleaned between patients.
	Other office areas are cleaned at least weekly.
	Medical equipment used on multiple patients is cleaned between patients.
	There is a procedure in place for cleaning up spills of bodily fluids.
	Waste is segregated and managed according to regulations and local bylaws.

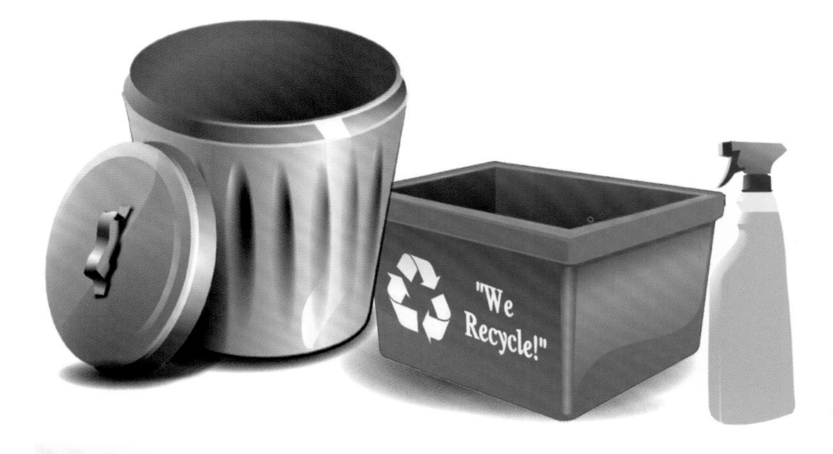

Medical Asepsis

Medical asepsis is the practice of killing germs after they leave the body in order to reduce the number of microorganisms present in an environment. This type of asepsis is known as the first line of defence as personal cleanliness and proper hygiene will prevent the carrying of infectious organisms between home and work. The purpose of medical asepsis is to eliminate the spread of microorganisms through facility practices.

***Medical asepsis:** The practice of killing germs after they leave the body in order to reduce the spread of microorganisms.*

Methods for maintaining medical asepsis:

- Leaving scrubs or lab coat at work instead of wearing it home
- Washing clothes regularly
- Keeping shoes clean
- Encouraging staff who are ill not to come into work
- Disinfecting countertops after tests
- Using a tissue when you cough or sneeze
- Disinfecting all items that come in contact with patients (e.g. the waiting room, exam bed, stethoscope, etc.)
- Disposing of garbage frequently
- Making sure the waiting area is well-ventilated
- Keeping small groupings of seats in the waiting area
- Removing samples to the storage area quickly and handling them with gloves

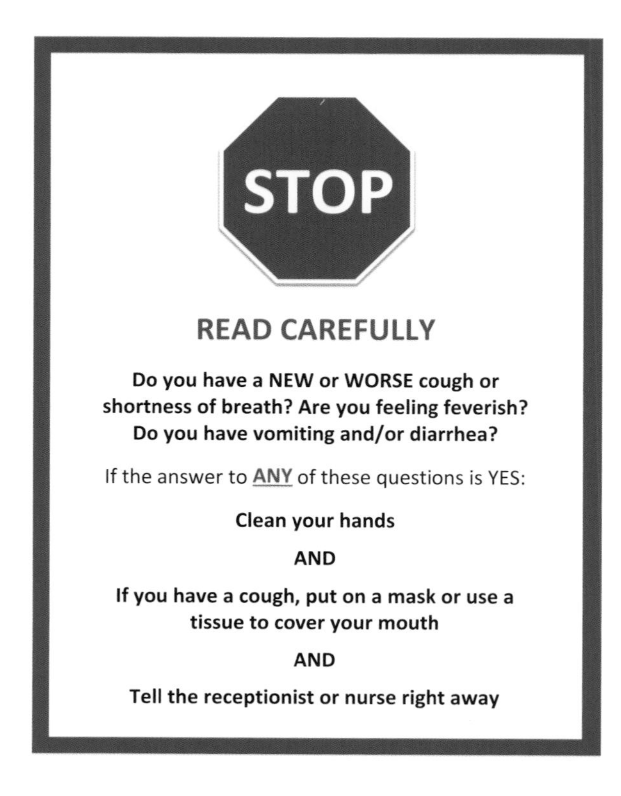

Sign from Public Health Ontario found at: https://www.publichealthontario.ca/en/eRepository/IPAC_Clinical_Office_Practice_Signage_Self-screening_2013.pdf

Public Health Ontario | Santé publique Ontario

PARTNERS FOR HEALTH | PARTENAIRES POUR LA SANTÉ

This is an excerpt from
Infection Prevention and Control for Clinical Office Practice

COVER YOUR COUGH

Stop the spread of **germs** that can make you and others sick!

Cover your mouth and nose with a tissue when you cough or sneeze. Put your used tissue in the waste basket.

If you don't have a tissue, cough or sneeze into your upper sleeve or elbow, not your hands.

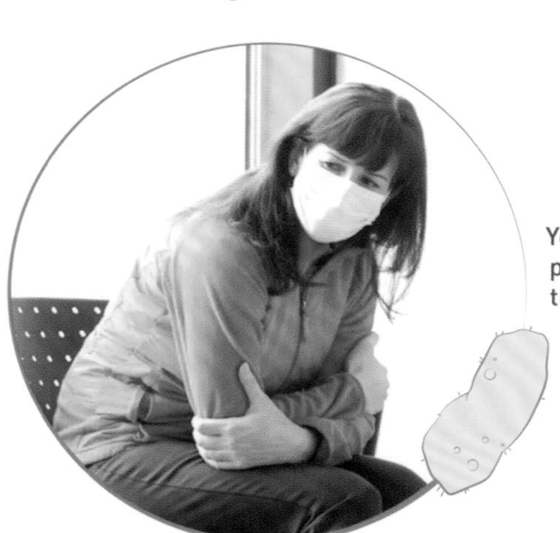

You may be asked to put on a facemask to protect others.

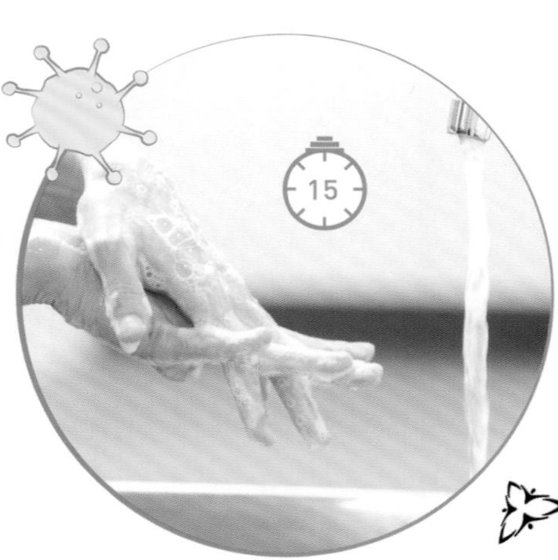

Wash hands often with soap and warm water for 15 seconds. If soap and water are not available, use an alcohol-based hand rub.

For more information please contact Public Health Ontario's Infection Prevention and Control Department at ipac@oahpp.ca or visit www.publichealthontario.ca

Ontario
Agency for Health Protection and Promotion
Agence de protection et de promotion de la santé

As a medical office assistant, it is important to practice good personal hygiene, exercise proper hand washing techniques, and to wear sterile gloves properly, especially when exposed to infectious organisms. Medical asepsis protects both patients and caregivers from becoming infected. All health care facilities have infection control policies and procedures that personnel must follow to control the spread of infection. Be familiar with these policies and procedures to properly maintain medical asepsis.

Facility Check List

	There is infection control signage at the entrance of the office or clinic.
	There are alcohol-based hand rub and masks available at reception, with signage for appropriate use.
	There are tissue boxes available.
	Reception staff is protected from patients by a barrier.
	Toys are properly cleaned in the waiting room.
	There are waste receptacles available in each room.
	There is a waiting area for patients that need to be segregated for acute infection.
	Gloves are available and used appropriately.
	Masks are available and used appropriately.
	There is a functional separation of clean storage and dirty utility areas.

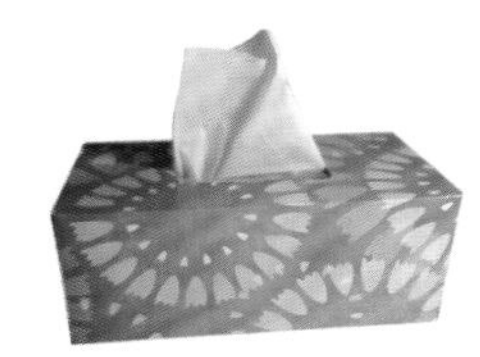

How to

PROPER HAND WASHING TECHNIQUE

In order to prevent the spread of pathogens, practice proper hand washing techniques to help you achieve asepsis. Washing your hands may become tedious when you have to do it countless times a day, but it is crucial for your health as well as your patients' health. Keeping a low level of contamination at your practice will lead to a healthier work environment.

Liquid antimicrobial soap, clean warm running water, paper towels, and a waste container are all that you need to properly wash your hands.

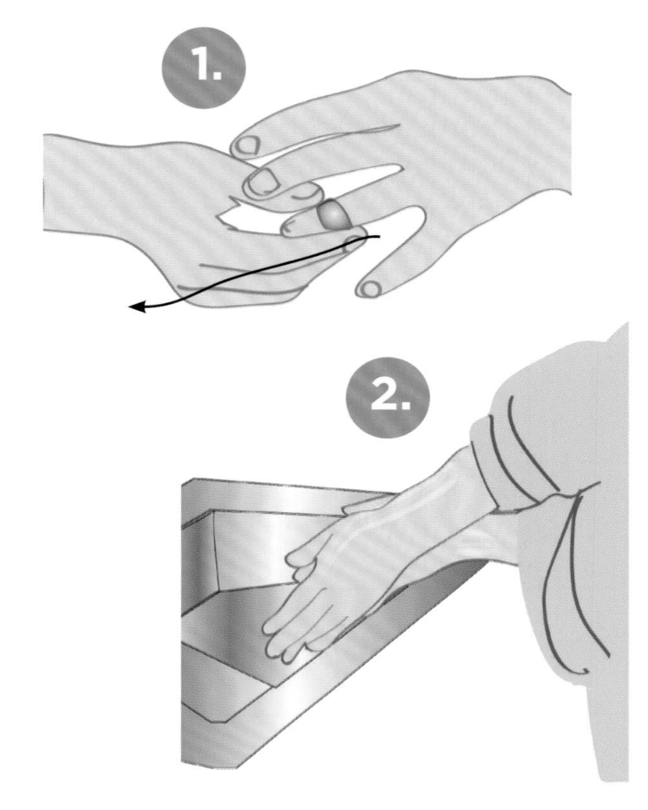

1. Before you begin to wash your hands, remove your watch or any pieces of jewellery on your hands or wrists and push your sleeves up on the forearm. Microorganisms can lodge in the grooves of rings.

2. Stand at the sink and avoid touching the basin. Microorganisms contaminate the basin, and if you or your uniform touches it, you can pick up and transfer these microorganisms to other locations in the practice.

3. Using a paper towel, turn on the faucets and adjust the water temperature to warm. Not only does warm water make the best suds with your antimicrobial soap, but water at extreme hot or cold temperatures may result in dry or cracked skin. Dry skin makes it easy for pathogens to enter your body or transfer to your patients.

4. Once you have turned the faucet on, discard the paper towel in the waste container as the paper towel is now considered contaminated.

5. Start by running your hands and forearms under the water, ensuring they are completely wet. Do not touch the inside of the sink, and keep your hands lower than your forearms so when you wash, the bacteria and dirt flows away from your body rather than towards it.

4.

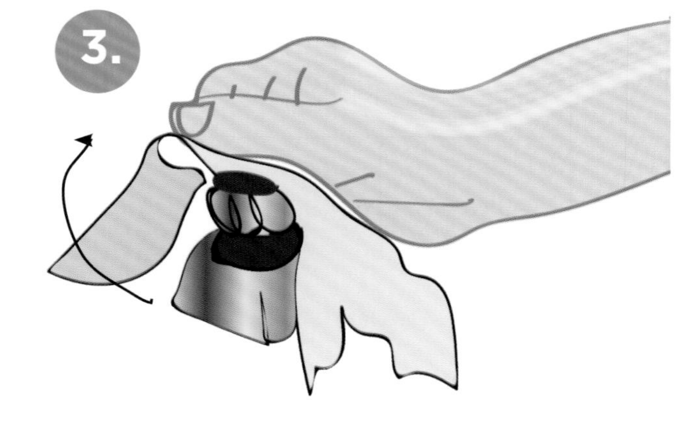

6. Apply one teaspoon of your antimicrobial soap to the palm of your hand. It should look like the size of a nickel. Wash your palms and the backs of your hands in a high friction, circular motion. This helps remove any microorganisms present on your hands.

7. Continue to use circular motions and wash your fingers 10 times for a minimum of 20 seconds, concentrating on your fingertips and fingernails. To help dislodge any remaining debris, interlace your fingers while rubbing them together.

8. Rinse well under running water and remember to hold your hands below your elbows to rinse off any leftover suds and debris.

9. Apply an additional teaspoon of antimicrobial soap and, using the same high friction, circular motion, wash your wrists and forearms.

10. Rinse your arms and hands well. Repeat the hand washing procedure as soon as your hands are contaminated, especially if they were exposed to blood or other potentially infectious materials.

11. Gently dry your hands and throw out the paper towel. Turn off the water with paper towels, as the sink is contaminated, and avoid touching the sink with your bare hands. Your hands are now medically aseptic.

12. Clean your fingernails with a manicure stick once a day, preferably soon after arriving at the practice. Dirt and microorganisms collect underneath the fingernails.

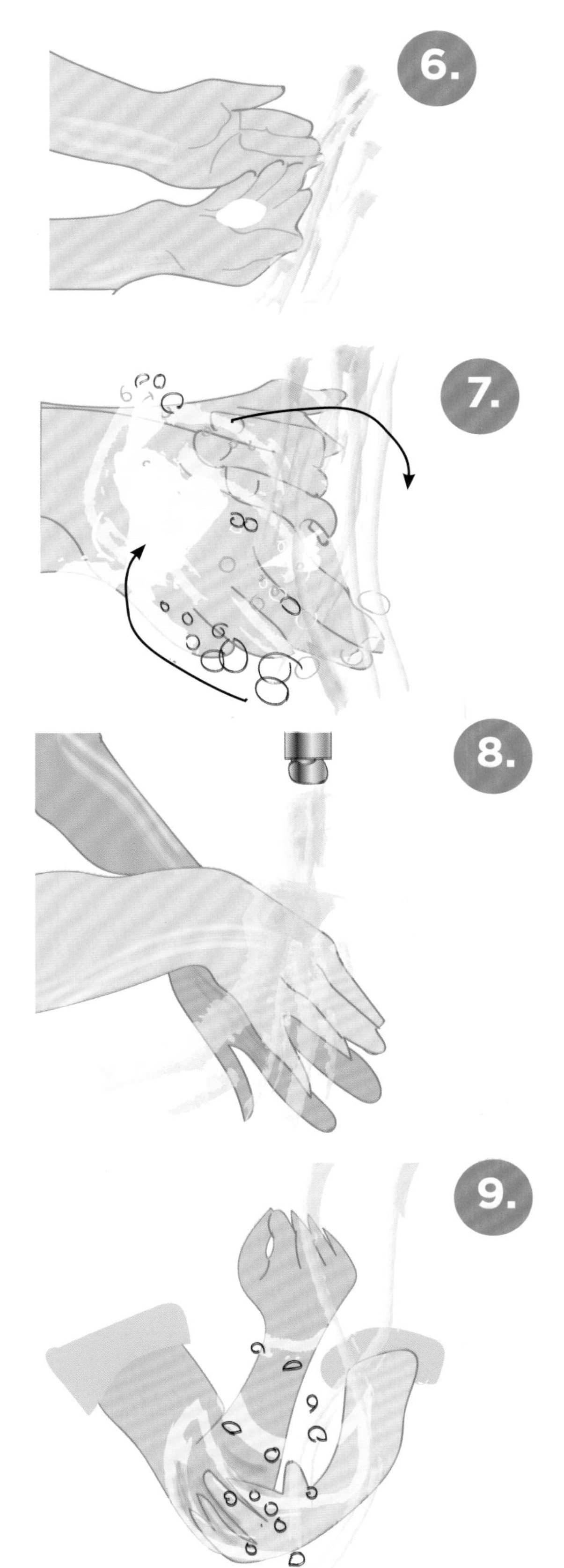

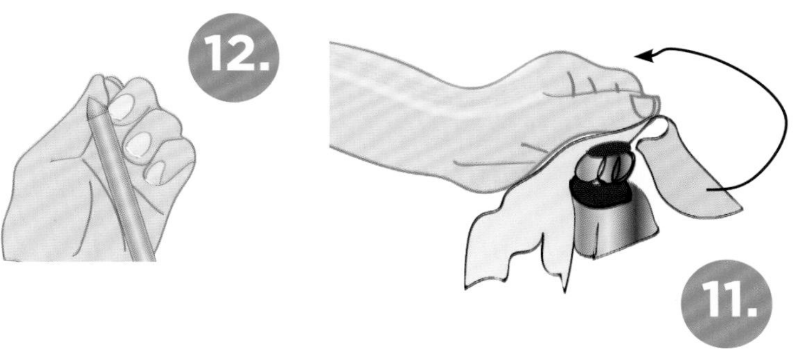

In order to ensure you clean your hands, wrists, and forearms properly, it is best to follow these steps each time you need to wash your hands. Help lower the chance of spreading microorganisms by practicing proper hand washing.

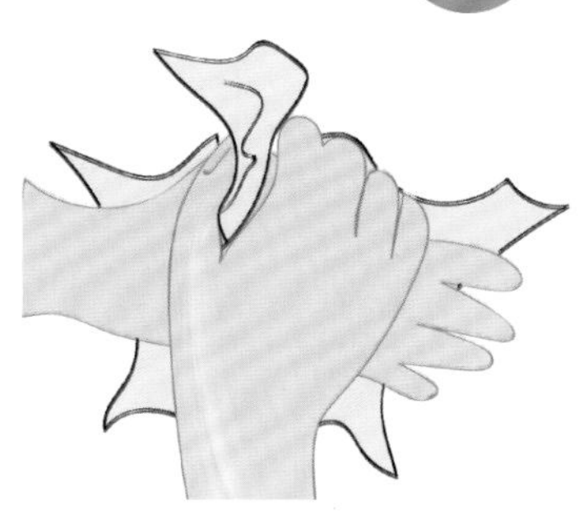

Activity

WHEN SHOULD YOU WASH OR SANITIZE?

Do you know when you should wash your hands or when using alcohol-based hand sanitizers are enough to destroy the pathogens on your skin?

Wash hands	Hand sanitizer	
		Before, during, and after preparing food
		Before eating food
		Between traveling in a car and entering into a meeting
		Before and after treating a cut or wound
		Before and after caring for someone who is sick
		While camping or outdoors
		After blowing your nose, coughing, or sneezing
		After working with something soiled or greasy
		After working in the garden
		After using the washroom
		After changing diapers or cleaning up a child who has used the washroom
		Before eating an in-flight meal or snack
		After touching an animal, or animal waste
		After handling pet food or a pet treat
		After touching garbage

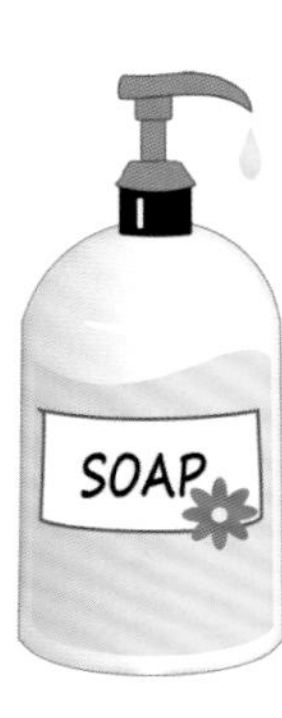

How to

PROPER GLOVING TECHNIQUE

Medical office assistants must wear sterile gloves to protect themselves and the patient when performing or assisting any procedure. In order to avoid contaminating clean hands with pathogens, the medical office assistant must not handle or directly contact patients with their bare hands.

Applying Sterile Gloves

1. Before washing your hands, remove all rings to prevent tearing of gloves, and select the right size gloves for your hands. Have the gloves ready to put on to avoid contamination.

2. Follow proper hand washing technique using anti-microbial soap, and open the glove package without touching the inside of the wrapper.

3. You will notice that the gloves are cuffed for sterile purposes and for easy gloving procedure. DO NOT TOUCH the outside of the glove with your bare hands, as your hands are considered contaminated.

4. With the fingers of the opposite hand, pick up the first glove on the inside of the cuff and put the glove on without touching the outside of the gloves. Use the cuff only to guide your fingers.

5. With your gloved hand now considered sterile, pick up the second glove by slipping your gloved fingers under the cuff and grasping the opposite side of the cuff with your thumb, as the cuff is sterile at this point.

6. Remove your thumb from the cuff and pull the glove on.

7. Reach under the cuff with the other gloved hand, and turn back the cuff of the first glove. Don't come into contact with the inside of the cuff.

8. Inspect the gloves for tears, and replace them if there are any present. Always follow the proper gloving technique to apply a new pair of sterile gloves.

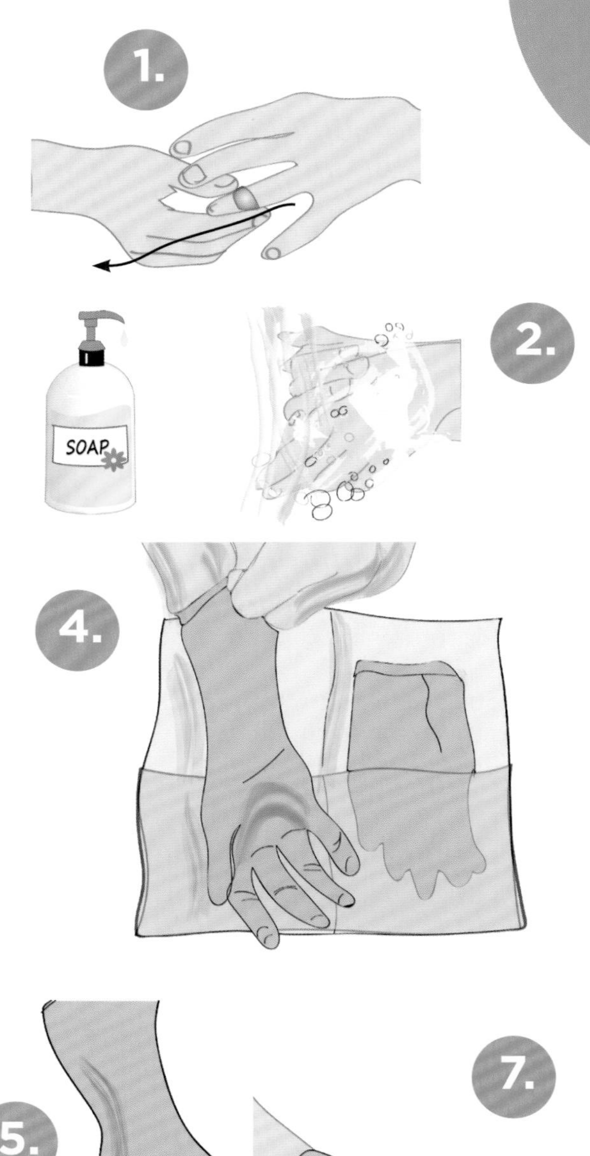

PROPER GLOVE REMOVAL TECHNIQUE

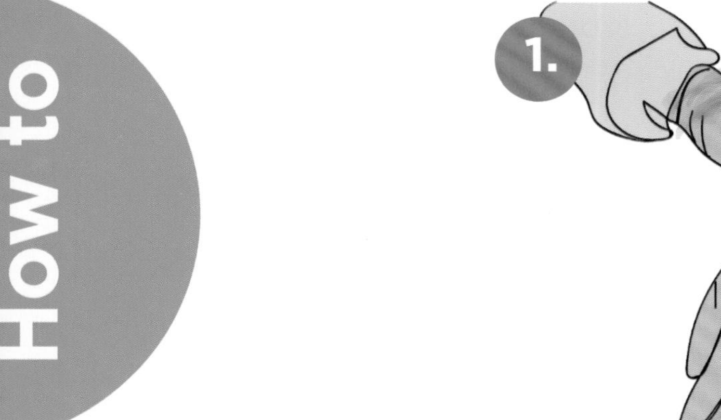

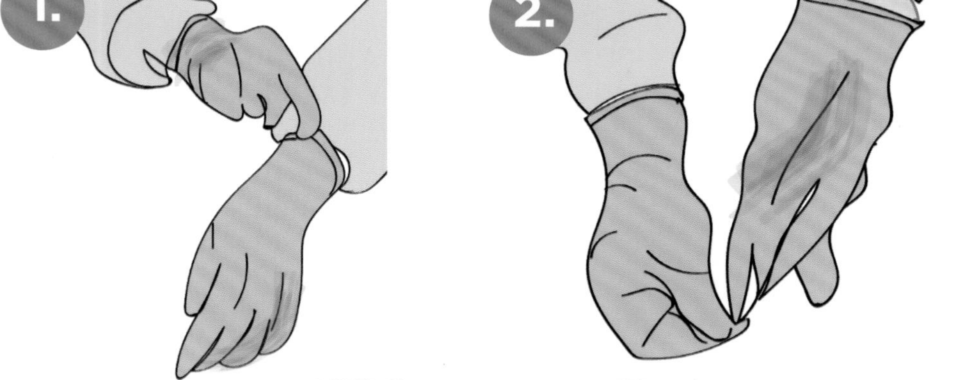

Removing Sterile or Contaminated Gloves

1. Choose the hand with which you want to start. Pinch the outside of the other glove, about two inches from the top, with two fingers.

2. Pull the glove away and off your hand slowly, until the glove comes off. Allow the glove to turn inside out as you remove it.

3. Once the glove is off your hand, scrunch it into a ball with your remaining gloved hand.

4. Place your index and middle fingers on the inside of the other glove without letting your clean hands touch the outside of the glove.

5. Slide your fingers inside the glove until you can turn the glove inside out while pulling the glove off your hand, enclosing the balled-up glove.

6. Discard both gloves in the appropriate waste disposal. If blood or other infectious material has contaminated your gloves, discard them in a biohazard container.

7. Wash your hands with the proper hand washing technique to make sure that you have removed any microorganisms that may have come into contact with your hands.

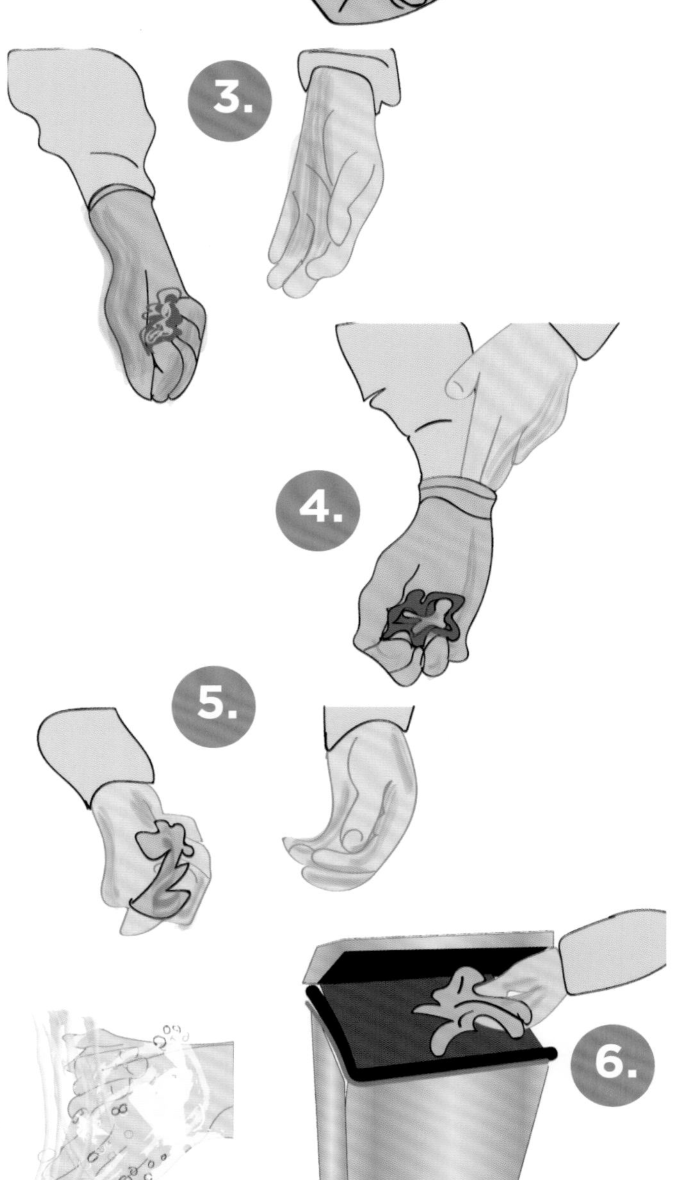

Surgical Asepsis

Surgical asepsis, also known as *sterile technique*, helps to protect you and your patients from pathogens that may cause disease should they enter the body. Surgical asepsis is maintained when medical offices keep objects and operating areas sterile and free from any living microorganisms and spores. In order to achieve a sterile state, offices use physical and chemical processes to remove all living organisms from any equipment and instruments that will come into contact with patients; this is also known as sterilization. Once items have been sterilized, it is important to practice sterile technique—avoid touching any part of the item that is considered sterile. The goal is to destroy pathogens before they have the chance to enter the body and infect someone.

***Surgical asepsis** (sterile technique): This is attained by maintaining sterility of objects and areas to limit sources of infection.*

Situations in which surgical asepsis is crucial include:

- Caring for open wounds, suture punctures, and other instances where the patient's skin is broken
- When a doctor or medical assistant penetrates the patient's skin, such as administering an injection (the needle must remain sterile)
- When the normally sterile body cavity is entered (e.g. inserting a urinary catheter or intravenous catheter to administer I.V. therapy)

Sterility is maintained by using disposable sterile tools and materials, or by properly sterilizing reusable instruments. If a sterile item touches an unsterile one in any way, it is immediately considered contaminated. It can no longer be used in a sterile procedure. Remove the object from the sterile field accordingly and replace it with a sterile version, if needed.

If there are any doubts regarding the sterility of a tool, operate under the assumption it is contaminated and replace with a sterile tool. Wear sterile gloves when working with articles during a sterile procedure in order to avoid the contamination of sterile articles.

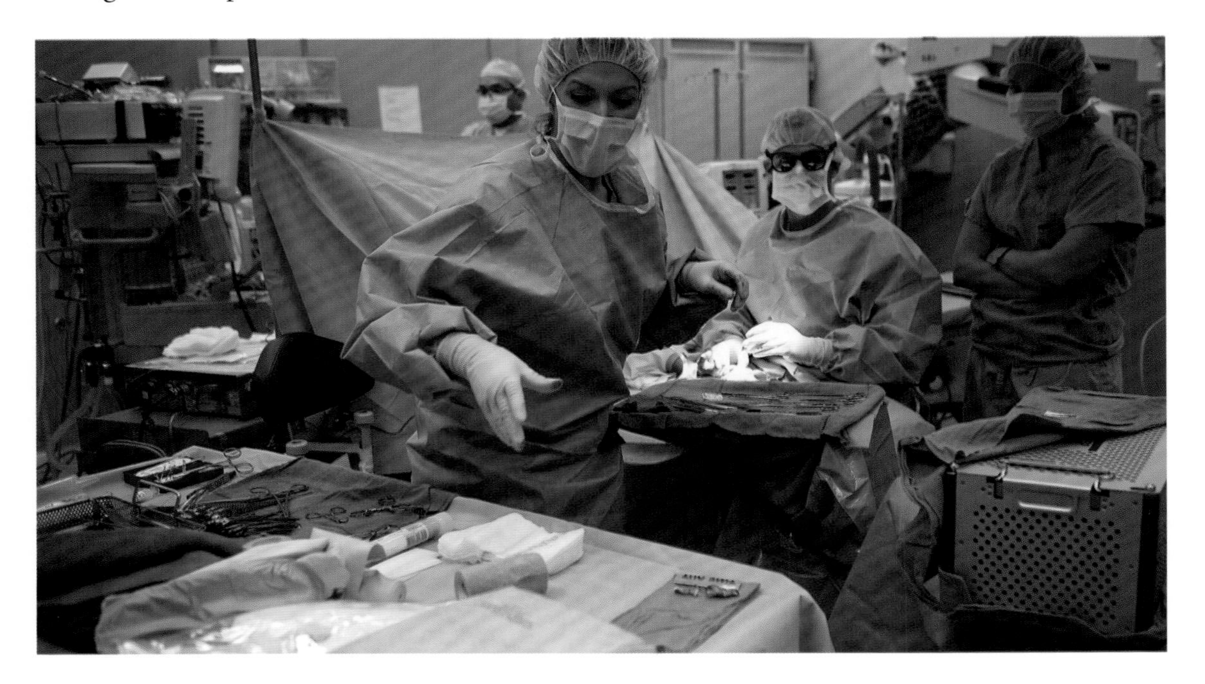

Specific guidelines should be followed and observed during a sterile procedure to maintain surgical asepsis. Only use single-use medical devices on one patient for a single procedure before discarding the device appropriately. Adhere to the following guidelines during a sterile procedure to maintain surgical asepsis.

Sterile field: *A microorganism-free area, that is also free of spores. The use of sterile gloves, gowns, and drapes helps maintain sterility by creating a barrier between the environment, the medical personnel, and the patient.*

1. Don't allow sterile packages to become wet. This may draw microorganisms into the package, resulting in contamination. Consider any wet packages contaminated. If they are reusable, rewrap and re-sterilize the package before using it. If it is a disposable package, discard immediately.
2. A one-inch border around the **sterile field** is considered contaminated, because it may have been contaminated during the setup process.
3. If you have to leave the room during a sterile procedure, place a sterile towel over the sterile field. Otherwise, be sure to always face the sterile field.
4. Hold everything in front of you without letting sterile items touch your uniform. Ensure all sterile items remain in your line of vision. Anything that leaves is no longer sterile.
5. All sterile items should be placed in the center of the sterile field and not around the edges. Only sterile items are used within the sterile field.
6. Do not spill water or solutions on or near the sterile field, as this will lead to contamination. Microorganisms can potentially be drawn up into the field by capillary action.
7. Any water vapour from your nose, mouth, or lungs will render the sterile field contaminated. Avoid talking, coughing, or sneezing over the sterile field.
8. Reaching over a sterile field may result in your clothing making contact with or dust falling into the sterile field. Both result in contamination. Never pass soiled items across the field for this reason.
9. Acknowledge if you or anyone else in the room contaminates the sterile field. Take the time to follow the proper steps to re-sterilize the field.

OPENING A STERILE PACKAGE

There are times when a medical office assistant needs to help open sterile packages for the physician ahead of time, or during a sterile procedure. It is crucial to learn the methods of removing sterile contents while maintaining sterility. Always sanitize your hands prior to opening any sterile packaging. Items displaying a manufacturer's expiration date should be considered unsafe for use after expiry. Confirm the expiration date prior to opening any packages intended for sterile purposes.

To open a commercially sterilized package, grasp each flap between a bent index finger and an extended thumb, and roll hands outwards to pull apart. Avoid touching the contents within the sterile package, particularly when you step back to eject the contents into the sterile field. As the medical assistant, you are in charge of opening the packs, and only the physician is allowed to remove the sterile contents with a sterile, gloved hand. The inside of the sterile peel-apart package can be used as a sterile field to hold scalpels or additional gauze, as long as it has not been contaminated.

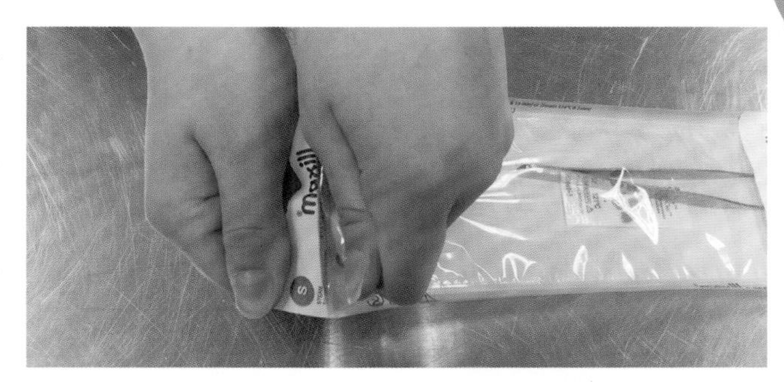

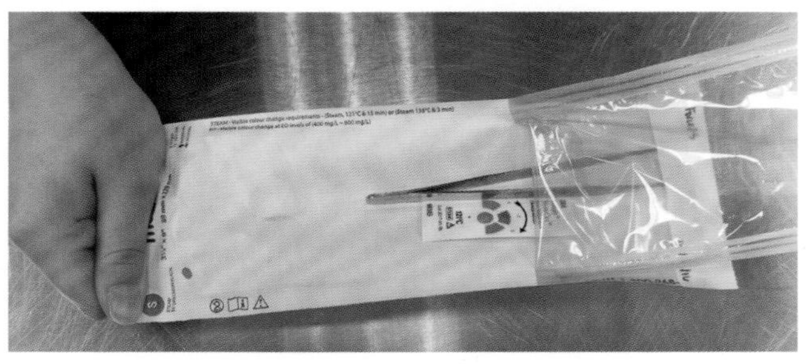

To open a wrapped sterile package, remove the sterilization indicator tape only after you have made sure that the pack is not wet, opened, or torn. These factors indicate that the pack is no longer sterilized, but contaminated and must not be used. Double check to make sure that the sterilization indicator tape has changed color, indicating a "pass" result.

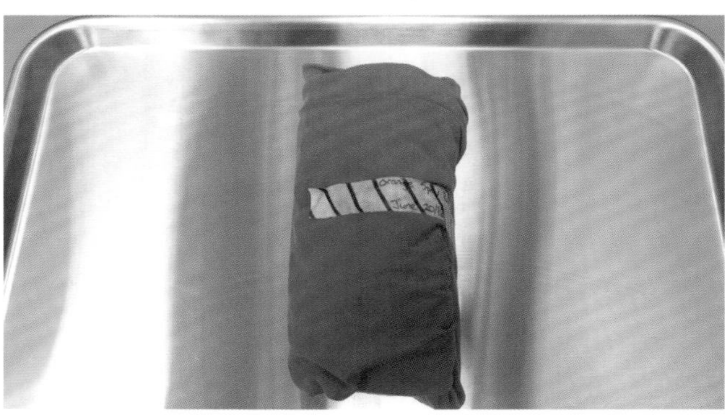

Place the package on a clean flat surface so that the top flap opens away from you. While facing the sterile field, open the first flap away from the body and handle only the outside of the wrapper. Avoid sneezing, talking, coughing, and laughing as you face the sterile field to avoid contamination. To avoid any lint or transfer of microorganisms that may be present on your clothing, don't reach over the sterile field or have your clothing drag over the sterile field.

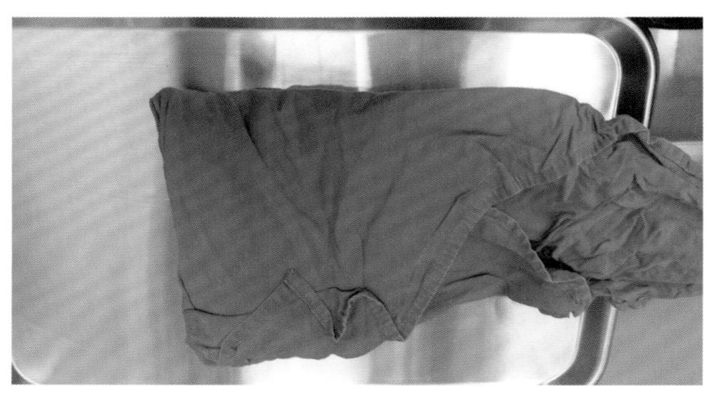

Once the first flap is opened away from you, open the left and right flaps. Lastly, lift the last flap closest to your body and avoid touching the contents inside. Adjust the wrapper by the corners on the tray or table to prevent having the tray knocked to the ground. Check the sterilization indicator to confirm that the contents in the pack are sterile.

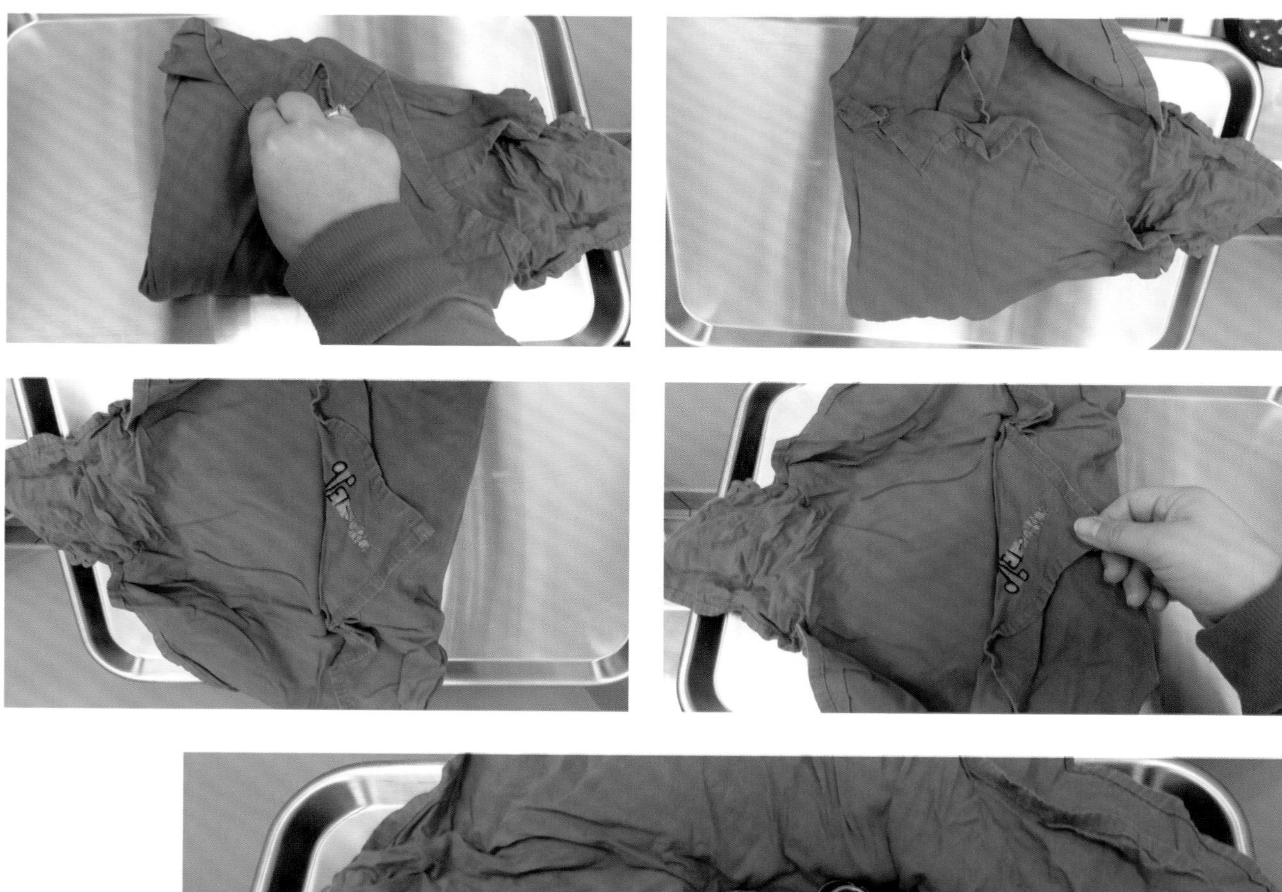

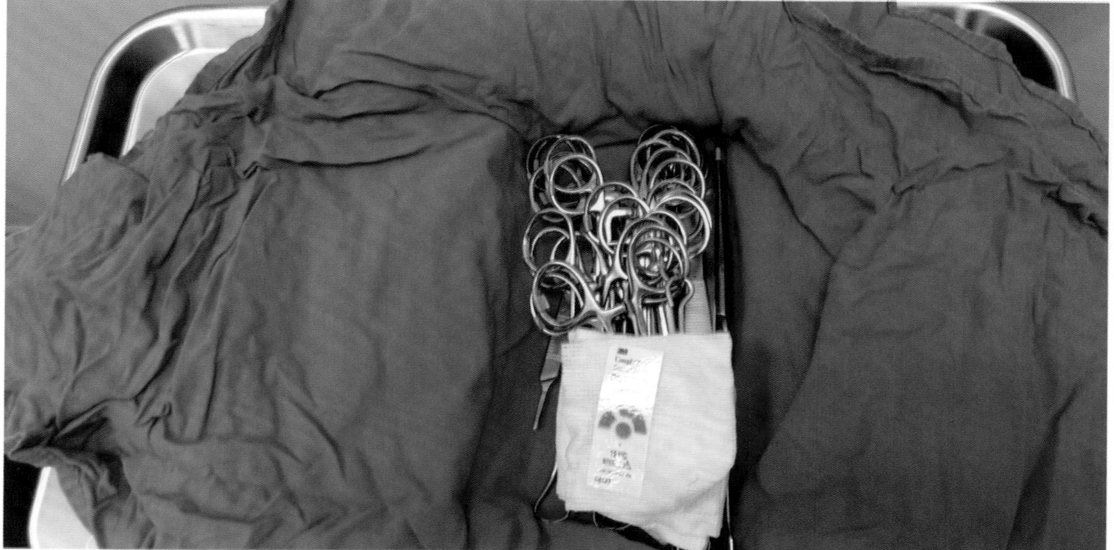

A medical office assistant should know how to open a sterile package, and how to keep the contents inside a wrapped package sterile. In order to prevent the transfer of microorganisms during a surgical procedure, physicians need to work in a sterile environment and sterile field, which the office assistant provides. This lowers the probability of transferring infectious diseases, and maintains a proper level of medical hygiene.

Activity

STERILITY EXERCISE

Identify whether sterile technique is required for the following procedures by checking yes or no:

Procedure	Sterile technique required?	
	Yes	No
Administering an injection		
Invasive surgical procedure		
Removing a peripheral IV line		
Taking blood pressure		
Inserting a peripheral IV line		
Wound dressing		
Assisting patient onto examination table		

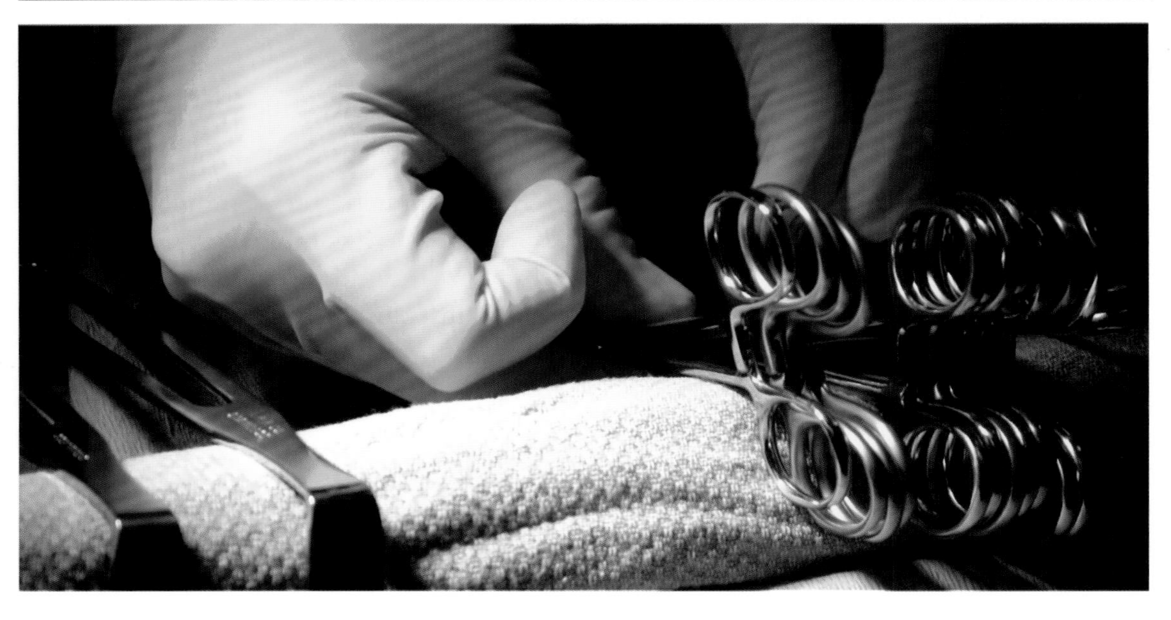

Three Levels of Hygiene

Maintaining a clean and safe health care environment is essential for the safety of patients, as well as medical personnel. Environmental cleaning and disinfection should be performed routinely for a safe and sanitary environment. There are three levels of hygiene that can be exercised in a medical office, depending on how sterile a particular instrument needs to be for its purpose.

Sanitization: *A process to remove organic matter from an article and to lower the number of microorganisms to a safe level as determined by public health management.*

1. **Sanitization:** Removal of some of the contaminants and microorganisms from instruments, skin, and so on.
2. **Disinfection:** More thorough removal of contaminants than sanitization, but less thorough than sterilization.
3. **Sterilization:** Complete removal of microorganisms and considered the highest level of medical hygiene.

Sanitization

Disinfection: *A more thorough removal of contaminants than sanitization, but less thorough than sterilization.*

The first step in the cleaning process is sanitization, which removes pathogenic organisms, as well as blood and tissue debris. Sanitization is often needed for objects that contact intact skin. Objects should be sanitized immediately so fluids don't dry on the object.

Sterilization: *Complete removal of microorganisms. Considered the highest level of medical hygiene.*

Sanitizers are specifically formulated, nonabrasive, low-sudsing detergents with a neutral pH. Hand sanitizers should not and cannot take the place of proper hand washing with soap and water. They should only act as a supplement. Alcohol-based hand sanitizers kill bacteria by dissolving important proteins in the cell membrane, while also stripping away the outer layer of oil on the skin. This prevents **commensal** bacteria from populating the surface of the hand.

Sanitizers: *Specially formulated, nonabrasive, low-sudsing detergents with a neutral pH.*

Guidelines and procedures to maintain a sanitary environment at the office involve:

- Rinsing thoroughly in warm, not hot, water
- Making sure you clean all surfaces
- Using proper cleaning devices
- Inspecting each instrument for defects and proper working condition
- Using proper cleaning agent and following instructions on labels

Commensal: *An interaction between an animal, plant, fungus, or other microorganism. The interaction involves living with, on, or in another, without injury to either.*

When sanitizing surgical instruments, wear heavy-duty, puncture-resistant gloves to protect against bloodborne pathogens. Use these especially when working with sharp instruments. Place each instrument on a mat or towel to dry— do not overlap the instruments to avoid entanglement and damage. Handle delicate instruments with care, and separate them from dull or sharp instruments.

The sanitation level of hygiene is considered a barrier to contamination, and is the first step towards prevention of contamination by microorganisms. Hand sanitizers should never replace proper soap and water hand washing, but should be used to supplement it.

Proper Application of Alcohol-Based Hand Sanitizer

When hand washing is unavailable, the medical office assistant may use an alcohol-based hand sanitizer until they have access to a sink, warm running water, and liquid antimicrobial soap. Again, the use of an alcohol-based hand sanitizer must never replace actual hand washing.

Properly applying hand sanitizer is important to avoid transmitting pathogens. The following steps will ensure appropriate application of alcohol-based hand sanitizer.

Friction from your hands and an alcohol-based hand sanitizer are all you need for this application.

1. Make sure that your hands are not visibly soiled or greasy. If they are, remove all visible organic matter from your hands before applying the sanitizer.
2. Apply a dime-sized amount of sanitizer to the palm of one hand.
3. Rub hands together briskly, covering all surfaces including the front and back of hands until hands are dry. Don't forget under the nails, as well as around and between fingers.
4. Rub until the hand sanitizer is absorbed. Do not wipe away any remaining product—let it air dry.

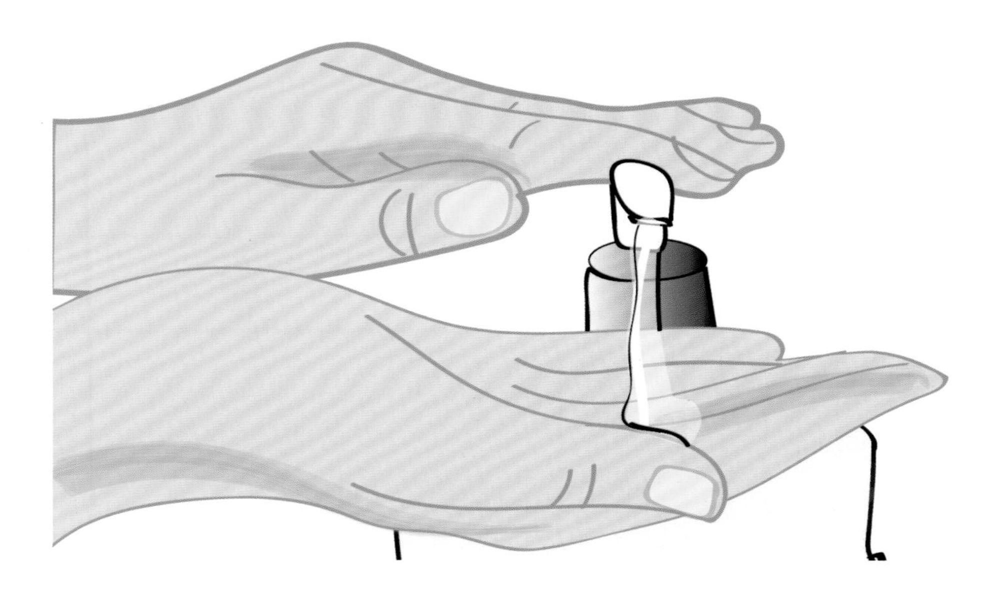

Activity

PROPER APPLICATION OF ALCOHOL-BASED HAND SANITIZER

Create a flow chart describing the steps on how to properly apply alcohol-based hand sanitizer.

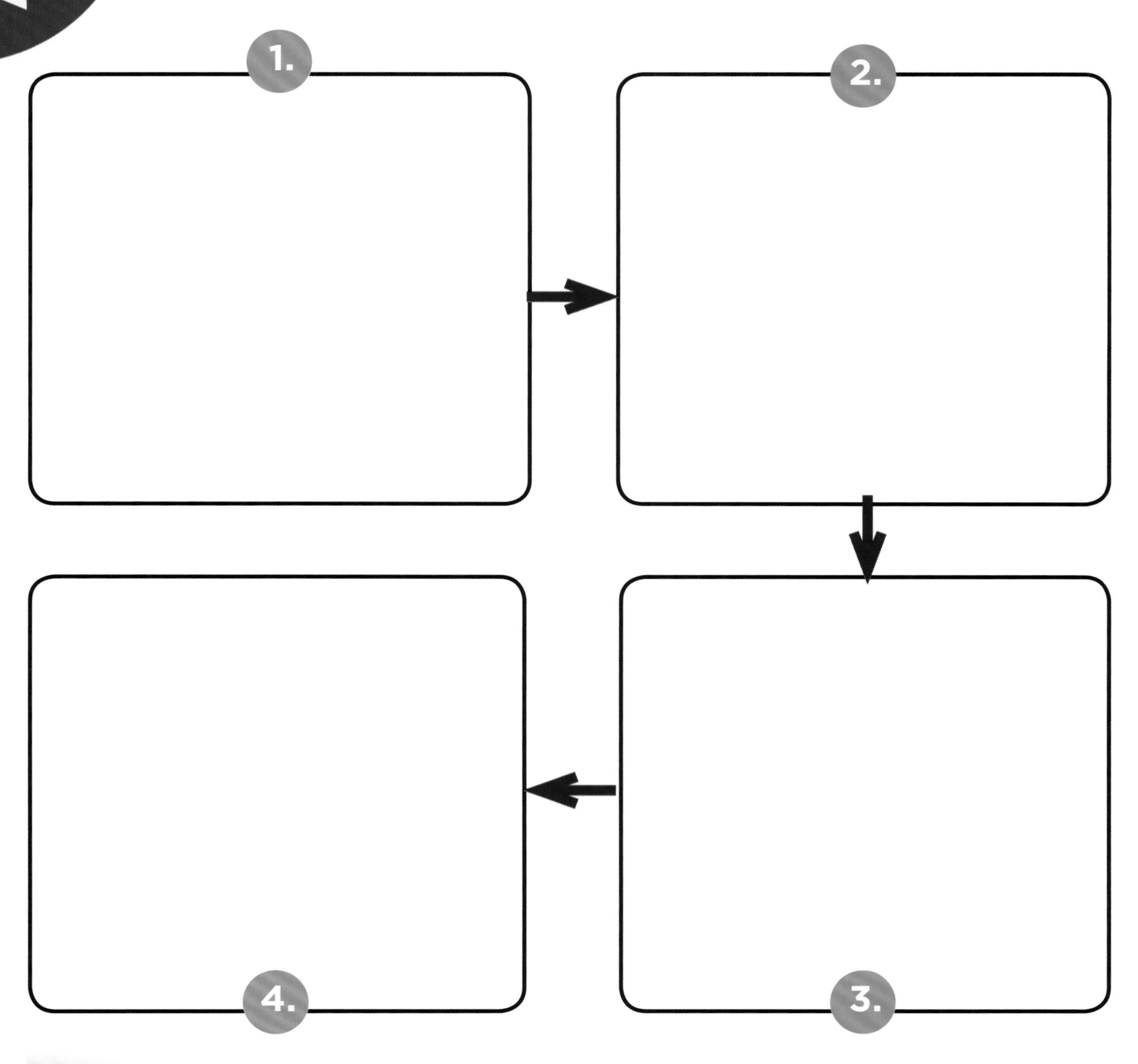

Disinfection

The second step in the cleaning process is disinfection and the final step for objects that do not require (or cannot withstand) sterilization. Frequently touched surfaces in the immediate vicinity of a patient may be a breeding ground for pathogens. Clean and disinfect a minimum of once each day, more frequently if the risk of contamination is higher.

Methods of disinfecting include:

- Ultraviolet (UV) light: environmentally safe and wide range of efficacy.
- Moist heat: boiling at a temperature of 100°C for 30 minutes. This method does not kill all pathogens.
- Antiseptics and disinfectant chemicals:
    - Disinfectants (such as bleach) are common but are often too harsh for use on human tissue – antiseptics such as isopropyl alcohol or betadine are gentler.
    - Disinfectants are **bactericidal,** which means that they destroy bacteria; antiseptics are **bacteriostatic**, which are agents that prevent the growth of bacteria or keep them in a stationary phase of growth.

Bactericidal: *Disinfectants that destroy bacteria.*

Bacteriostatic: *Agents that prevent the growth of bacteria or keep them in the stationary phase of growth.*

Disinfectant chemicals come in various strengths, with low-level disinfectants killing most bacteria, some fungi, and some inactive viruses. This low-strength is useful for linens, or instruments that contact intact skin. Disinfectants destroy pathogenic microorganisms, but do not kill the resistant bacterial spores.

Intermediate level disinfectants are effective against most viruses and fungi. They will kill most bacteria, but are not effective against spores. They are useful for items that come in contact with a patient's mucous membrane, such as the specula. The highest level of disinfectant is used for articles that need the highest possible level of pathogen reduction, but cannot withstand the sterilization process, such as anesthetic, respiratory, and endoscopic equipment.

Sterilization

Part of the last step in the cleaning process, sterilization methods can vary, depending on the level of disinfection or sterilization and the intended use of the object.

For example, critical items (such as a surgical instrument that comes into contact with sterile tissue) require a high level of sterilization, whereas noncritical items (such as stethoscopes that only come into contact with skin) are considered a low level sterilization.

The purpose of sterilization is to decrease the risk of introducing pathogenic microbes that could lead to infection. In a medical office environment, the spread of infection can be transferred between people directly or through inanimate objects (also known as fomites). For example, the waiting room of the office is known as a primary source of communicable diseases between patients or employees.

Sterile: *An item or object that is free of all living microorganisms and spores.*

Critical item*: All instruments and items that come into contact with sterile tissue or vascular systems that must be sterilized prior to use to avoid infection.*

Semi-critical items: *Instruments or objects that come into contact with non-intact skin or with intact mucous membranes and can be chemically disinfected using a high-level disinfectant.*

An item or object is deemed **sterile** if it is free of all living microorganisms and spores. All instruments and items that come into contact with sterile tissue or vascular systems are considered **critical items.** They must be sterilized prior to use to avoid infection.

Semi-critical items are instruments or objects that come into contact with non-intact skin or intact mucous membranes. These instruments can be chemically disinfected using a high-level disinfectant. Semi-critical items, such as vaginal and nasal specula, can be autoclaved without damage and sterilized using steam under pressure, instead of being sterilized chemically.

The nature of the item to be sterilized decides on the method to achieve sterilization. Physical methods and chemical methods are two classes of sterilization with advantages as well as disadvantages.

Methods of Sterilization

Physical methods include autoclave, dry heat oven, and radiation. Autoclaves are convenient, effective, safe, and inexpensive to use for destroying microorganisms. Unlike chemical disinfectants that can be expensive and hazardous to use, autoclaves don't create issues with proper disposal.

Steam **autoclaves** use pressurized steam at 121°C to 132°C for 30 or 40 minutes. Items to be autoclaved are wrapped with autoclave tape, which indicates that an item was brought to the correct temperature with indicator marks. If they are to be stored for long periods of time, autoclaved wrapped packs should be routinely checked to make sure they stay dry and sealed with the date of when it was sterilized. Chemical and biological indicators can be used to show that the appropriate temperature was reached for the appropriate length of time, and to prove sterilization was achieved.

The **dry heat method** exposes objects to temperatures of 160°C to 170°C for at least two hours. Dry heat is used for objects that cannot withstand moisture. Dry heat is less corrosive than moist heat, and doesn't erode ground-glass surfaces of reusable syringes. Dry heat ovens operate relatively the same to household cooking ovens.

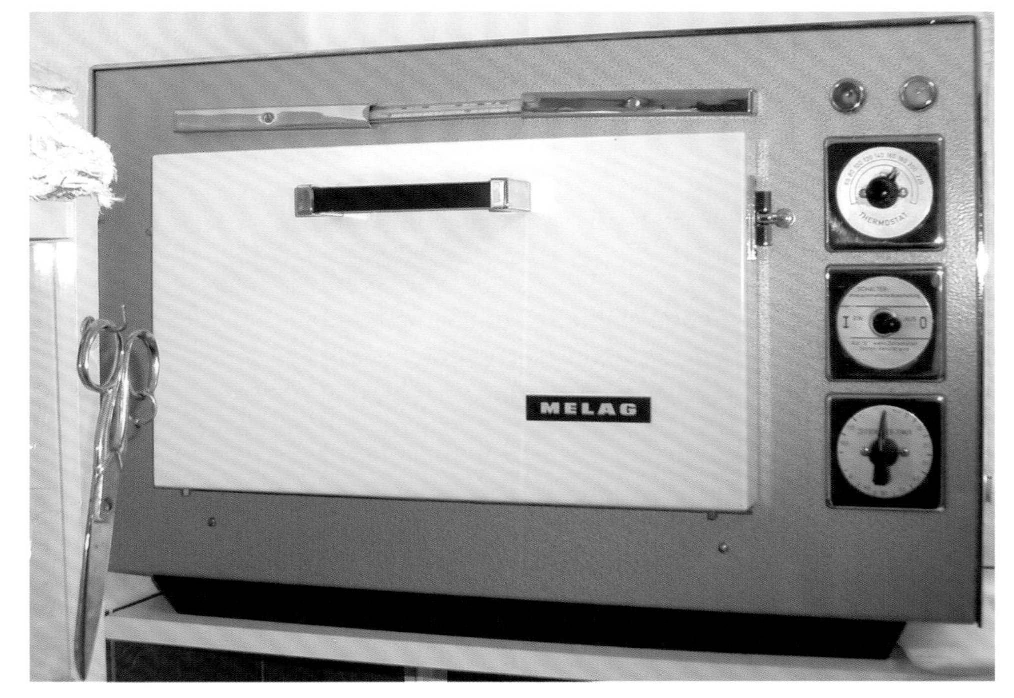

By R-E-AL (talk | contribs | Gallery) (German Wikipedia) - English: This Photo has been taken with a Casio Exilim EX-Z3 camera.,

Aluminum foil wrapping is the ideal material for this method of sterilization because of its conductive properties and protection against recontamination during handling.

Oil, petroleum jelly, and powder cannot be penetrated by steam, making the dry heat method the best for sterilizing these items. Microorganisms and spores are more resistant to dry heat due to slow and uneven distribution compared to moist heat. Always check dry heat sterilization indicators to determine the efficacy of the sterilization process.

Radiation, uses high-energy ionized radiation to sterilize articles and is often the method that medical manufacturers use to sterilize pre-packaged surgical equipment that cannot be sterilized by heat or chemicals.

Chemical methods include the use of ethylene oxide gas and cold sterilization for equipment that is heat sensitive. It involves the use of a substance known as a **sterilant**—a mixture of chlorine and Cidex—which needs to be handled with caution.

Gas sterilization uses toxic gasses to destroy living organisms within the chamber. It is only used with extreme caution and for items that cannot be sterilized any other way. Ethylene oxide gas is colourless, toxic, and flammable. Heat sensitive instruments, as well as items that cannot be autoclaved, use the ethylene oxide gas sterilization process.

It is complex and expensive to use this chemical method, which is why it is used mostly in the medical manufacturing industry for sterilizing pre-packaged and pre-sterilized disposable items such as syringes, sutures, catheters, and surgical packs.

Cold sterilization involves the use of a chemical agent preapproved as a sterilant by the U.S. Environmental Protection Agency (EPA). The chemical agent will have a clear label marking it as a sterilant on the bottle. These are the only chemical agents you can use for sterilization.

To effectively sterilize articles, completely submerge them in the sterilant, following the manufacturer's specific instructions regarding the length of time. For the most part, this time varies between 6 to 24 hours. However, keep in mind that you must restart the clock whenever you add additional tools into the sterilant. This process is more arduous and hazardous, so only use cold sterilization if you are unable to use other methods such as the autoclave for sterilizing tools.

The cleaning process reduces infections associated with contaminated patient-care items. Sterilization is the highest level of cleanliness that can be achieved. All medical procedures that require sterile instruments run the risk of introducing pathogenic microbes, which can lead to infection. In order to prevent this, protocols must be established and followed to minimize, maintain, and control the spread of infectious diseases in a medical office environment.

Dry heat method: *A method of sterilization where objects are exposed to temperatures of 160°C to 170°C for at least two hours and used for objects that cannot withstand moisture.*

Radiation Sterilization: *The use of high-energy ionized radiation to sterilize articles.*

Sterilant: *A chemical method to achieve sterility that involves a mixure of chlorine and Cidex. Sterilants need to be handled with caution.*

How to

WRAPPING SURGICAL PACKS

Supplies/Equipment needed:

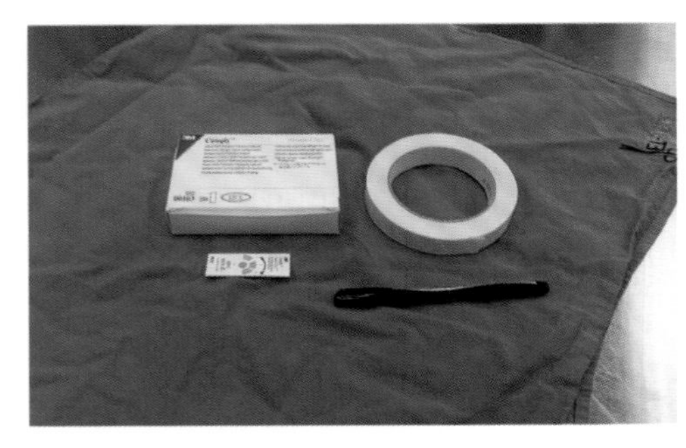

- **Autoclave tape**
- **Autoclave indicator**
- **Sanitized instruments**
- **Two appropriate sized wrapping materials** (sterilization paper or muslin)
- **Any additional materials needed to complete the surgical pack** (i.e., gauze, drapes, etc.)
- **Permanent marker or pen**

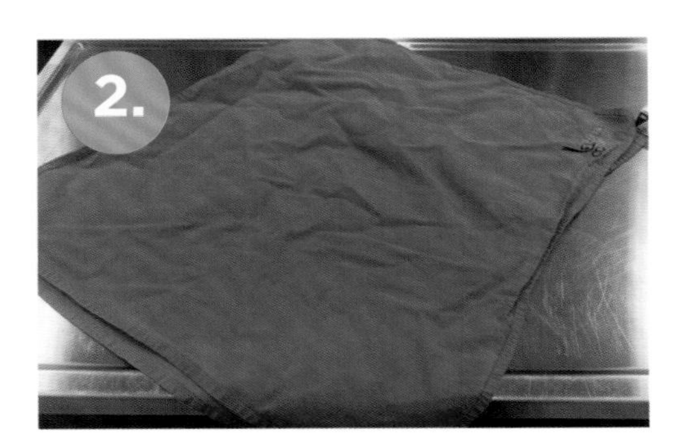

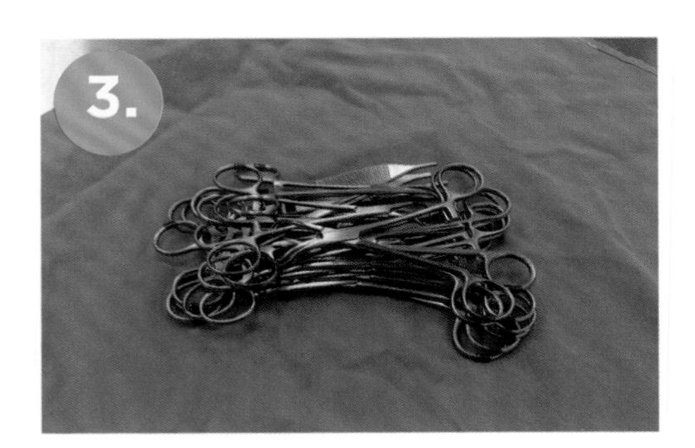

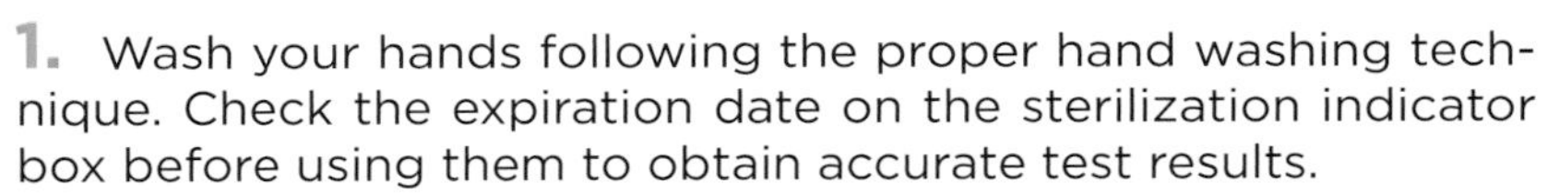

1. Wash your hands following the proper hand washing technique. Check the expiration date on the sterilization indicator box before using them to obtain accurate test results.

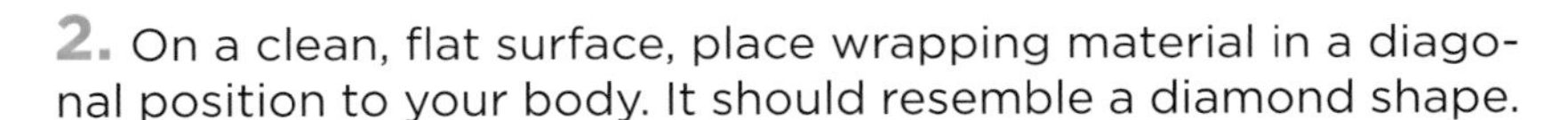

2. On a clean, flat surface, place wrapping material in a diagonal position to your body. It should resemble a diamond shape.

3. Place sanitized instruments in the middle of the inner drape, placing longer instruments on a diagonal. For instruments with hinges, slightly open the instruments before placing them on the wrap. If necessary, use square gauze to keep the instruments in this position. This allows the steam to reach every part of the instrument. It also prevents cracks at the weak points of instruments when exposed to high temperatures.

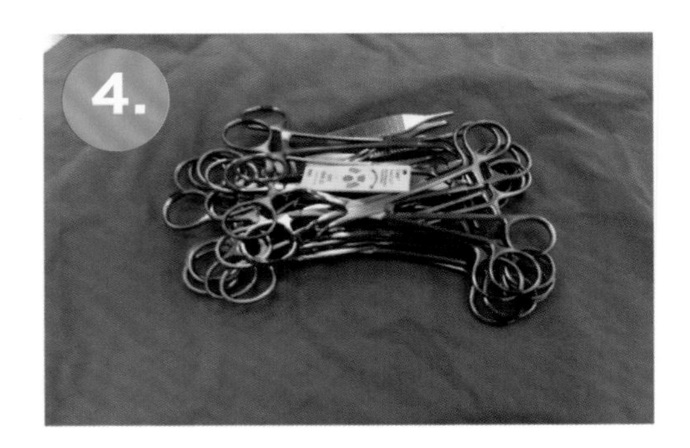

4. Place a sterilization indicator in the centre of the pack. This will verify that the sterilization process is effective.

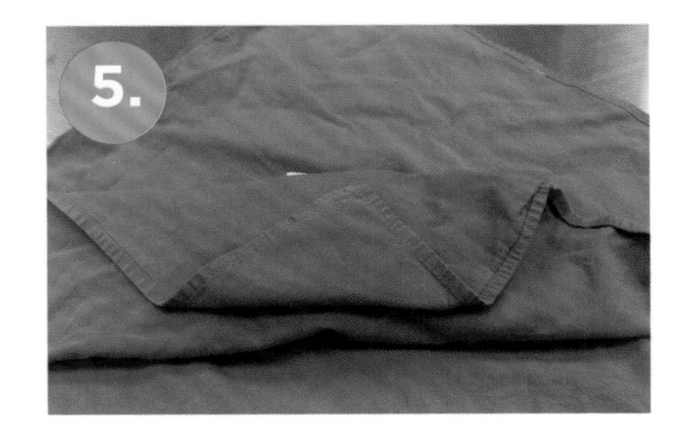

5. Start at the bottom corner closest to you and fold the drape upwards. Double-back the corner and make sure the folds are tight to prevent contamination.

6. Fold over the other two edges of the wrapping material and double back the corner.

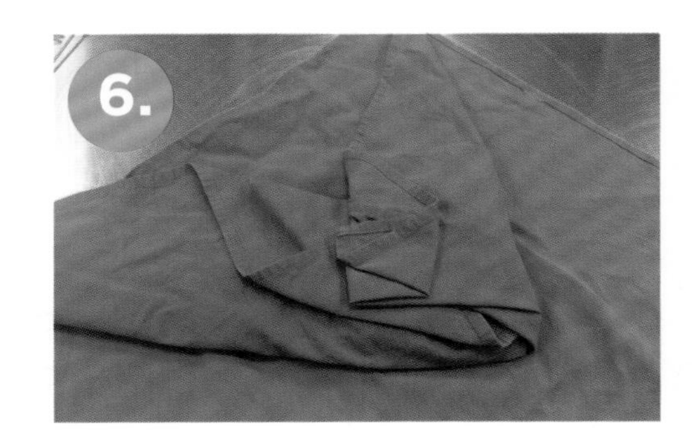

7. Fold the pack up from the bottom and pull the top flap down.

8. Using your second sheet, repeat Steps 2 to 7, but place the wrapped parcel in the centre instead. Wrap the pack up tightly to avoid water retention after the autoclave process, but loose enough to permit steam circulation in the autoclave.

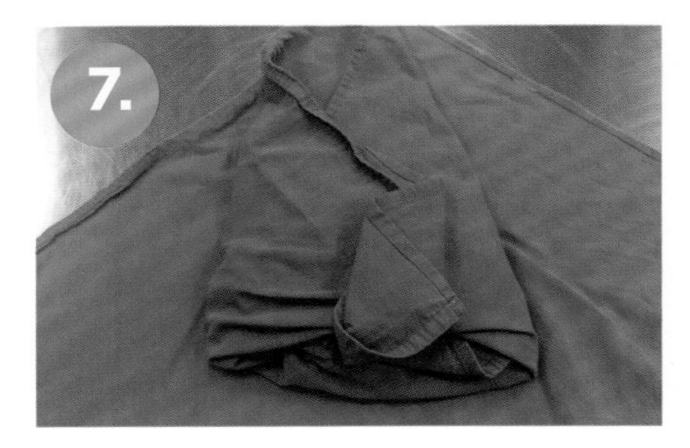

9. Secure the neat and tightly wrapped pack with the autoclave tape where its indicator will become visible and easily read. This indicates that the parcel has been autoclaved.

10. With a marker or pen, label the pack according to its contents. Write your initials and the date of when the contents were autoclaved. Sterilize the pack in the autoclave following proper autoclave procedure.

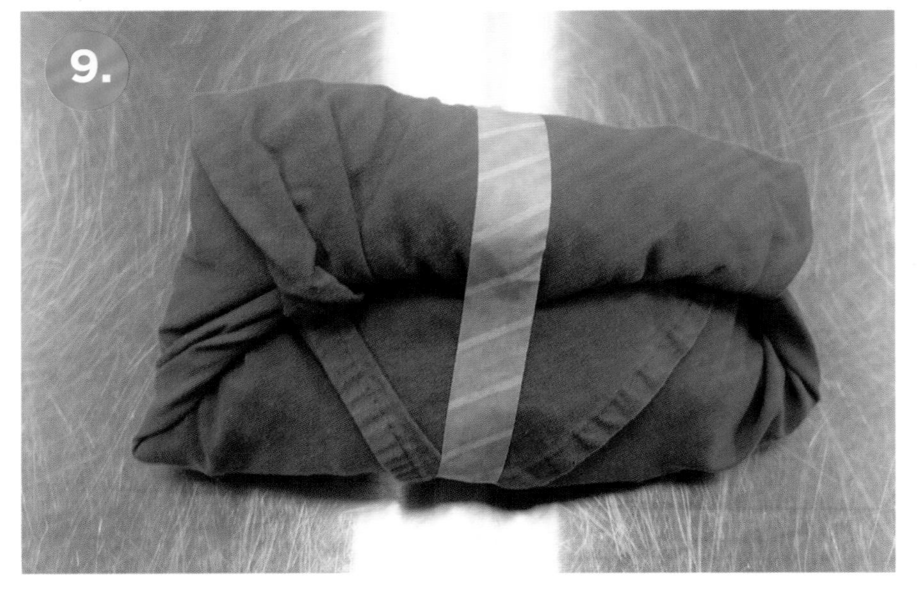

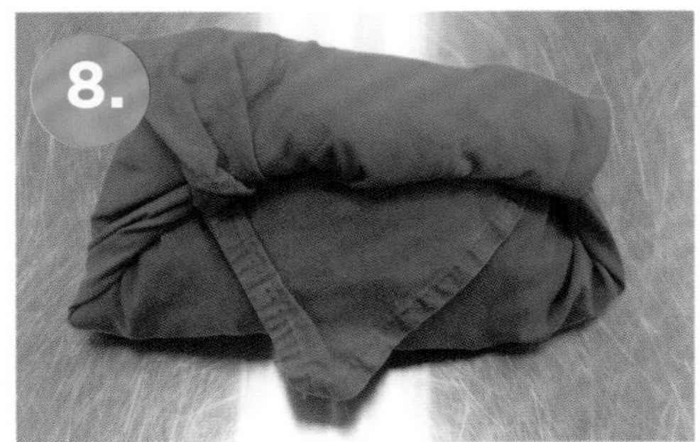

How to

WRAPPING INSTRUMENTS USING A POUCH

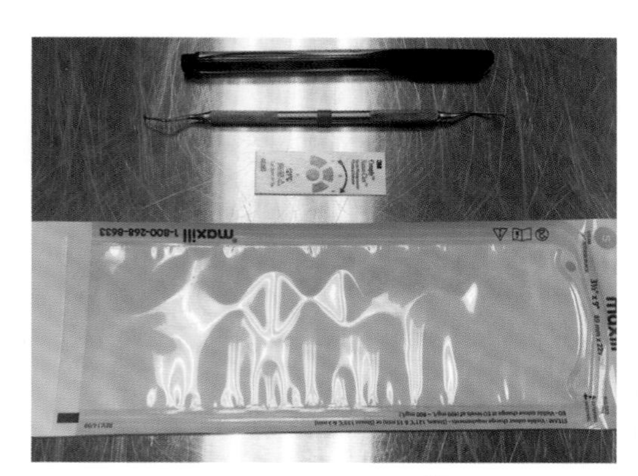

Supplies/Equipment needed:

- **Sterilization indicator strip**
- **Sanitized instruments**
- **Appropriate-sized sterilization pouch**
- **Permanent marker or pen**

1. Wash your hands following the proper hand washing technique.

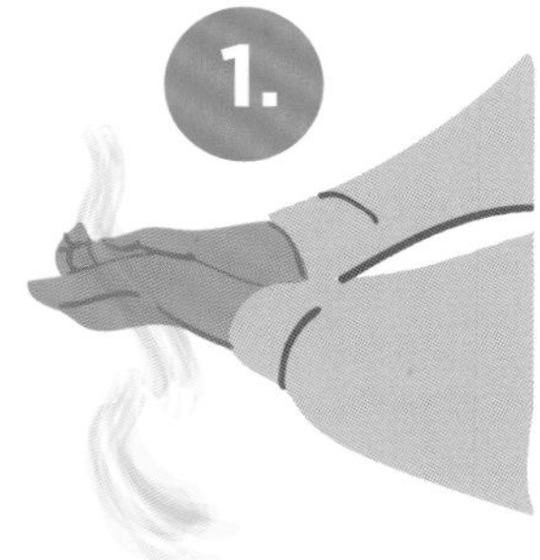

2. Place the sterilization pouches on a clean, flat surface.

3. Gather the sanitized instruments and choose the appropriate-sized sterilization pouch. For hinged instruments, select a pouch that allows the instrument to remain in a slightly open position. Use square gauze to hold the instrument open.

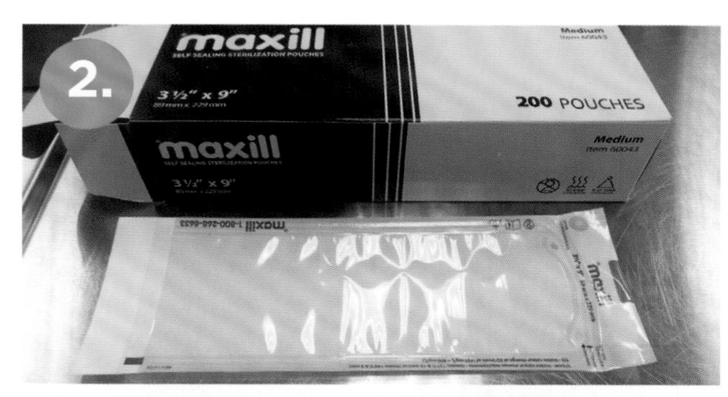

4. Insert the sanitized instruments in the pouch, along with sterilization indicator strip facing up, so that you can easily see if the pouch has been effectively sanitized once opened.

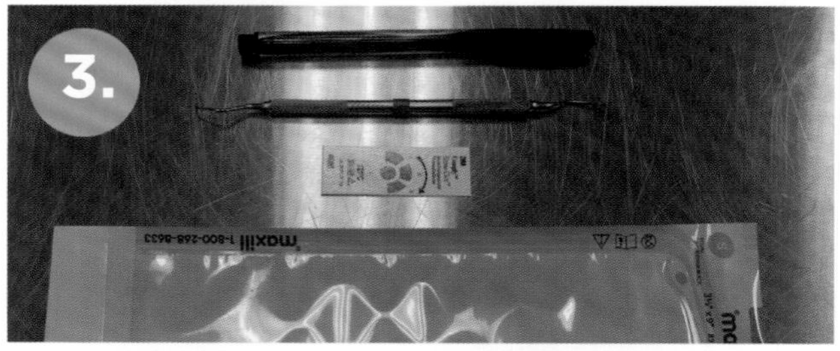

5. Remove the paper strip located above the perforation to expose the adhesive and fold along the perforation. Press firmly to seal the pouch with your fingers starting at the center and work your way to the sides of the pouch.

6. Label the pack according to the contents inside and mark the pack with the date of sterilization, along with your initials.

7. Sterilize the pouch in the autoclave.

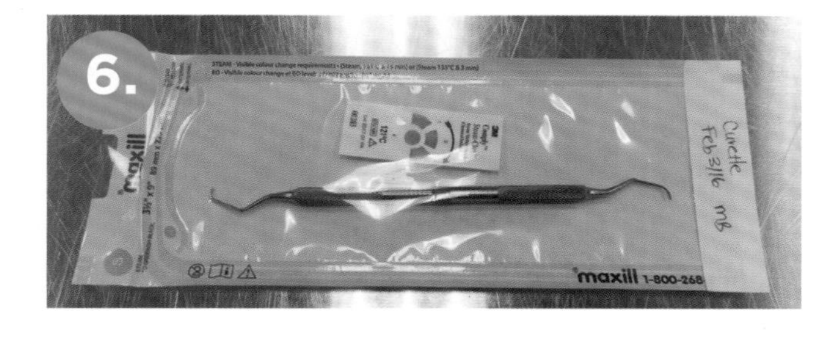

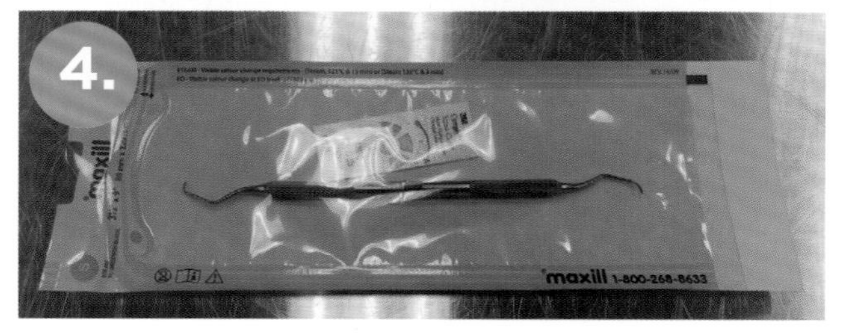

STERILIZATION USING AN AUTOCLAVE

Supplies/Equipment needed:

- **Autoclave and instruction manual**
- **Distilled water**
- **Wrapped articles**
- **Heat-resistant gloves**

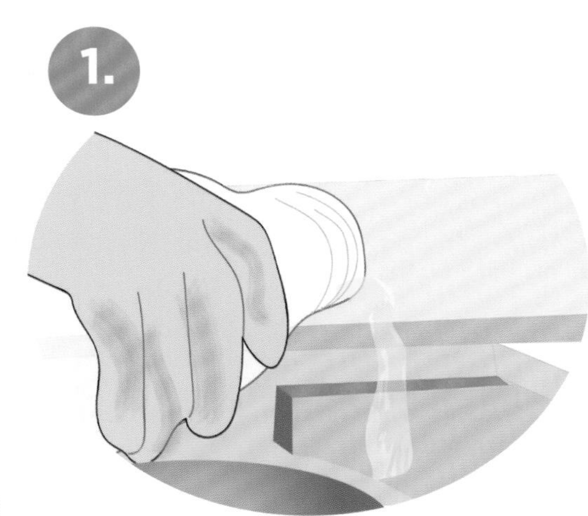

1. Assemble the equipment accordingly and check the level of water in the autoclave. Add distilled water ONLY if needed.

- *Note: Water in the reservoir of the autoclave becomes steam during the sterilization process. The use of distilled water prevents corrosion of the autoclave's stainless steel chamber.*

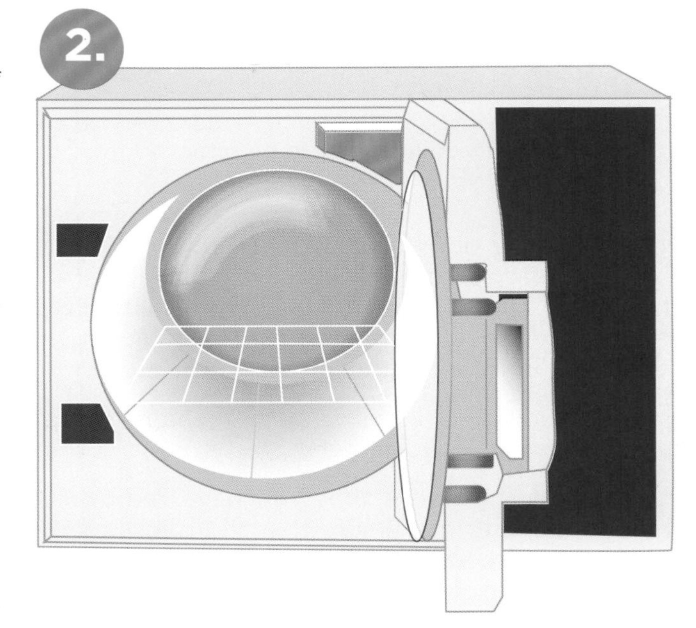

2. Load the autoclave with the following precautions in mind. Improper loading of the autoclave will lead to inadequate steam penetration:

- Do not overload the chamber. Place smaller packs one to three inches apart from each other, and larger packs two to four inches apart. Do not let the packs touch the chamber walls. This allows steam to reach the entire pack and allows for proper ventilation after sterilization, when the packs are cooling down.
- Leave at least one inch between autoclave trays to allow airflow.
- Place jars and glassware on their sides to prevent anything from rolling out when the door to the autoclave pops open.
- Place dressings in a vertical position and on the top shelf if sterilizing with hard goods. Place hard goods on the lower shelf of the autoclave.
- When sterilizing pouches, set pouches on their side to maximize steam circulation and facilitate drying.

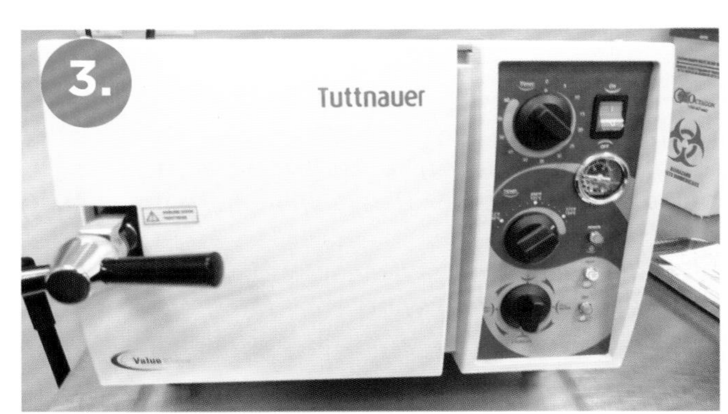

3. For automatically operated autoclaves, securely close the door to the autoclave. Turn on the autoclave.

4. Operate the autoclave according to the procedures described in its manual and set the autoclave to sterilize the appropriate articles. You will see the option for sterilizing pouches, wrapped packs, and unwrapped instruments. Determine the appropriate program to use to sterilize the articles that you've loaded.

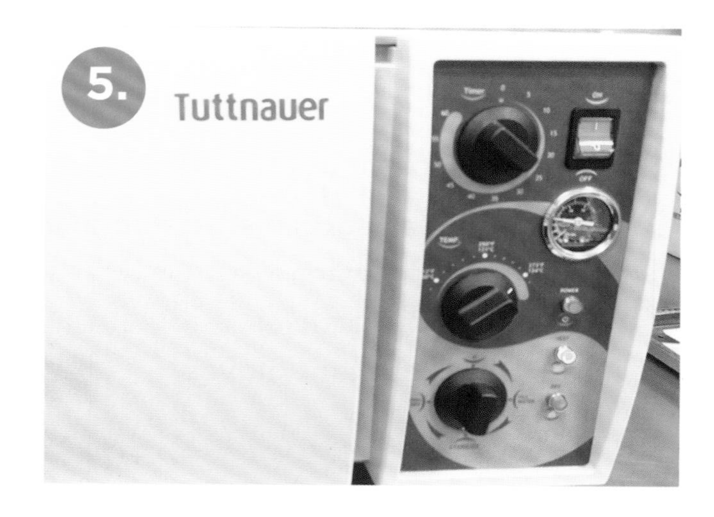

5. Press the start button. Indicators on the front of the autoclave will tell you what is happening in the autoclave.

- *Filling indicator:* lights up when the chamber is filing with water
- *Sterilizing indicator:* lights up during the heat-up and sterilization phases of the cycle
- *Temperature display*: digital display of the temperature in the autoclave
- *Time display:* digital countdown of the time remaining in the sterilization program
- *Drying indicator:* lights up during the drying phase of the cycle
- *Complete or Ready indicator:* illuminates when the autoclave has completed the cycle and the sterilized articles can be removed from the autoclave.

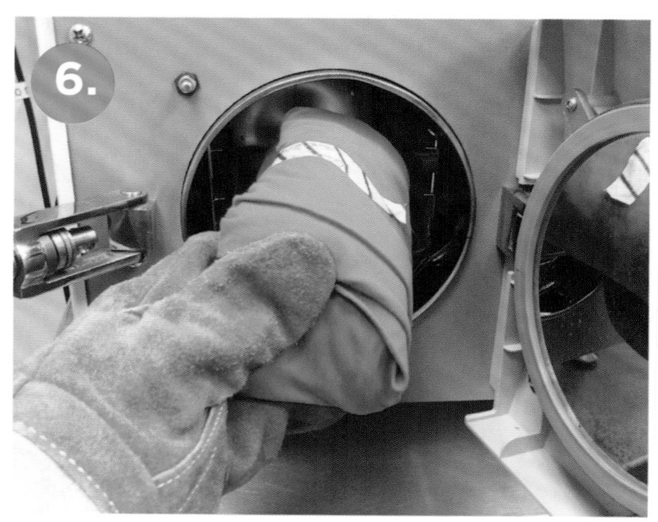

6. Leave the door open a crack to air out and dry the load. The autoclave will turn off or indicate when the drying cycle is done. Turn off the autoclave and remove the articles with heat-resistant gloves. Do not touch the inner chamber of the autoclave with your bare hands—the autoclave will be hot enough to burn unprotected skin.

7. Inspect the packs that you have removed from the autoclave to make sure that the packs are dry to the touch and not damp or soggy. If there are any holes, tears, or other damages to the packs, the articles should be re-wrapped and undergo the autoclave process once again.

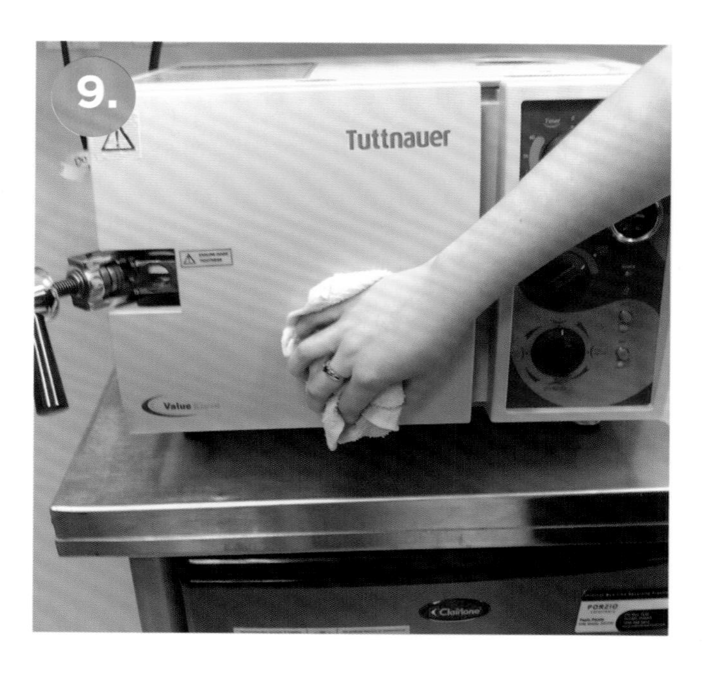

8. Store the autoclaved packs in a dry, clean, and dustproof place with other recently sterilized packs. Place the most recently sterilized packs behind previously sterilized ones. Packs will expire if not used.

9. Keep the autoclave clean and properly maintained with daily care following the manufacturer's recommendations in order for the autoclave to work efficiently.

Waste Disposal

There are two categories of waste that need special attention, and it is necessary to understand the differences between these two types so that medical personnel can separate the waste, and make arrangements for its appropriate disposal. To avoid the spread of infection from biohazardous materials, it is important to know the different categories of waste disposal.

Biomedical waste disposal includes anatomical waste and non-anatomical waste. Anatomical waste consists of tissues, organs, and body parts, but does not include teeth, hair, and nails. Non-anatomical waste consists of human liquid blood, semi-liquid blood, and blood products.

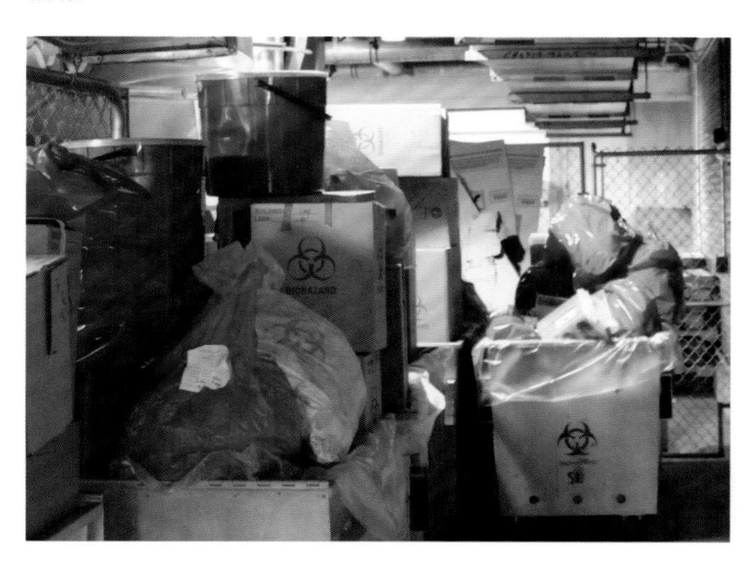

(Far left) By MFERMION - Own work, CC BY-SA

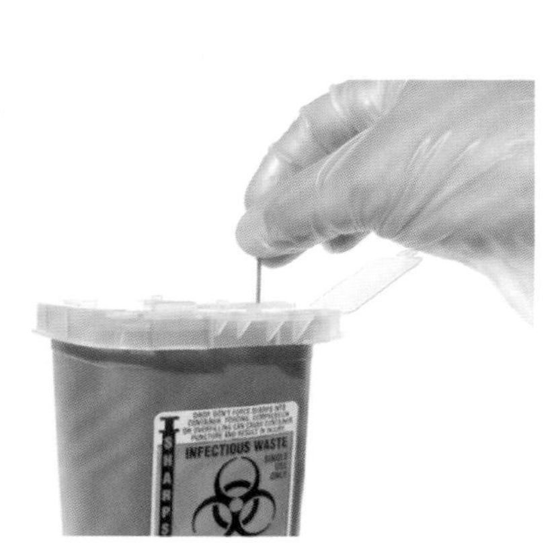

(photo at left)Photographed by William Rafti of the William Rafti Institute. - "The Body Piercing Encyclopedia Vol. 1" by William Rafti

Items that release liquid or semi-liquid blood if compressed are considered non-anatomical waste. In the course of surgery or treatment, any bodily fluids removed, excluding urine and feces, fall under the non-anatomical waste category as well.

Sharps disposal is required for anything that can puncture or tear, especially if it has encountered biomedical waste such as blood. Sharps are non-anatomical waste and include:

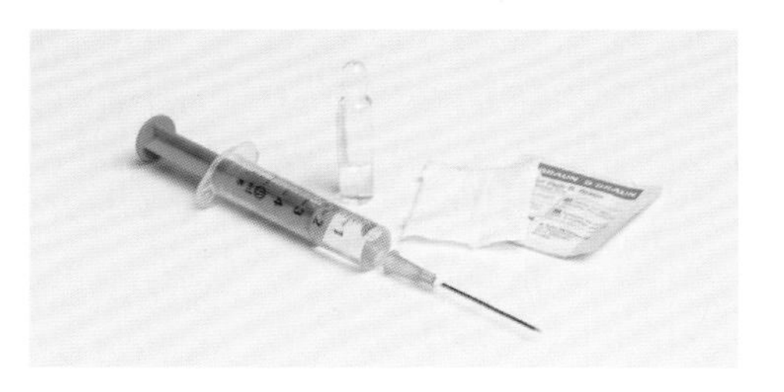

- Needles or needles attached to syringes
- Blades
- Glass (broken or unbroken) or other materials capable of causing punctures or cuts when in contact with human blood or body fluids

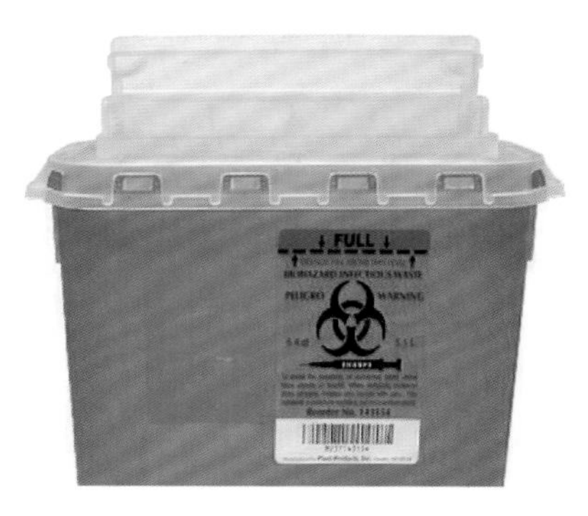

Sharps containers are rigid and resistant, as well as leak-proof. They are specially designed to have lids that cannot be easily removed and can be locked down when full. Sharps containers should be checked frequently for damage and never filled beyond the "full" line.

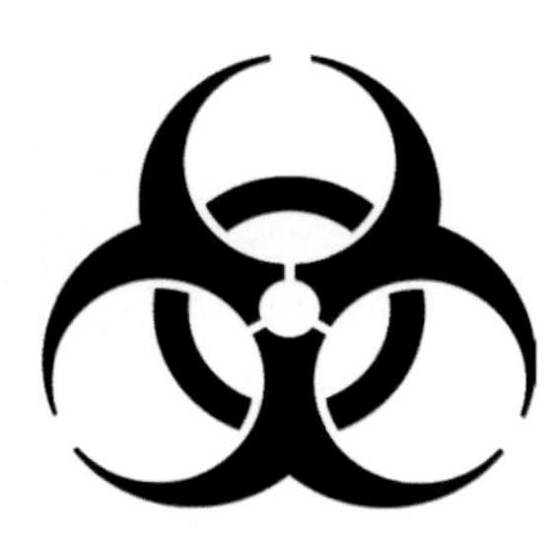

Universal Biohazard Symbol

The physician will place sharps into the container after they are finished with them. For sharp instruments, it is safest to have as few people handling them as possible. Needles should never be recapped or removed from syringes—the entire unit can be placed into the sharps container.

Biomedical waste must go into a rigid container or bag that is marked with the universal biohazard symbol. There are two colours of bags for biomedical waste, red and yellow. The yellow bag is for waste such as personal protective equipment, plastic tubing, disposable sharps containers, and gloves, bandages, or gauze that are soiled with blood.

Place all infectious or anatomical waste into a red bag and make sure the opening is tightly sealed. Infectious or anatomical waste is any human or animal waste involving tissue or blood potentially contaminated with infectious organisms. The red bag indicates a potential for pathogen transfer and special precautions need to be observed for the protection of anyone dealing with the waste. Red bag waste is disposed of through incineration.

Many facilities contract disposal companies to remove the sharps and biohazardous waste from the premises. Pharmacies can also accept full sharps containers for disposal. By law, only a licenced biomedical waste company can transport biomedical waste for disposal, but trained non-licenced personnel may transport small amounts of waste to a hospital or lab for disposal.

Includes personal protective equipment, plastic tubing, disposable sharps containers, and gloves, bandages, or gauze that are soiled with blood.

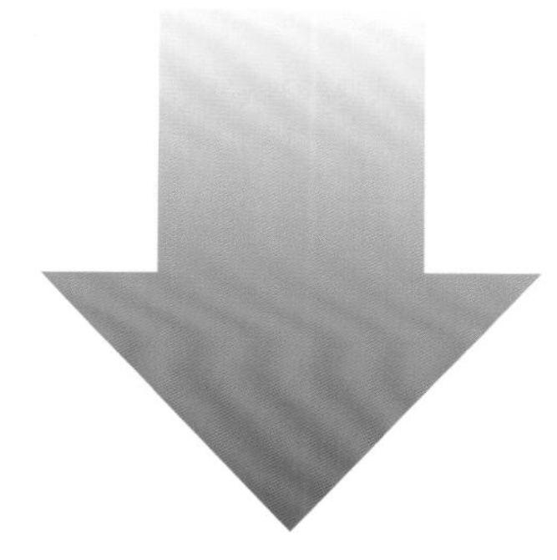

When there is a potential for pathogen transfer and special precautions need to be observed for the protection of anyone dealing with this waste.

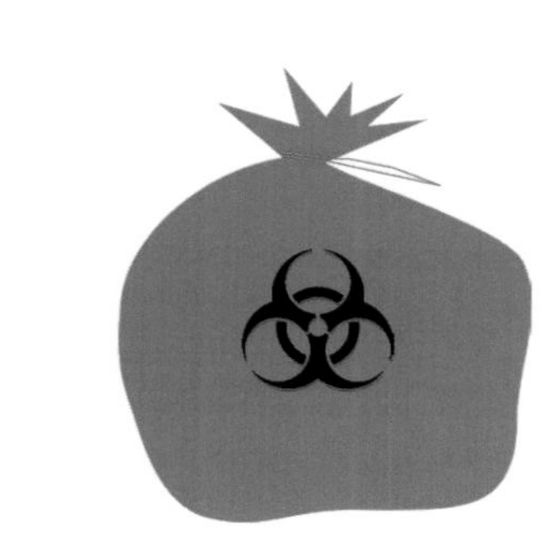

In the medical office, store biomedical waste in a safe spot until it can be transported to an appropriate facility for disposal by incineration, autoclaving, chemical treatment, or other necessary means.

What about garbage that does not fall into any of these categories? General office waste requiring no specific disposal method, still requires careful containment during disposal and removal. Ensure that all garbage containers are waterproof and have tight-fitting lids—ideally, containers that operate with a foot pedal. Do not overfill garbage containers, and empty receptacles as soon as they are full or scheduled for emptying.

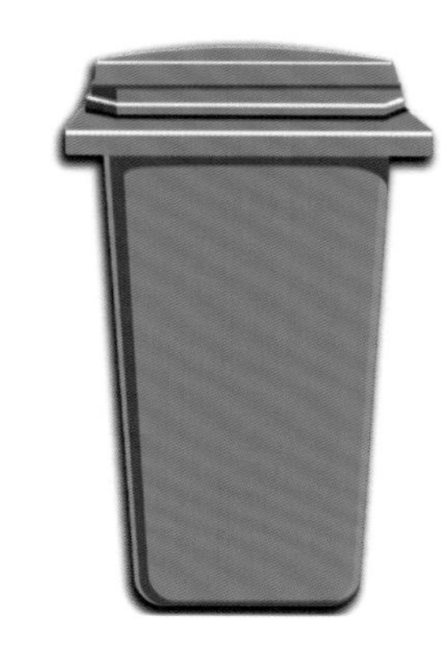

Proper disposal of biomedical waste is another of the many responsibilities of a medical office assistant. To avoid the spread of infections through careless disposal of biohazardous material, all medical personnel in the medical office must follow protocols and safety standards. A medical assistant must keep up to date with new safety standards or protocols that are implemented in the office.

Activity

IDENTIFYING WASTE CONTAINERS

Identify which waste container each of the following items should be placed into:

1. Yellow biomedical container
2. Red biomedical container
3. Sharps container
4. Regular waste container

Item	Container
Alcohol swab used to clean patient's skin prior to drawing blood	
Tissue or cotton ball saturated with blood	
Blood-soaked gloves	
Used bandage with dried blood	
Used face mask	
Cotton swab	
Used urine pregnancy test	
Urinalysis specimen container – specimen contained blood	
Urinalysis specimen container – specimen did not contain blood	
Used urinalysis reagent strip that was positive for hemoglobin	
Used syringe	
Empty glass serum bottle	
Broken glass vial	
Disposable scalpel	
Metal skewer that had punctured a patient's skin and was removed	
Tube of blood drawn by mistake	
Clippings from a patient's nails	
Tooth that had fallen out of a patient's mouth	
Used baby diaper	
Used adult diaper	
Needle removed from a syringe	
Saliva soaked gauze	
Gloves with minimal traces of blood	
Polyp removed from patient's respiratory tract	
Used lancet	

Quiz

CHAPTER 2 QUIZ

1. Define asepsis and why it is important. Explain the two principal types.

____

____

____

____

____

____

____

____

____

2. True or false? When applying sterile gloves, your hands are considered sterile and can reach inside the cuff of the second glove, but you should dispose of any gloves if tears are present.

3. Fill in the blank: In order to prevent the spread of pathogens, practicing proper hand washing techniques can help you achieve __________________.

4. When opening a sterile package, which of the following is part of keeping sterility?

    a. Do not reach over the sterile field

    b. Place the package on a clean surface at low hip level so that you can easily access everything

    c. Check to make sure the sterilization indicator tape shows a "pass" result

    d. Do not use packs that are wet on the outside, but if the wrap inside is dry it is fine

    e. More than one of the above

    f. None of the above

5. Why should only distilled water be used in the water reservoir of an autoclave?

____

____

____

____

____

____

____

6. True or false? Disinfectants are good for destroying bacteria and are safe for human use, including keeping stationary phase growth on human tissue.

7. Of the three levels of hygiene, the complete removal of microorganisms and the highest level of medical hygiene is:

   a. Sanitization

   b. Disinfection

   c. Sterilization

   d. None of the above

8. Of the three levels of hygiene, the removal of contaminants and microorganisms from instruments and skin is:

   a. Sanitization

   b. Disinfection

   c. Sterilization

   d. None of the above

9. Fill in the blank: ________________ is a more thorough removal of contaminants, but less thorough than sterilization.

10. The ________________ method is similar to ordinary cooking ovens, though it is less corrosive than moist heat and non-erosive surfaces.

11. Describe two out of the six indicators on the front of an autoclave that tell you what is happening.

____

____

____

____

____

____

____

____

12. Biomedical waste includes all of the following except:

    a. Tissues

    b. Organs and body parts

    c. Human liquid and blood

    d. Teeth, hair, and nails

    e. Semi-liquid blood

13. Sharp disposal includes anything that can puncture or tear, including the following:

    a. Needles or needles with syringes

    b. Blades

    c. Syringes or other sharps

    d. All of the above

14. How should general office waste be disposed?

____

____

____

____

____

____

____

____

Chapter 3

Standards and Safety

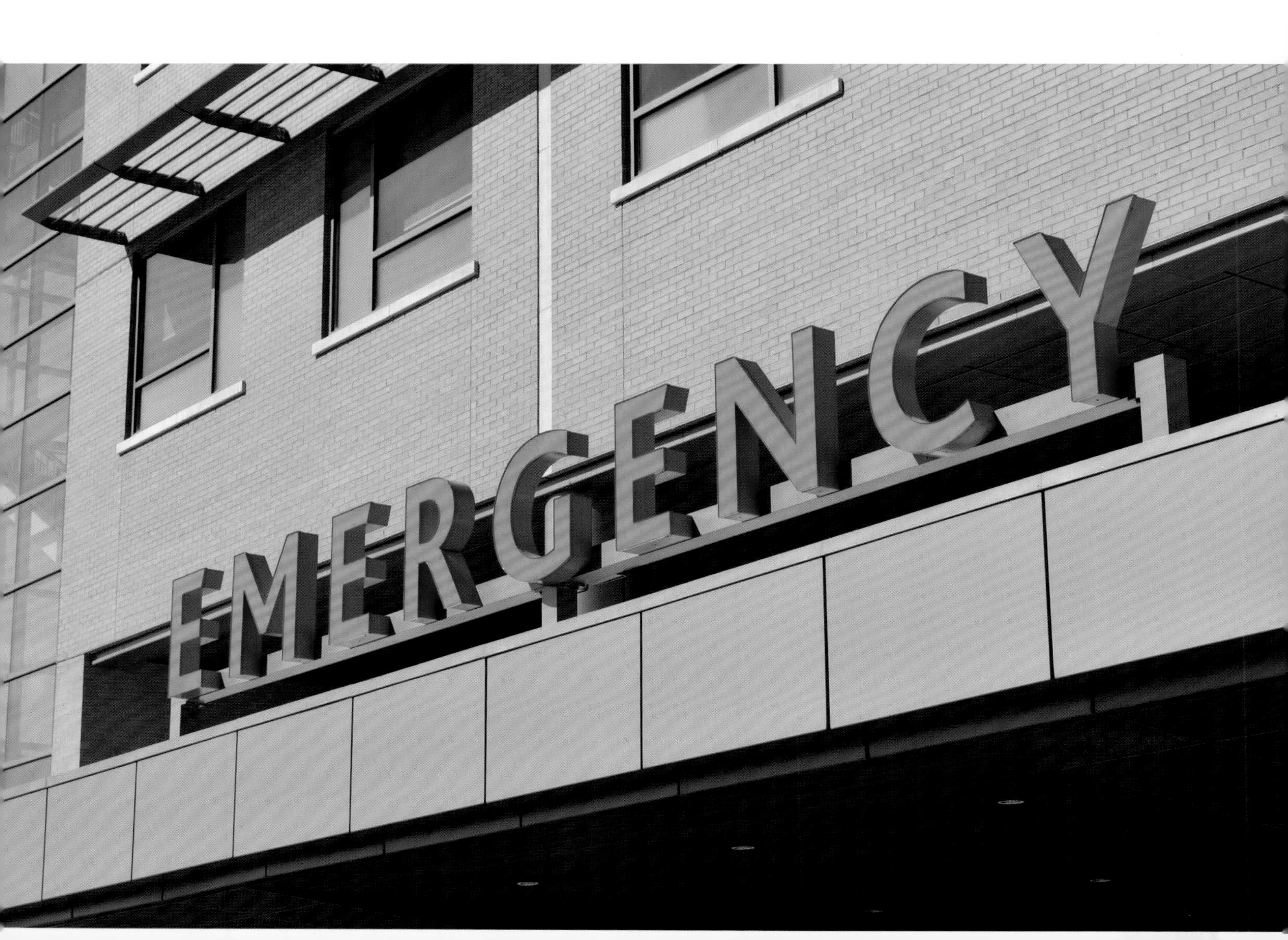

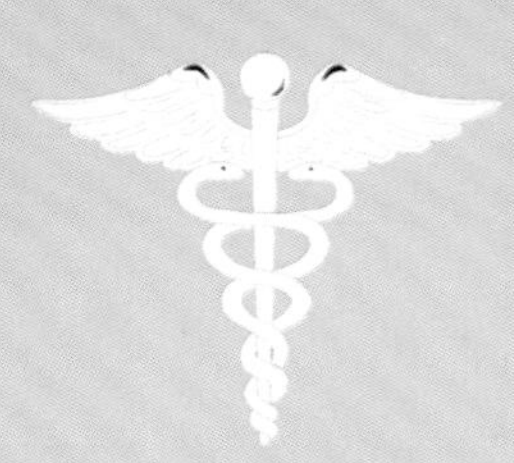

CHAPTER THREE LEARNING OBJECTIVES

After completing this chapter, you should be able to:

- ❑ Understand the standards of health care and quality assurance
- ❑ Describe the rights and responsibilities of medical personnel
- ❑ Define and explain WHMIS
- ❑ Understand the Occupational Health and Safety Act (OHSA), Exposure Control Plan, Needlestick and Sharps Injuries, and OHSA labelling requirements
- ❑ Understand and implement communication of hazards to employees

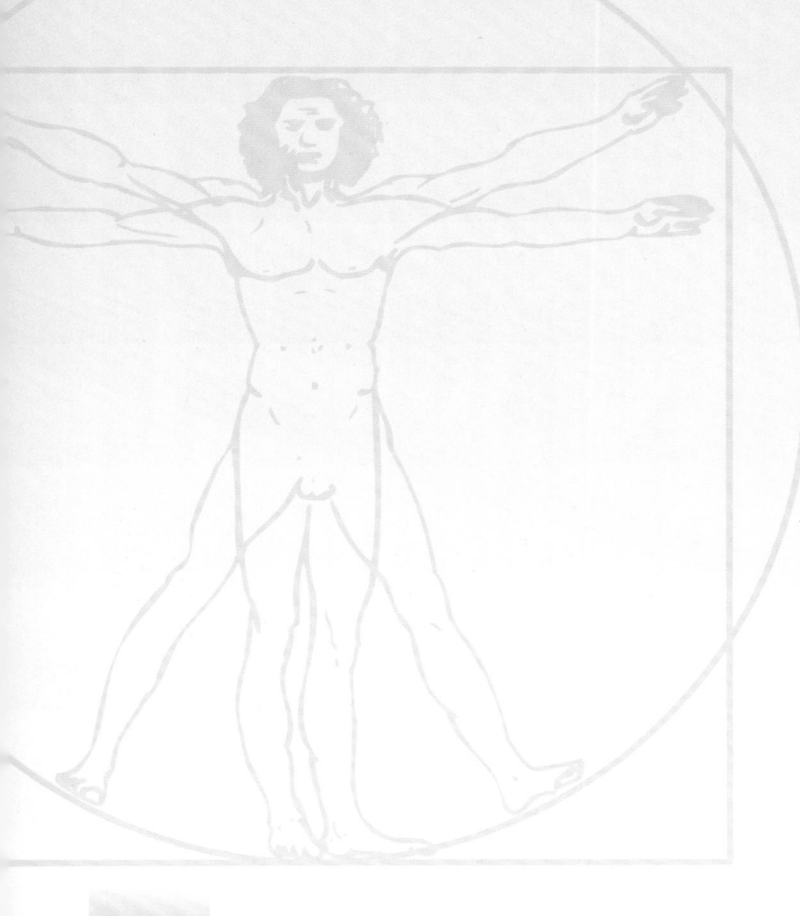

Standards of Care

A business has the responsibility to provide good service to its clients—the physician provides a service to a **client**. The medical office assistant acts as a liaison between the physician and client, while adopting a supportive role at the office.

Client: *A patient who receives health care.*

Clients of a physician or health care facility have a reasonable expectation that standards of care and service will be met. However, where does one turn when these standards of health care are compromised? First, let's look at the standards themselves.

Standards in Ontario Health Care

What standards exist in health care?

- Prompt treatment
- Prompt preparation and evaluation of diagnostic reports
- Accurate prescriptions
- Reasonable waiting times
- Direction regarding emergencies
- Pleasant communication
- Proper follow-up
- Safe environment

Quality assurance: *The systematic process of checking whether a product or service is meeting specific requirements.*

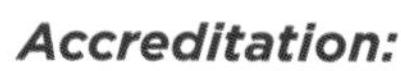

Accreditation: *Results from a detailed comparison of an organization's services against a national standard to ensure consistent standards of care.*

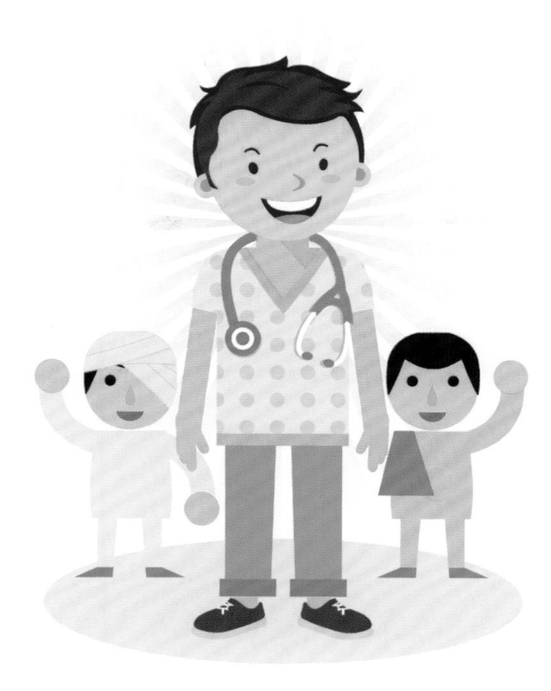

Quality assurance is the systematic process of ensuring that a product or service meets specified requirements.

Hospital **accreditation** is a process that compares an organization's services with a national standard. It allows a facility to demonstrate their ability to meet standards of care. A commonly known organization for accreditation of different types of health care facilities is Accreditation Canada, at https://www.accreditation.ca/. Accreditation has a significant impact on a health care facility by establishing an expected performance standard—this is important for both clients and the facility itself.

Credentialing: *Comparing a health care provider's education and experience against a national standard.*

Review: *A formal examination or assessment with the possibility or intention of instituting change if necessary, such as office protocols.*

Credentialing is a comparison of a health care provider's education and experience against a national standard. Health care organizations and hospitals evaluate documentation regarding a medical provider's detailed history before allowing the provider to practice. The medical provider's education, training, work history, licence, malpractice history, and regulatory compliance record all undergo examination before approving their credentials.

If a medical professional cannot obtain proper credentialing, they are not permitted to perform or provide medical services. Insurance providers will not reimburse for visits by professionals who have not been properly credentialed. Medical personnel practicing without credentials can result in financial losses—sometimes ranging in the thousands.

Reviews are conducted by the office itself to implement and monitor appropriate actions that arise from the re-evaluation of policies, procedures, and other office protocols. Patient safety training falls under this category and ensures that organization leaders, team members, and volunteers focus on areas of specific patient safety. Areas of focus include safe medication use, reporting patient safety incidents, techniques for effective communication, equipment and facility sterilization, hand washing hygiene, and infection prevention and control.

Reviews occur whenever any of the following incidents arise, but are not limited to:

- Death in the hospital
- Client readmitted too soon after discharge
- Unscheduled return to surgery
- Infection that was contracted in the hospital
- Falls and injuries
- Medication errors

In health care offices, there are usually no formal quality assurance plans in place and quality is handled informally as needed. Policies or procedures may need to be reviewed when there are errors in relaying prescription information, when specimens are mislabelled, if patients are frequently found waiting for long periods, or if phone calls and lab reports are delayed. Policies and procedures must also be revisited when charting is incomplete or inaccurate.

Incident reports are filed whenever there are any falls or injuries in the workplace. Incident reports are formal documentations of any lapses of procedure—they are commonly seen in large facilities, but are also useful in smaller offices. Included in incident reports are:

- A summary of events
- A detailed event history
- A list of who was present at time of event
- Any actions taken at time of event
- Any recommendations for preventing a similar occurrence

Rights and Responsibilities

All medical personnel should know their rights and responsibilities in the workplace. Most workplace injuries occur when people are new to a job, so thorough training is crucial. This is also the case when new equipment is introduced. Safety protocols and procedures should be reviewed annually in a refresher training course for relevant skills. For example, first aiders must attend a refresher training course every three years in order for their certification to remain valid.

If work procedures change, or if new equipment is introduced to the workplace, training is required to minimize the risk of workplace injuries. Although not compulsory, it is a good idea to keep training records with health and safety documentation stating that all employees have received proper training in their particular field of employment. Make sure that all employees have completed Worker Health and Safety Training prior to starting their position.

Globally Harmonized System (GHS)

The Globally Harmonized System of Classification and Labelling of Chemicals (GHS) helps define and classify the hazards of chemical products.

The Hazardous Products Act (HPA) has been amended. Requirements for WHMIS hazard classification and communication set in the *Controlled Product Regulations* (CPR) and the Ingredient Disclosure List are repealed. It has been replaced with new regulations, known as *Hazardous Products Regulations* (HPR). The modified WHMIS is referred to as WHMIS 2015.

The HPA and HPR regulate suppliers of hazardous products. Federal, provincial, and territorial occupational health and safety (FPTOHS) authorities regulate the employer requirements of WHMIS in workplaces.

To implement WHMIS 2015 fully into the workplace, changes to the FPTOHS for labels and safety data sheets are required.

Canada has implemented the GHS to give suppliers, employers, and workers time to adjust to the new system over a three-stage transition period that synchronizes across federal, provincial, and territorial jurisdictions.

During the initial stage, suppliers can use either WHMIS 1988 (repealed CPR/old HPA) or WHMIS 2015 (HPR/new HPA) to classify and communicate the hazards of their products. The classification, label, and material safety data sheet (MSDS) must comply with the specific law and regulation chosen, and not as a combination of the two WHMIS systems.

If a hazardous product is noncompliant with the CPR during the transition process, modifications must be made to reach compliance. Otherwise, the supplier will be required to comply with the HPR, no matter which transitional phase applies at that time. See the table of Transition Phases for more detail regarding the implementation of WHMIS 2015.

Acronyms

CPR—*Controlled Products Regulations*

FPTOHS—*Federal, Provincial, and Territorial Occupational Health and Safety*

GHS— *Globally Harmonized System of Classification and Labelling of Chemicals*

HPR—*Hazardous Products Regulations*

HPA—*Hazardous Products Act*

MSDS—*Material Safety Data Sheet*

WHMIS—*Workplace Hazardous Materials Information System*

Transition Phases

Phases	Timing	Suppliers		Employers
		Manufacturers and Importers	**Distributors**	
Phase 1	From coming-into-force to May 31, 2017	Comply with CPR or HPR requirements	Comply with CPR or HPR requirements	Consult FPT OSH regulator
Phase 2	From June 1, 2017 to May 31, 2018	Comply with HPR requirements	Comply with CPR or HPR requirements	Comply with CPR or HPR requirements
Phase 3	From June 1, 2018 to November 30, 2018	Comply with HPR requirements	Comply with HPR requirements	Comply with CPR or HPR requirements
Completion	December 1, 2018	Comply with HPR requirements	Comply with HPR requirements	Comply with HPR requirements

Table obtained from Health Canada (www.hc-sc.gc.ca)

http://www.hc-sc.gc.ca/ewh-semt/occup-travail/whmis-simdut/transition/index-eng.php

Workplace Hazardous Materials Information System (WHMIS)

The **Workplace Hazardous Materials Information System** (WHMIS) is a Canada-wide system designed to inform and ensure that both employers and employees are educated about hazardous materials in the workplace. The purpose of WHMIS is to provide information on the safe usage of hazardous materials—this information includes proper use, storage, and disposal of all hazardous materials within the workplace. Suppliers, employers, and employees must all participate in proper use of the WHMIS system.

WHMIS: *A Canada-wide system designed to inform and ensure that both employers and employees are educated about hazardous materials in the workplace.*

In Canada, many workers encounter hazardous materials on the job. Before this system was in place, workers and employers were potentially unaware of the hazardous materials in their workplace. As such, precautions were set in place to ensure a safe work environment for all employees. From the development of WHMIS and its successful implementation of training, the workplace has seen a reduction in occurrence of illnesses and injuries.

Proper classification is essential for storing, managing, using, and safely disposing of controlled materials. These procedures increase the safety of the workplace. The pictograms on the following page can be found in WHMIS 2015 and were taken from the Canadian Centre for Occupational Health and Safety.

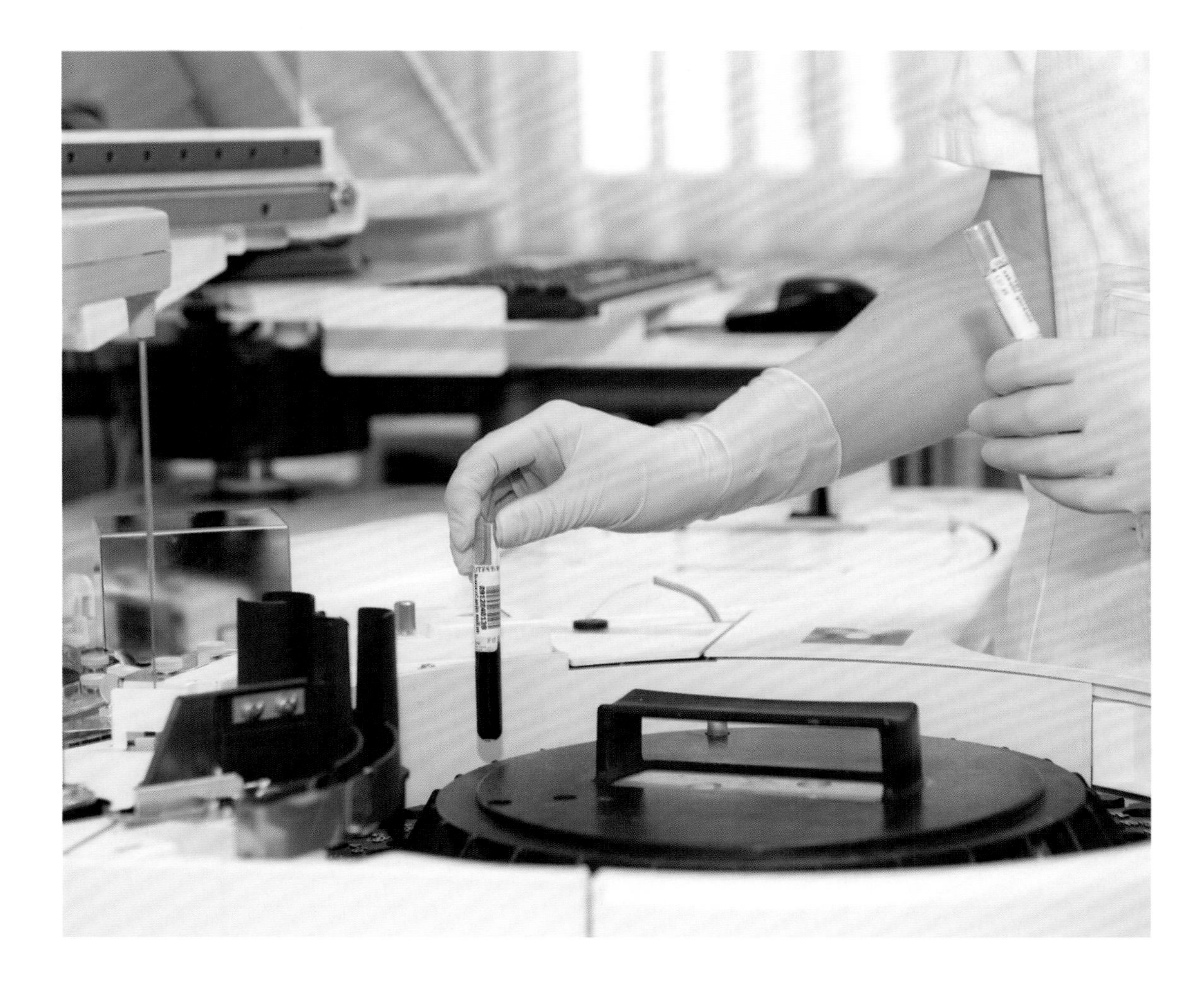

Gas Cylinder: Gases under pressure.	
Flame: Fire hazards. Flammables (gases, aerosols, liquids, and solids), pyrophoric (liquids, solids, and gases), self-reactive substances and mixtures, self-heating substances and mixtures, substances and mixtures which, in contact with water, emit flammable gases, and organic peroxides.	
Flame over circle: Oxidizing hazards (liquids, solids, gases).	
Skull and Crossbones: Material can cause death or toxicity with short exposure to small amounts - acute toxicity (fatal or toxic).	
Biohazardous infectious materials: Organisms or toxins that can cause diseases in people or animals.	
Corrosive: Can cause corrosive damage to metals, as well as serious skin and eye damage.	
Exploding bomb: Self-reactive substances and mixtures, organic peroxides.	
Health hazard: Carcinogenicity, germ cell mutagenicity, respiratory sensitization, reproductive toxicity, specific target organ toxicity (single exposure and/or repeated exposure) aspiration hazard. May cause or suspected of causing serious health effects.	
Exclamation mark: May cause less serious health effects or damage the ozone layer. Acute toxicity (harmful), skin irritation, eye irritation, skin sensitization, and specific target organ toxicity—single exposure (respiratory irritation or drowsiness or dizziness).	
Environment: May cause damage to the aquatic environment. This group and its classes were not adopted in WHMIS 2015 even though it is defined in the GHS system, but you may see the environmental class listed on labels and SDS. Including information about environmental hazards is allowed by WHMIS 2015.	

Supplier

The supplier plays a major role in WHMIS duties and contributes greatly to implementing WHMIS into the work environment. The major roles of the supplier include accurate classification of materials and the determination of which products are controlled materials. Suppliers need to determine which products are controlled materials and designate how hazardous materials are managed, including the use and storage of the material.

The supplier of the materials must provide a label on every controlled product, as it is crucial for those who are exposed to the material to be able to properly manage the product. The label should include:

- Name of the product
- Name of the supplier
- Reference to a material safety sheet which provides further information on the material
- Hazard symbol to identify each material with the classification it belongs to
- Risk and precautionary phrases that describe the hazard affiliated with the product
- First aid measures in regards to how to safely avoid and handle the possible hazard

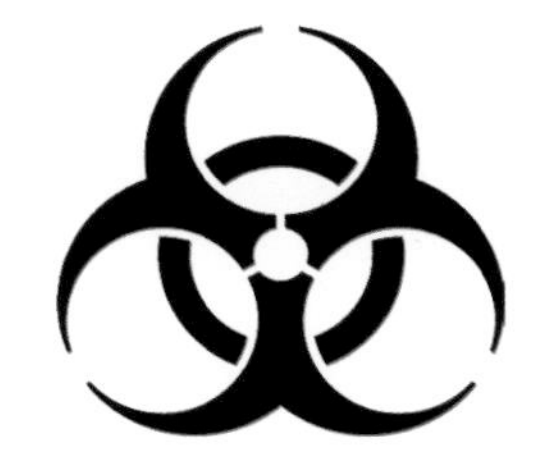

With each shipment of hazardous materials, the supplier must always provide a **Material Safety Data Sheet** (MSDS). MSDS are important documents that provide further information on the health and safety of the controlled product, which in turn, will help the user to understand the product and the management of it.

***Material Safety Data Sheet** (MSDS): Documents that provide further information on the health and safety of the controlled product to help understand the product and the management of it.*

Employers

The employer has the most crucial role in the WHMIS and workplace safety process. The employer must obtain and maintain the MSDS supplied for each controlled product, ensure that products are properly labeled and identified, and educate employees to ensure that wants and needs align.

The employer must ensure that each product has the correct label. If the employer finds that the supplier did not provide an appropriate label, they need to contact the supplier in order to request another label for the product. If the employer cannot reach the supplier, the employer must then notify the ministry of labour in writing about the missing label.

If a label was removed or has gone missing, the employer has two options. The first is to request a replacement label or use an extra label that may be on hand. An alternative is to create a workplace label that will identify the product, provide the necessary information for the safe handling of the product, and a statement that the MSDS is available.

A MSDS must be obtained for each product, and this is the responsibility of the employer. In most cases, the supplier is required to provide the MSDS before (or on the day of) the first shipment. The MSDS cannot be expired, and it must match the products received in the shipment. If the employer has not received a MSDS with the product, or the MSDS has expired, the employer must attempt to retrieve an up-to-date MSDS from the supplier.

The most critical function of WHMIS is educating employees, and this should include the proper handling of hazardous products. The employer's responsibility is to educate and train any employee who is exposed to, or is likely to be exposed to, any type of hazardous material within the workplace.

Employees should be educated on topics that involve the following:

- Identifying products without using labels
- MSDS
- Procedures for safe use
- Storage, handling and disposal of the materials
- Procedures when emissions are present
- The procedures in case of emergency involving a controlled product

Employees

Employees have the right to refuse unsafe work, and the right to be aware of any safety risks involved with a particular job. In the workplace, employees always have the right to know about hazardous materials they may be exposed to. This must include the ability to review labels for hazardous materials, review MSDS, and to receive the proper training for handling hazardous materials. Employees also have the right to participate, and that may include being consulted regarding the development and implementation of the training program offered to them.

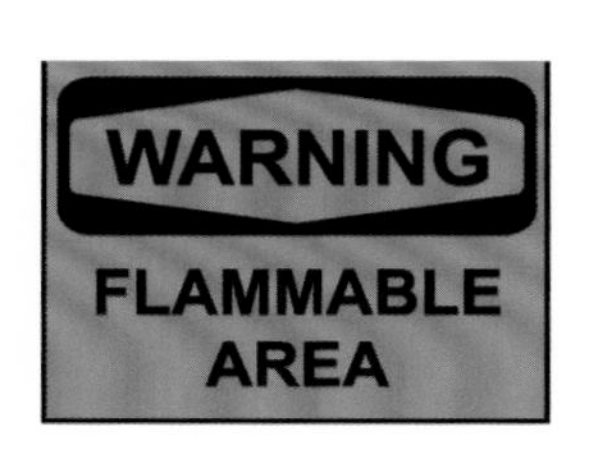

Employees are responsible for their own safety, as well as the safety of others in order for WHMIS to be effective in the work place. All violations of the WHMIS Act must be reported. Violations by employees should be brought to the attention of the employer, while violations by employers may be reported directly to the ministry of labour.

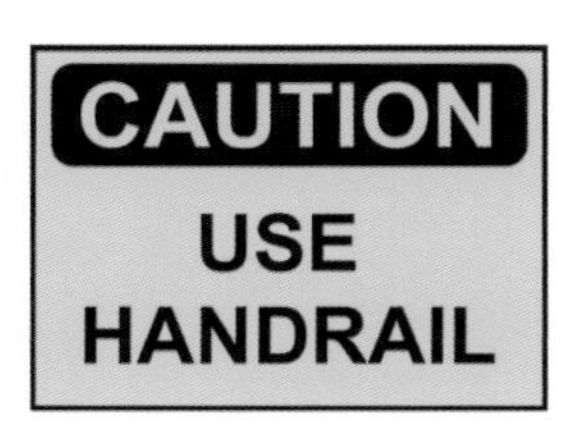

In order to implement WHMIS in a workplace, all suppliers, employers, and employees must ensure that the necessary duties and responsibilities are followed. Successful implementation of WHIMIS will decrease or prevent risks that occur around the workplace, especially for those who handle hazardous materials and chemicals.

Safety Checklist

	There are written Infection Prevention and Control (IPAC) policies and procedures.
	Employees are aware of the location of IPAC policies and procedures.
	All employers and employees follow IPAC policies and procedures.
	All employees are immunized appropriately.
	Employees and employers who wear N95 respirators are fit-tested.

Occupational Health and Safety Act (OHSA)

Workers in health care face the same challenges as any clerical worker, such as repetitive strain injury and falls, in addition to the risk of infection or contamination. Exposure to ionizing radiation, bloodborne pathogens, and other infections or diseases exposes employees to dangerous situations. To protect people in the workplace, federal and provincial legislation has developed a set of regulations. The Occupational Health and Safety Act (OHSA) guidelines include the Occupational Exposure to Bloodborne Pathogens Standard.

The OHSA came into effect in 1992 and is designed to reduce the risk of exposure to infectious diseases. Controlled in Ontario by the Ministry of Labour, these regulations must be followed by any employee with occupational exposure to pathogens, regardless of the place of employment. Each violation of the OHSA standard has a maximum penalty of $7,000. If an employee fails to comply repeatedly, the maximum penalty is $70,000.

The OHSA was created to help employers and employees reduce the frequency of injuries, illnesses, and deaths as a result of workplace hazards. Workplace duties and the rights of any parties in the workplace are outlined in the OHSA, which is enforceable by law.

OHSA does not apply to workplaces that fall under federal jurisdiction, although federal authorities accept that outside contractors and their employees, while in federal workplaces, are under provincial jurisdiction.

Regulations made under OHSA, Revised Statutes of Ontario, 1990, Chapter O.1 as amended can be found at: http://www.ontario.ca/laws/statute/90o01#_ga=1.61066473.496925131.1432578680

A complete table of regulations can be found at:

http://www.ontario.ca/laws#_ga=1.64078058.496925131.1432578680

Components of the OHSA Standard

Medical offices are required to develop an exposure control plan in compliance with the OHSA standard act. This is a written document outlining the protective measures necessary to eliminate or reduce employee exposure to bloodborne pathogens and infectious material. As a medical office assistant, this Act needs to be understood and followed to prevent workplace injuries. All employers and employees should review an annual refresher of OHSA.

All injuries in the workplace must be reported, and a Workplace Safety and Insurance Board (WSIB) form must be filled out immediately. If an injury is caused by workplace hazards, or if the patient's current condition is a recurrence of a previous work-related injury, a WSIB form must be completed and processed.

my notes

Exposure Control Plan (ECP)

The Exposure Control Plan is a "living" document that can be used as a source of information for answering questions should an employee be exposed to a harmful material, such as bloodborne pathogens. It will also contain protocol for what should be done in the event of exposure.

This document must include the following elements:

1. Determine an exposure
2. Method of compliance
3. Post-exposure evaluation and follow-up procedures

Determine an Exposure

In order to determine a potential exposure, compile a list of all job classifications in which the employees are likely to have occupational exposure, such as physicians, medical assistants, and laboratory technicians. Include any job classifications, such as an office custodian, for which only some will have occupational exposure. The complete list will help you identify every employee who requires protection in accordance with the OHSA Bloodborne Pathogens Standard. Examples of protections include training, protective equipment, and hepatitis vaccinations.

Method of Compliance

This component of the ECP outlines the specific health and safety control measures in place within a medical office to eliminate or reduce the risk of occupational exposure. These measures are important for medical assistants to reduce the risk of infectious disease. Divide the control measures into the following six categories: engineering controls, work practice controls, personal protective equipment, housekeeping, hepatitis B vaccination, and universal precautions.

1. **Engineering controls**: These are all of the measures taken and devices used to isolate or remove bloodborne pathogen hazards from the workplace. To ensure the effectiveness of engineering controls, inspections are required for repairs or maintenance to avoid faulty equipment. Engineering controls include autoclaves, safer medical devices, readily accessible hand washing facilities, biohazard bags, and biohazard sharps containers.
2. **Work practice controls:** Techniques and methods should be altered to reduce the likelihood of exposure to existing injuries, such as bandaging cuts before gloving, sanitizing hands as soon as possible after removing gloves, and placing contaminated sharps into biohazard sharp containers. Apply first aid measures immediately when exposed to blood, and report the incident to the physician so that post-exposure prophylaxis (PEP) can be instituted. It is strongly advised to avoid eating and drinking in areas exposed to blood or other infectious materials.

3. **Personal protective equipment:** Appropriate protective equipment must be worn to protect a person from contact with blood or other infectious material, depending on the degree of exposure anticipated. For example, gloves, masks, protective eyewear, laboratory coats, and gowns are all considered personal protective equipment.
4. **Housekeeping:** As part of the OHSA's required housekeeping procedures, the medical office must create and adhere to a written schedule for cleaning and decontaminating areas in which exposure occurs. Clearly indicate the specific cleaning method for each task. Build the protocol based on the type of surface, the present contaminations, and the procedure performed in the area.
5. **Hepatitis B vaccination:** Employers are required to offer hepatitis B vaccines free of charge to all medical office personnel who experience occupational exposure within 10 days of initial position assignment. If the employee has previously received the vaccination, the employee is not required to have the vaccine, but can instead determine immunity to hepatitis B through antibody testing. Alternately, if the vaccine is contraindicated for medical reasons, the employee is not forced to accept the vaccine.
6. Any medical office personnel who decline the vaccination must sign a waiver form for documentation and filing in the employee's OHSA records. An employee has the right to request and opt in to have the vaccination series done at a later time.
7. **Universal precautions:** All human blood and bodily fluids are to be treated as though they contain infectious pathogens such as HIV, HBV, HCV, or any other bloodborne pathogens.

Post-exposure Evaluation and Follow-up Procedures

In an ideal world, exposure to harmful chemicals would not happen, but should an exposure occur in the medical office, there should be a plan to deal with it. These procedures should include how to record and investigate the incident and the events afterwards, as well as the medical treatment available to the employee affected during the incident.

According to OHSA requirements, employers must review and make necessary updates to their ECP at least once a year, and update as new or altered tasks affecting exposure are introduced. This ensures the plan follows the latest information regarding the elimination of exposure to pathogens. All employers and employees must be aware of any reviews or updates that are made to the ECP.

Needlestick and Sharps Injuries

The Centre for Communicable Diseases and Infection Control—part of the Public Health Agency of Canada (PHAC)—reviews, publishes, and updates guidelines to protect staff from exposure to all infection causing agents within health care settings. A guideline, titled *Routine Practices and Additional Precautions for Preventing the Transmission of Infection in Healthcare Settings*, is in place to prevent injuries from sharps and needlesticks. This guideline is considered a part of the "routine practices" used by health care workers.

Needlestick injuries are wounds caused by needles that inadvertantly puncture the skin. This can occur when removing or replacing a needle cap, drawing up vaccines, puncturing a vial, or while injecting a patient.

Sharps include needles, as well as items such as scalpels, lancets, razor blades, scissors, metal wire, retractors, clamps, pins, staples, cutters, and glass items. Any object that is able to cut the skin is a sharp.

In response to the frequency and severity of health issues associated with exposure to blood-borne pathogens, PHAC has implemented the Needlestick and Sharps Injuries guidelines. To reduce needlestick and sharps injuries among health care workers, employers must identify and make use of safe medical devices.

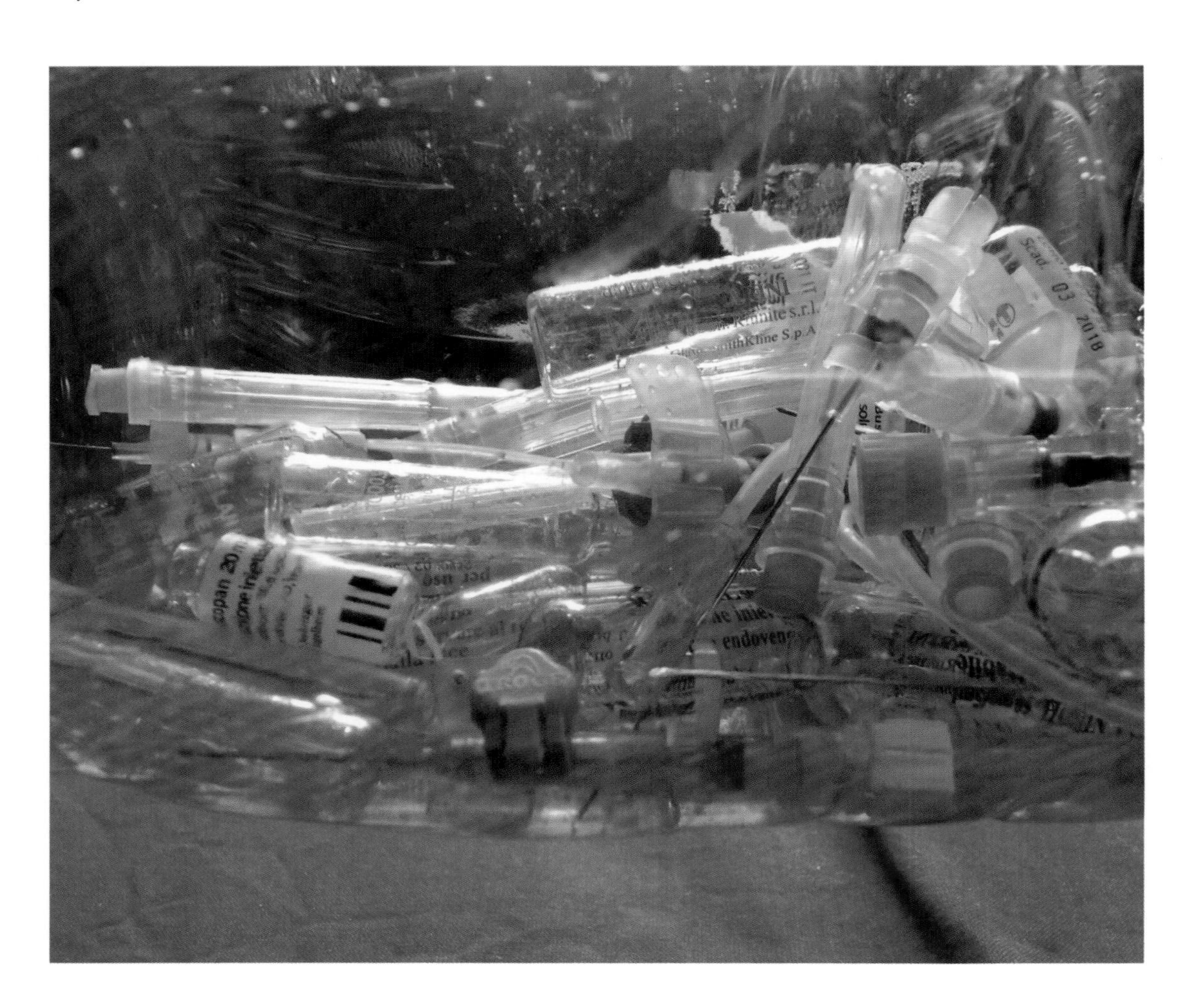

Employees should be educated in how to use sharp instruments safely, and to keep others who may encounter the device safe, either during or after its use.

Taken from the Canadian Centre for Occupational Health and Safety (CCOHS), PHAC recommends that:

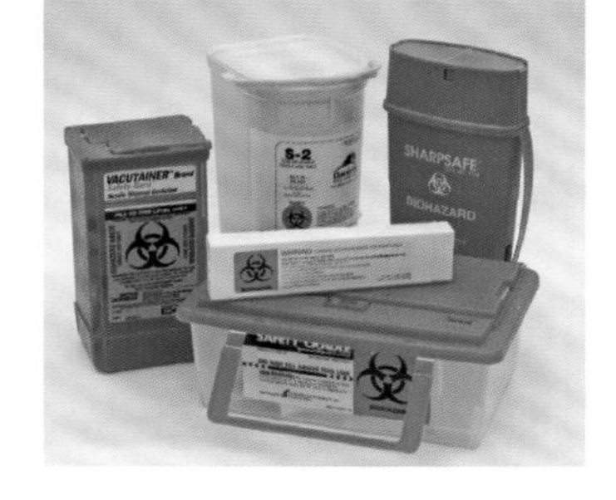

- Needles should not be recapped—used items should be placed immediately in a sharps container that is easily accessible at the point-of-care.
- Health care workers should cover open skin areas or lesions with a dry dressing at all times. Hand hygiene is essential, so review the procedure with a supervisor if the dressing interferes with the procedure.
- A worker's eyes, nose, and mouth should be protected, especially if blood or body fluid are being handled.
- First aid should be immediate if a worker is exposed to blood or body fluids. Report to the employer and follow the employer's procedure for further testing. The site should be thoroughly, and immediately, cleaned.

In situations where recapping is deemed necessary, all employees should follow safe procedure to avoid needlestick injuries. Recap the needle by laying the cap on a flat surface, and scoop it onto the tip of the needle. Keep the other hand away from the sheath and well behind the exposed needle. The health care worker should never move an exposed needle tip towards an unprotected hand.

Examination Room Checklist

	There are hand washing sinks with liquid soap available in each clinic area.
	Alcohol-based hand rub is available in each examination room.
	Puncture-resistant sharps containers are provided in each exam room or clinic area.
	Sharps are discarded directly into sharps containers.
	Sharps containers are not overfilled past the fill line.
	Personal protective equipment (PPE) is available and is worn when necessary and appropriate.
	Supplies (other than cleaning supplies) are not stored under, or on counters adjacent to, hand washing sinks.
	The examination rooms are well ventilated and well lit.

The OHSA Bloodborne Pathogens Standard states that all containers with biohazardous materials must be clearly labelled with a biohazard warning. The label itself must adhere to the following: orange-red or fluorescent orange for consistency and visibility, include the biohazard symbol at an appropriate size, and include "BIOHAZARD" in a contrasting colour such as black. The warning should be obvious to anyone, not just those in the medical field.

Examples of cases in which medical offices must include a biohazard warning label include:

1. Containers of regulated waste
2. Refrigerators and freezers storing blood or other potentially infectious materials
3. All containers and bags used to store, transport, or ship blood or other potentially infectious materials

These labels make employees aware of potential exposure, particularly when they are unable to identify the nature of the material inside the container. If the medical office does not have access to biohazard labels, use red bags or containers until labels are found. All efforts should be made to identify and minimize the risk to all those that might be exposed.

Communicating Hazards to Employees

Employers must provide all medical office employees at risk of exposure with a training program in order to adhere to OHSA standards. An Exposure Control Plan (ECP) must be in place alongside the medical office safety measures program. Employers must provide this training the first time they encounter the employee, and make that training available a minimum of once every year following that.

Record all training sessions and keep them for at least three years afterwards. In these recordings, include the session dates, content, names of trainers and their qualifications, as well as the names and job titles of the employees involved in the sessions.

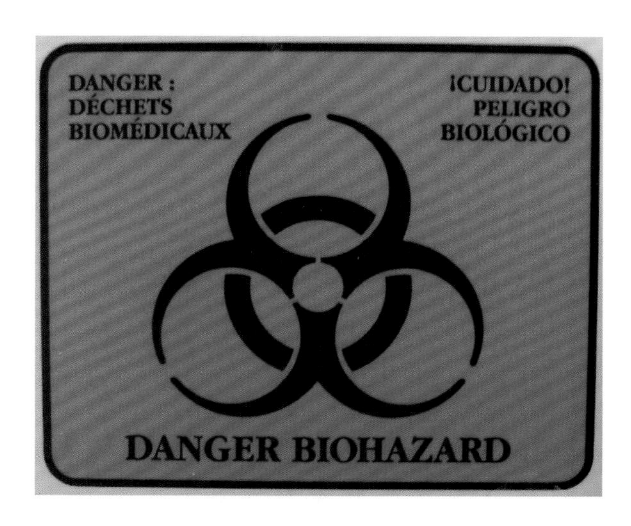

Quiz

CHAPTER 3 QUIZ

1. What does MSDS stand for?
    a. Material Safety Day Sheets
    b. Material Safety Data Standard
    c. Material Safety Data Sheets
    d. Material Standard Data Sheets

2. Fill in the blank: The systematic process of checking to see whether a product or service is meeting specified requirements is known as ____________________.

3. Define credentialing.

____

____

____

____

4. True or false? A medical provider can still practice as long as they can obtain proper credentialing at a later date. Insurance carriers will reimburse any medical office bills once proof can be given for proper credentialing.

5. Fill in the blanks: Office reviews are conducted to ________________ and ____________________ appropriate actions that arise from the re-evaluation of policies, procedures, and other office protocols.

6. What does OHSA acronym stand for?
    a. Occupation Health and Standard Act
    b. Operational Health and Safety Act
    c. Occupational Health and Safety Act
    d. Operational Health and Standard Act

7. Incident reports include the following, except for:
    a. Summary of events
    b. Detailed event history
    c. List of who was present at time of event
    d. Any actions that weren't taken at time of event

8. What does WHMIS stand for and why was it implemented in the work place?

____

____

____

____

____

____

____

____

9. True or false? GHS defines the Environment pictogram, but this group was not adopted in WHMIS 2015. However, you may see the environmental classes listed on labels and SDS.

10. Which pictogram will describe the probability of causing death or toxicity with short exposure to small amounts?

a. Flame

b. Skull and Crossbones

c. Flame over circle

d. Health hazard

11. Which pictogram will describe oxidizing hazards?

a. Flame

b. Skull and Crossbones

c. Flame over circle

d. Health hazard

12. True or false? The employer must ensure that each product has a proper label attached and must notify the ministry of labour immediately regarding any missing labels if a supplier does not provide an appropriate label.

13. Fill in the blank: The ______________________________ is a written document which includes the following elements: determine an exposure, method of compliance, post-exposure evaluation, and follow-up procedures.

14. List the six categories under the method of compliance.

____

____

____

____

____

____

____

____

15. True or false? After the initial refusal to receive the hepatitis B vaccination, the employee can change their mind later and have the employer provide them with the vaccination series even after a waiver form has been signed.

16. What are needlestick injuries and were they integrated with OHSA?

____

____

____

____

____

____

____

17. A warning label must be attached to which of the following?

a. Containers of regulated waste and potentially infectious materials

b. Sharp containers

c. All containers and bags used to store, transport, or ship blood

d. Two of the above

e. None of the above

Chapter 4

Drugs, Prescription, and Handling Patient Prescription Requests

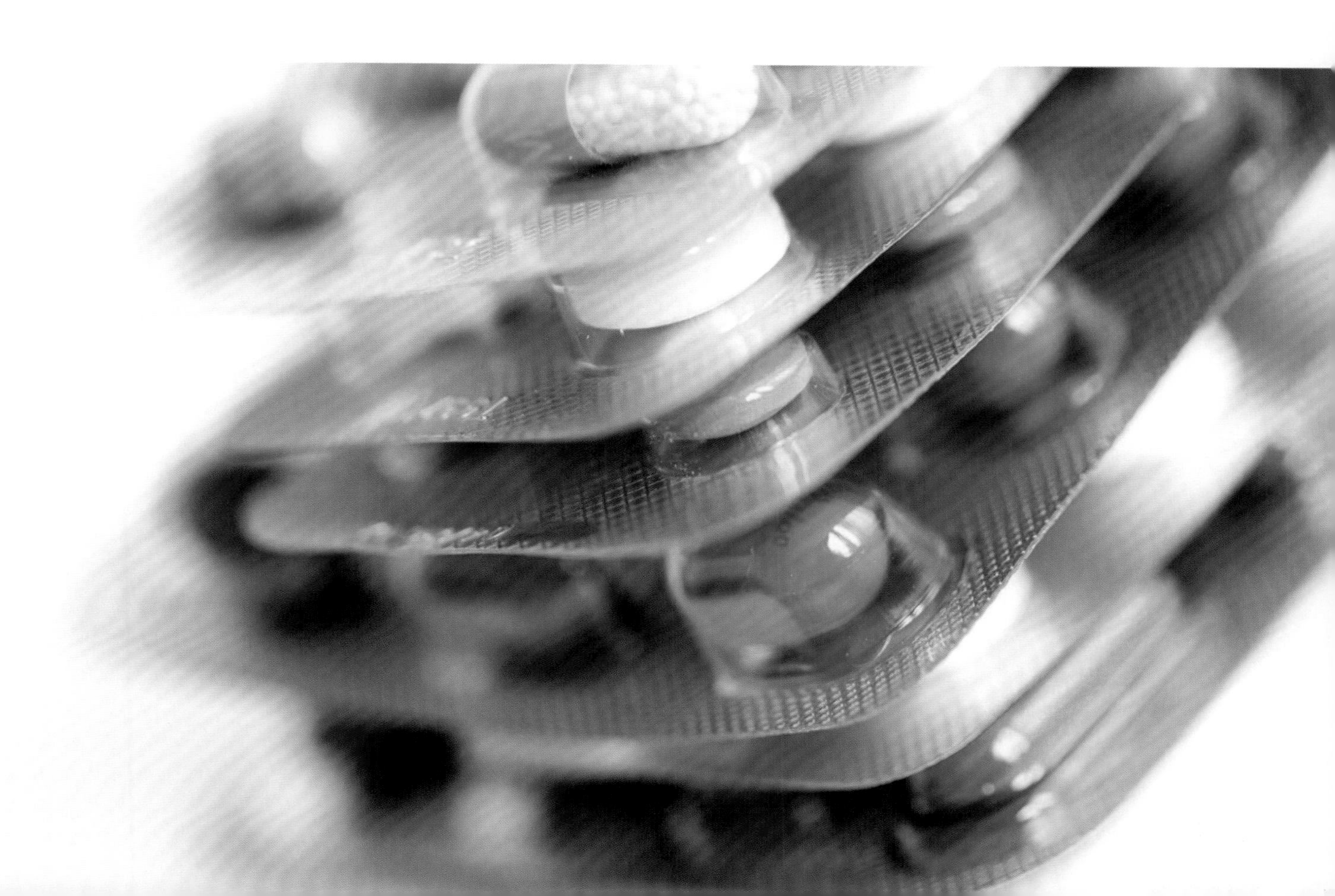

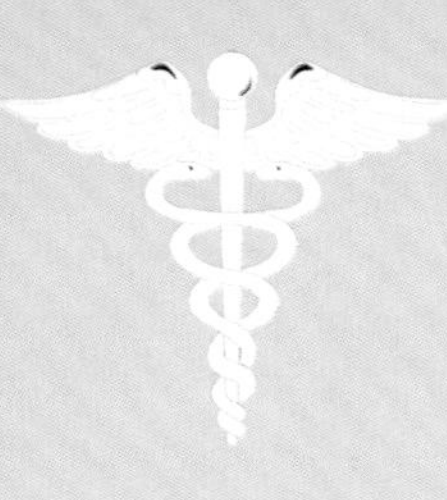

CHAPTER FOUR LEARNING OBJECTIVES

After completing this chapter, you should be able to:

- ❑ Define the term prescription and identify which drugs can be sold over-the-counter
- ❑ Understand the practice of prescribing medication to patients
- ❑ Explain and implement steps to provide prescription security
- ❑ Recognize and define parts of a prescription
- ❑ Define prescription abbreviations
- ❑ Calculate and understand drug measurements
- ❑ Understand the importance of patient compliance, especially with antibiotics
- ❑ Understand and explain the available drug benefit programs
- ❑ Distinguish between prescription repeats and renewals
- ❑ Understand how to handle phoned or faxed-in prescription requests
- ❑ Understand the deterioration of drugs
- ❑ Comprehend and implement safe drug handling protocols
- ❑ Identify and avoid drug errors
- ❑ Understand how to handle controlled drugs
- ❑ Identify and understand how to prevent drug abuse

Dispensing Drugs

According to the College of Physicians and Surgeons of Ontario, physicians can only prescribe medication within the context of a physician-patient relationship and must only act in the patient's best interest. Medication can be dispensed to patients in two methods: prescription medication and over-the-counter medication.

***Dispense:** To prepare and distribute medicine, usually by prescription.*

Medical office assistants should know which types of medication can only be obtained with a prescription written by a physician, and the protocols for filling certain types of medication. In the case of over-the-counter medication, patients can be directed to the closest pharmacy to purchase the required medication.

Over-the-Counter (OTC)

Drugs that are considered safe to take without specific advice from a physician and do not require a medical prescription can be dispensed over-the-counter. Patients have access to these drugs without having to schedule an appointment with their physician, but can ask the pharmacist any questions. Over-the-counter drugs can be found in the following three categories:

***Over-the-counter drugs:** Medication that can be obtained from a pharmacy and does not require a medical prescription.*

1. Pharmacy only: Restricted Access (Schedule II)

These drugs are kept behind the counter, under the control of the pharmacist. The pharmacist may be required to record the sale in the patient's profile.

By law, the pharmacist must ask questions and provide counseling to anyone that is purchasing one of these medications because these are drugs that can be abused. Their use should be monitored and the pharmacist fills this role.

Examples include: charcoal, vaccines, dextrose, epinephrine and its salts, ephedrine and its salts in single entity products, fibrin, insulin, influenza vaccine, lidocaine and its salts, etc.

2. Pharmacy only: Under Supervision (Schedule III)

These medications are in the self-serve section of pharmacies. While a pharmacist does not need to control the access, these medications must be locked when the pharmacy is closed. The medicine can only be sold in a pharmacy when a pharmacist is present. This is to ensure that the pharmacist is available to discuss proper use should a patient have a question before purchasing.

These drugs treat conditions that can resolve on their own like a cold, diarrhea, indigestion, or a headache.

Examples include: acetaminophen in sustained release formulations, acetylsalicylic acid and its salts, famotidine and its salts, fluoride and its salts, ibuprofen, lactic acid, naproxen, etc.

3. Sold anywhere: No Restrictions (Unscheduled)

These medications have no restriction on their sale and can be found in retail stores without a pharmacy. These drugs often pose little risk because their use is common for most patients.

Be aware, though, that many unscheduled drugs still pose a harmful risk to patients if used incorrectly. Acetaminophen is a common pain-relieving medication but an unsafe dose has the potential to be fatal. In fact, many individuals die each year from accidental or intentional overdose.

Examples include: acetaminophen in sustained release formulations, acetylsalicylic acid and its salts, benzoyl peroxide, bioflavonoids, charcoal (activated), famotidine and its salts, glutamic acid and its salts, ibuprofen and its salts, niacin, pepsin, etc.

It is important to take medicine correctly and it should never be taken longer or in higher doses than the drug label recommends. If a patient is taking a medication for longer than indicated but still has symptoms, the patient should see a physician. Some medications interact with other medicines, supplements, foods, and drinks and may create problems for people with unrelated medical conditions.

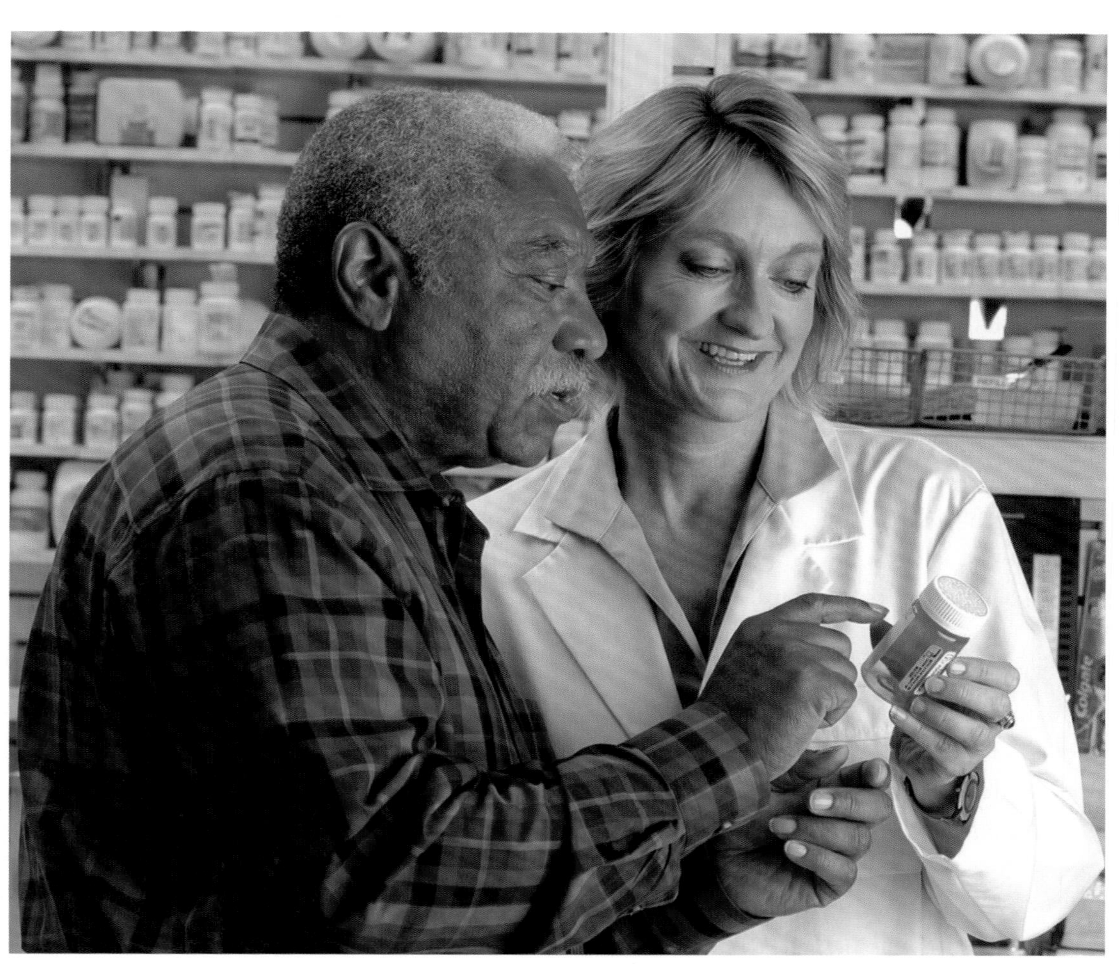

Photo By Rhoda Baer (Photographer) [Public domain], via Wikimedia Commons

Important Reminder!

A supplement is a product intended for ingestion only to supply a nutritional deficiency, or reinforce or extend a whole diet.
Supplements can reduce the risk of disease and come in many forms such as tablets, capsules, liquids, or powders. A supplement may be one, or any combination, of the following substances:
A vitamin
A mineral
An herb or other botanical
An amino acid
A dietary substance for use by people to supplement the diet by increasing the total dietary intake
A concentrate, metabolite, constituent, or extract

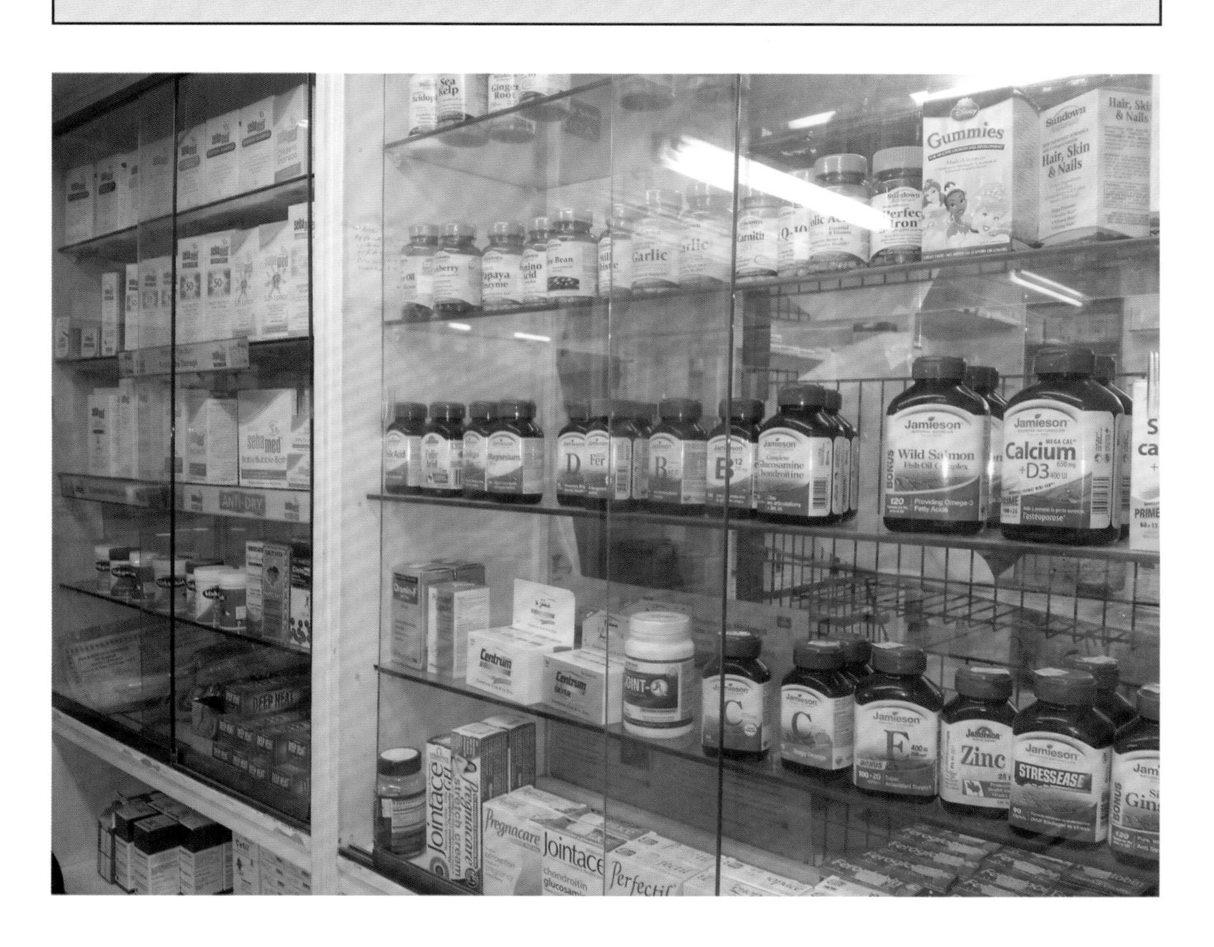

Dispensing prescriptions and over-the-counter medications have very different procedures. Drugs defined by the federal government to be dangerous, powerful, or habit-forming are only available by physician's order and correspond to NAPRA (National Association of Pharmacy Regulatory Authorities) Schedule I. Unlike over-the-counter medications, a pharmacist must have a signed prescription from a physician before providing it to a patient (e.g. narcotics).

What is a Prescription?

Prescription: *An order for medication created by a medical practitioner for dispensing to a patient from a pharmacy.*

A **prescription** is an order created by an MD for dispensing a particular medication to a patient. It can be relayed orally (directly from physician to pharmacist), hand-written, computer-generated, telephoned directly, or faxed directly to a pharmacy.

Practice of Prescribing

- **Rx Decided:** The physician writes the prescription on a notepad, and makes a note of the order in the patient's chart.
- **Rx Ordered:** Depending on the practice, prescriptions can be faxed to the pharmacy so the medication can be ready and waiting for the patient.
- **Rx Recorded:** Long-term prescriptions should be added to the patient's medication profile. If needed, short-term medications should be recorded to keep a detailed record of the patient's medical history.

Security of Prescriptions

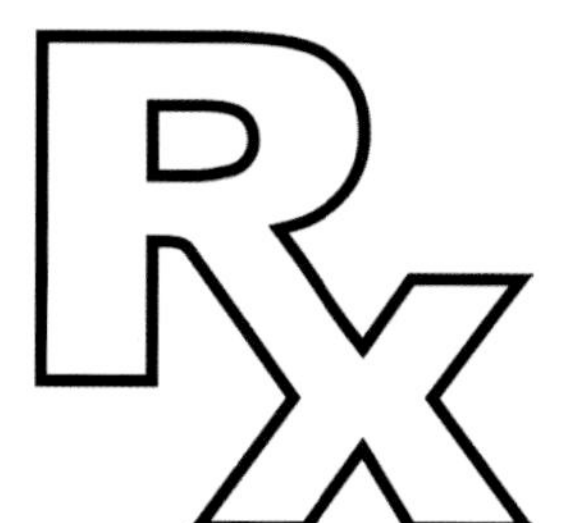

Prescription pads must be kept secure to avoid theft and forgery. When the physician is absent or the office is closed, prescription pads should be locked in a secure place. There are a number of things a medical office assistant can do to ensure that a prescription pad is not misused.

When ordering more prescription pads, pads should be labeled with the physician's name, address, and telephone number. One way to detect loss is to number the prescription pads sequentially—this helps to avoid stolen or forged prescriptions for the purpose of medication abuse.

Pads should be locked up and a physician should only use one pad at a time.

- **Physicians should never pre-sign prescription forms**
- **Prescription pads should never be used as notepaper**

In order to prevent changes to the prescription after it is written and signed by the physician, use tinted pads so alteration by erasers will be obvious. Physicians should draw a diagonal line across any empty spaces on the written prescription to prevent forgery.

Any discarded prescription orders should be shredded and disposed of properly to prevent forgery and to protect patient confidentiality.

If faxes are used to submit prescriptions, fax machines in the physician's office and the pharmacy should be kept secure in case of a breach in patient confidentiality or prescription tampering. Fax machines should be kept in an area where the public cannot easily access the machine or be able to see patient information from a distance. The medical office assistant should not stray from the fax machine while faxing a prescription—this will ensure that the fax goes through and will avoid misplacing the prescription.

Faxes should have a cover sheet that includes all physician information (including all identifiers), the date and time of transmission, the pharmacy address and phone number, and any other required contact information.

Parts of a Prescription

1. Heading

- **Physician's information** (usually pre-printed)
    - This area has information unique to the physician or the practice so the pharmacist can identify the source should he or she have any questions about the prescription. This must include the address and phone number of the clinic or office.
- **Accurate date and time**
    - A pharmacist cannot fill a prescription unless the date of issue is clearly stated. Prescription orders are only valid for a short time.
- **The patient's information (name, address, any other required contact information)**
    - The patient's name and address are needed for insurance billing purposes and for properly dispensing the medication.

2. Superscription

- Represented by the Rx symbol—which means "take thus" or "take"

3. Inscription

- Name of the drug, form, strength
- Most drugs are available in various doses—it is important to prescribe the correct dose.

4. Subscription (Mitte)

- Directions for the pharmacist (size of dose, the number of doses, amount to dispense)
- The quantity to be dispensed should be indicated numerically and spelt out to prevent a prescription from being altered illegally (e.g. #30 [thirty])

5. Signa

- Directions for the patient to be printed on the label (when and how many to take)

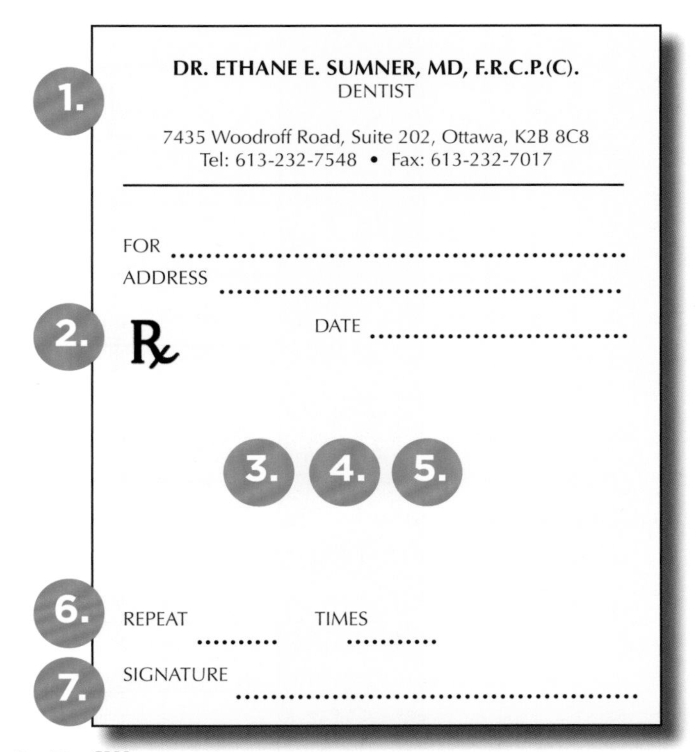

6. Refill

- Number of times a refill is allowed on a script

7. Signature

- Signature and identifier of the ordering physician
- The Narcotics Safety and Awareness Act, 2010 regulation came into force November 1, 2011. This act requires prescribers to include their registration number—issued to the prescriber by the College of which he or she is a member—for prescriptions of monitored drugs. The identification number of the patient and the type of identification used, such as a health card or driver's licence, must be recorded on the prescription. The version code on the patient's health card is not required to be included on the prescription. This process improves the accuracy and completeness of prescription data collection, leading to better patient outcomes.

Activity

PRESCRIPTION ABBREVIATIONS

Fill in what each prescription abbreviation means and explain why you have to be careful when it comes to using abbreviations with an asterisk(*) beside it.

a.c.	
p.c.	
gtt(s)	
b.i.d.	
t.i.d.	
q.i.d.	
q.4h.	
q.h.	
p.r.n.	
h.s.	
stat	
p.o.	
caps	
agit	
SL	
ad lib.	
OD(*)	
OS(*)	
AS	
AD	
Rx	

Do Not Use

Dangerous Abbreviations, Symbols, and Dose Designations

In July of 2006, the Food and Drugs Act (FDA) and the Institute for Safe Medical Practices (ISMP) embarked on a joint campaign to eliminate the use of potentially confusing abbreviations, symbols, and dose designations. Industry shorthand can create barriers to effective communication, resulting in potential harm to patients. The abbreviations, symbols, and dose designations found in this table have been reported as being frequently misinterpreted, so they should never be used when communicating medication information.

This list has been adapted from ISMP Canada's List of Error-Prone Abbreviations, Symbols, and Dose Designations 2006.

Avoid	Use instead	Problem
U	Unit	Can resemble "0" (zero), "4", or cc.
IU	International unit	Can resemble "IV" (intravenous) or 10 in roman numerals.
Abbreviations for drug names	Full drug names	Many drugs have similar abbreviations; e.g., MSO4 (morphine sulphate), MgSO4 (magnesium sulphate)
QD **QOD**	Every day (daily) Every other day	QD and QOD may be mistaken for each other, or as 'qid.'
OD	Every day (daily)	Mistaken for "right eye" (OD = oculus dexter).
OS, OD, OU	Left eye, right eye, both eyes	May be confused with dosing frequencies.
D/C	Discharge	Can be read as "discontinue."
cc	ml or millilitre	Mistaken for "u" (units).
µg	Microgram	Mistaken for "mg" (milligram) resulting in one thousand-fold overdose.
@	At	Mistaken for "2" (two) or "5" (five).
< >	Greater than, Less than	Mistaken for "7" (seven) or the letter "L." Confused with each other.
Zero after decimal point (x.0 mg)	x mg (omit zero)	A 10-fold dose error occurs if the decimal point is missed.
Missing zero before decimal point (.x mg)	0.x mg (include zero)	A 10-fold dose error occurs if the decimal point is missed.

Drug Measurements

Measuring drugs is serious business. As mentioned with the list of error-prone dose designations, a miscalculation in drug dosing can have disastrous results. While it is the responsibility of the physician to ensure dosing of drugs is clear, it often falls on the medical office assistant to explain to the patient how to measure out medication. Especially when providing medications in liquid form.

For example, a patient's prescription might recommend they take 15 mL of syrup medication and they may ask if they can measure it using a teaspoon. The physician and pharmacist should be available to clear up dosing confusion, but the medical office assistant may also have the task of explaining the instructions.

There are three systems of measurement in use in the medical field. The most common and most important to learn to use is the metric system. This system is widely used around the world and is the system that Canada—as well as the drug industry—has adopted.

The two other measurement systems (British imperial and British apothecaries') have fallen out of use and are not standard. However, it is still important to learn them and understand how to make conversions between the systems.

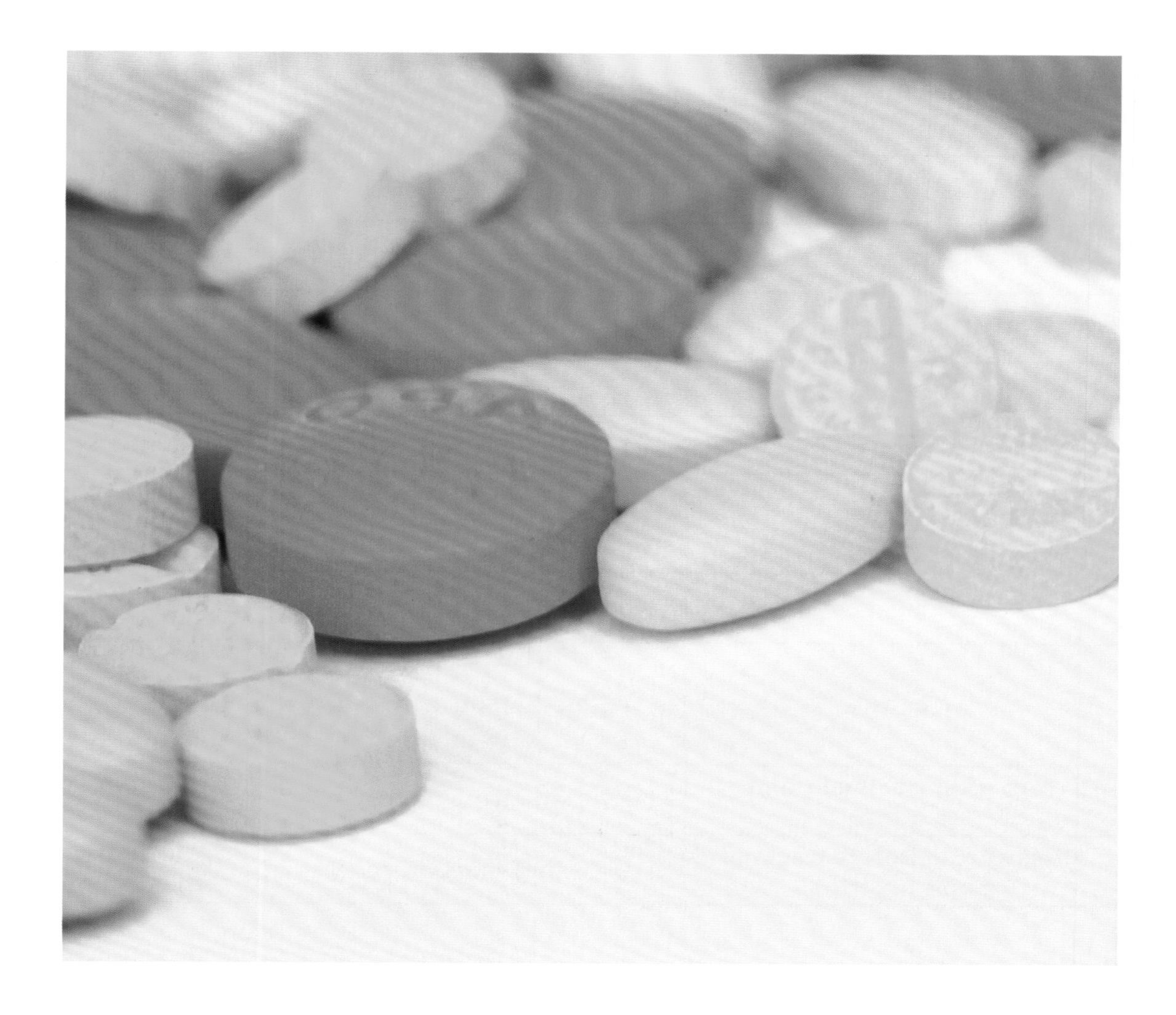

Metric System

Widely used around the world, the metric system has become the standard for measurement of most, if not all, medications. Although it is widely used in Canada, the metric system was not adopted by the Canadian Government until the 1970s despite having been developed nearly 200 years earlier by the First French Republic (France).

Canadian schools began teaching the metric system in the mid-1970s. This means many people born prior to the 1970s learnt to use the British Imperial system of measurement. As a result, many people identify and have a higher comprehension of the imperial system. To this day, miles, gallons, pounds, and degrees Fahrenheit are still commonly used.

Canada, as well as much of the world, adopted the metric system because of its relative simplicity and consistency. By standardizing the prefixes and suffixes and working in base10, the metric system reduces confusion and likelihood of error, especially when language barriers exist.

The system begins with a base unit. The most common base units are gram, litre, and metre. By adding a suffix, you designate the proportion of this unit. For example, *"milli"* is a prefix that means thousandth. Therefore, one *milli*metre is one-thousandth (1/1000) of a metre. This logic follows for milligram (thousandth of a gram) and millilitre (thousandth of a litre).

Some prefixes are more common than others and so it is likely that you have already encountered many of them. Below is a list of some prefixes and their relationship with the base unit:

Less than 1	Nano- (n)	1/1,000,000,000 (billionth)
	Micro- (μ)	1/1,000,000 (millionth)
	Milli- (m)	1/1,000 (thousandth)
	Centi- (c)	1/100 (hundredth)
	Deci- (d)	1/10 (tenth)
Base unit		
More than 1	Deca- (da)	10 (ten)
	Hecto- (h)	100 (hundred)
	Kilo- (k)	1,000 (thousand)
	Mega- (M)	1,000,000 (million)
	Giga- (G)	1,000,000,000 (billion)

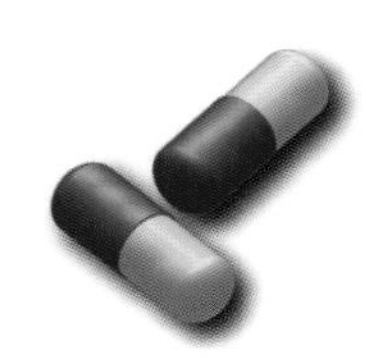

Medications are often in small amounts, so milli- and micro- are important to distinguish. Pharmacology companies measure solid medications in milligrams and micrograms, and liquid medications in millilitres and microlitres.

Be aware that the measure of volume (litres) is derived from the measure of length (metres). One millilitre (mL) is the equivalent to one cubic centimetre (cm^2). In other words, a cube with each side measuring one centimetre in length will contain 1 mL.

Syringes and some medications may be measured by cubic centimetres, or cc's. Those in the medical field should understand that cc is interchangeable with mL as they are the same amount. Interestingly, 1 ml or cc of water is also equal to 1 gram in weight (1 litre weighs 1 kg).

Avoid using cc's when discussing amounts with patients. This can create unnecessary confusion so it is best to use mL for the sake of simplicity.

Imperial (Household) Measurement

The British imperial measurement system is no longer the system used in Canada. Nevertheless, many Canadians grew up using the units: ounces, teaspoons, pounds, etc. A medical office assistant must be able to use these units of measurement with those individuals who are unfamiliar with the metric system. Imperial measurements will most likely be used when discussing dosing or measurements with patients. When conversing with a pharmacist or physician, it is best to be familiar with, and use, the metric system.

Older patients and patients from countries that have not adopted the metric system—such as the United States—may be restricted in their understanding to household measurements. Mistakes in drug dosing can be disastrous, so be sure instructions are clear to avoid confusion or errors. If a patient is only familiar with imperial units, be aware of areas in which miscommunications and misunderstandings can occur.

Volume measurements need to be extremely clear when discussing dosing of liquid measurements. Physicians usually prescribe liquid drugs in controlled amounts. For example, a liquid antibiotic may suggest a dose of 5 mL every 8 hours. The patient may not be able to make that measurement if they are constrained by the tools they have in their home. Also, be aware that imperial units differ between the British imperial and the US imperial systems.

The table on the following page is a guide for converting from metric to imperial. In Canada, a patient might have the tools to measure volumes in British imperial and US imperial in their home. US imperial is more common since most people are familiar with these measurements from using cooking recipes from the United States. These values have been rounded to the nearest millilitre.

Measurement	British imperial --> mL	US imperial --> mL
1 teaspoon	6	5
1 tablespoon	18	15
1 fluid ounce	28	30
¼ cup	71	59
⅓ cup	95	79
1 cup	284	237
1 pint	568	473
1 quart	1137	946
1 gallon	4546	3785

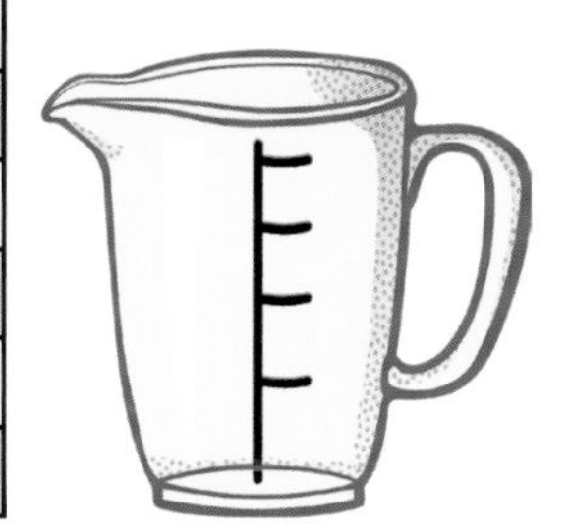

The imperial measurements should rarely, if ever, be used in the medical field. The household measurement system is notoriously inaccurate and the presence of two different systems (UK and US) compounds the problem. Only use it as a guideline to make sure that patients are not over dosing on medications.

If a physician gives a patient a prescription that needs to be measured, the medical office assistant should be ready to teach and explain the importance of accurate drug measurements. Measurement tools available to a patient should be reviewed and explained, especially when managing drugs that are taken at low doses. The lower the amount of medicine, the easier it is to make a mistake when measuring.

Apothecaries' Measure

The third measurement system commonly used for drugs is the apothecaries' measure. Used regularly in the UK during the 1800s, this system measures weight and volume.

The British apothecaries' volume measures are no longer recommended in the US or Canada, but it is still occasionally used in medicine. Some older medications may still use this notation, but presently, it is unlikely that a medical office assistant will ever need to work with this system.

Because of this, should the apothecaries' measure be encountered, any conversions or measurements should be left for the physician or pharmacist.

Pharmacists are comfortable making the conversions and explaining the dosing to patients. If a patient has any questions, direct them to their physician or pharmacist.

Quick Common Conversions

Some conversions may be worth remembering. Oftentimes, patient measurements such as height or weight need to be converted from imperial to metric. For exact values, a conversion calculator should be referenced but a quick mental calculation could be useful in preliminary information gathering.

The following table provides simplified conversions for a quick mental calculation from imperial to metric.

Convert	Use the equation	Opposite direction, Use the equation
Weight		
Pounds-->kilograms	1 lbs = 0.45 kg	1 kg = 2.2 lbs
Length		
Feet-->metres	1 foot = 0.305 m	1 m = 3.28 feet
Inches-->centimetres	1 inch = 2.54 cm	1 cm = 0.394 inches
Miles-->kilometres	1 mile = 1.61 km	1 km = 0.62 mile
Volume		
British Gallons-->litres	1 Gal = 4.55 L	1 L = 0.22 Gal
U.S. Gallons-->litres	1 Gal = 3.18 L	1 L = 0.26 Gal
Misc.		
Temperature: °F-->°C	°F = (°C x 2) + 30	°C = (°F-30) / 2
Energy: Joules->cal	1 J = 0.24 cal	1 cal = 4.184 J

my notes

Patient Compliance

Physicians prescribe medication for patients with an overall sense of the medication's desired outcome, as well as objectives in managing the diseases or conditions. No matter how good the intentions and efforts of the medical professional are, it is up to the patient to decide if they will adhere to the treatment.

Convincing patients to follow their treatment plan can be difficult, especially for patients with a chronic illness. Non-compliance with medical interventions is a problem that medical professionals face on a daily basis. Non-compliance impacts a client's quality of life, and results in major health problems when pain management and symptoms cannot be controlled.

Forgetfulness and the Importance of Reminders

Life can become hectic and forgetting to take prescribed medication at the required times is an honest mistake that patients sometimes make. There are solutions to remind patients when it is time to take their medication. For those that carry a daily planner, patients can write reminders of the date and time they need to take their medication. Some medications come with reminder stickers that patients can stick on their calendar.

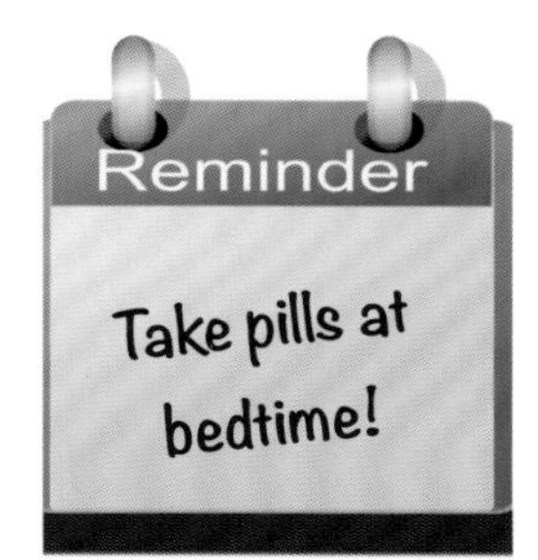

It can be challenging to remember to take a certain medication if it is not required every day. In this case, setting a reminder on a phone or even having the medication set out ahead of time in a pill organizer can be useful.

When medical office assistants receive prescription refill requests, it is important they ask the patient how often they are taking the medication to see if they are actually adhering to the prescription. Instead of relaying information and asking if the patient is taking x amount x times per day, it is better for the patient themselves to provide medical assistants with that information so that they can determine if the patient fully understands the directions.

This is the perfect opportunity to discuss with patients the importance of taking the medication as prescribed by the physician. It is a good idea to check the patient's file beforehand to see if they are due for any re-check appointments with the physician. If the physician requires a re-check appointment or would like a follow-up appointment, either schedule one before the patient leaves or set a reminder to contact the patient closer to the date of their appointment.

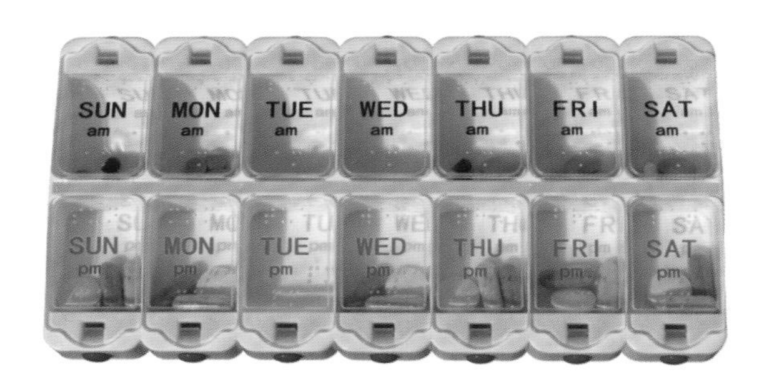

Antibiotics

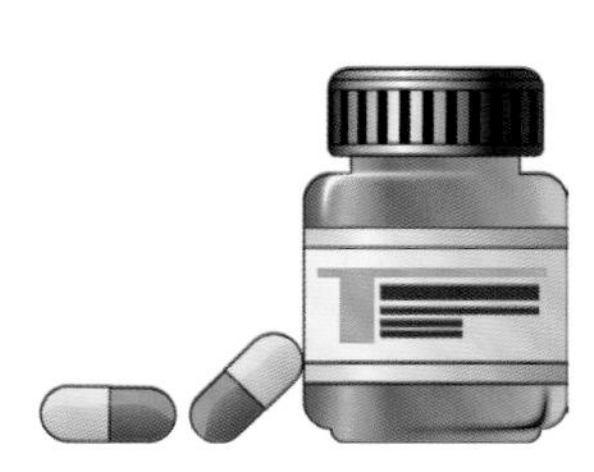

Patients placed on antibiotics may stop taking their medication once symptoms appear to clear up. They may believe they are no longer infected, but this is false—it is important for patients to adhere to the physician's orders regarding the length of time that antibiotics are taken. Antibiotics can be effective when treating bacterial infections, but can increase the likelihood of drug-resistant bacteria if patients misuse a course of antibiotics.

Patients who have followed the physician's orders on the frequency and length of antibiotics taken should not have any antibiotics left. The prescription filled is the exact number needed to complete an entire course of treatment. Patients should not take antibiotics from previous prescriptions or from someone else's prescription—a full treatment prescribed by the physician is the treatment needed to kill the disease-causing bacteria.

Antibiotics that were once used as standard treatments for bacterial infections are now less effective or don't work at all, as a result of bacteria growing resistant to antibiotics. The overuse and misuse of antibiotics are the key factors that contribute to the problem of antibiotic resistance—it is part of your responsibility as the medical office assistant to ensure patients are properly taking antibiotics to minimize the development of antibiotic resistance.

Bacteria become resistant to a drug when they have mutated to either protect it from the action of the drug or neutralize the drug. The mutated bacteria that carry the resistance can survive and pass on its resistant properties through replication or transferring it to other bacteria. The development of resistance to a drug is normal and expected of a bacteria, but the way that drugs are used affects how rapidly and to what extent drug resistance occurs.

If a patient calls to inquire about stopping their medication even though the physician has required the patient to finish the full treatment, the medical office assistant should encourage the physician's orders. If the patient relays that they are experiencing mild side effects, advise the patient to continue taking the antibiotics and schedule them to see the physician.

If the patient is experiencing an allergic reaction, instruct them to immediately stop taking any further antibiotics and to see a physician right away. An allergic reaction to medication can cause serious health effects and is potentially life threatening. Prompt treatment is necessary and timing is crucial for the patient.

Unsatisfied Patients

Patients not adhering to their treatment plans results in unsatisfactory clinical results and an overall lack of improvement in their condition. In cases where the patient's condition is worsening, chronic and non-communicable diseases can impact the patient's overall quality of life. Ultimately, it is the patient that has to decide whether or not they are compliant after being duly informed and advised by medical professionals.

Solutions to Non-Compliance

As a medical office assistant, it is crucial to educate patients on the importance of following a doctor's orders. The focus is on patient-care health compliance—this includes preventative medicine, awareness strategies, medication intake, diet control, therapeutic drug monitoring, and living an overall healthy lifestyle. Factors that affect patient compliance rely mostly on a patient's attitude rather than on medical resources or facilities.

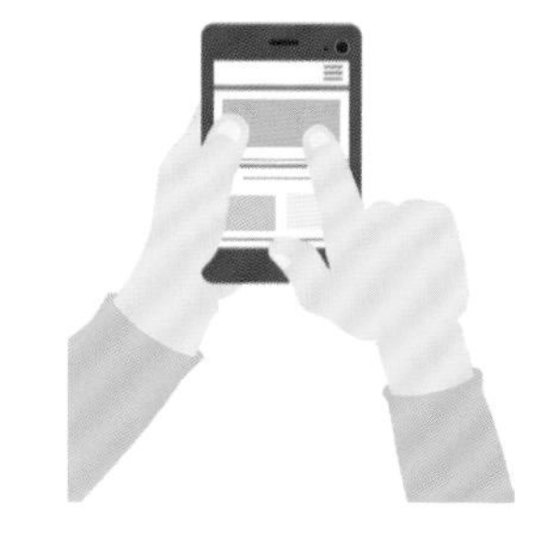

One way of establishing patient compliance is through patient-focused attention and encouraging positive behaviour. A potentially effective solution is using a smartphone calendar or reminders app, such as **Medisafe Medication Reminder and Pill Organizer** by **MediSafe Inc.,** that keeps patients on track and accountable for their condition. Many people keep their cell phone within reach and having an app a patient can update and track will encourage them to follow treatment.

Physicians need to build strong doctor-patient relationships to improve overall patient care. Medical office assistants play a crucial role in educating patients on the importance of adhering to a physician's orders and taking medication accordingly. In order to prevent poor patient welfare and the perception of poor medical services, the patient must follow medical prescriptions as well as their doctor's advice to improve. For chronic patients, improvement may not be possible, but following orders can control illness through therapeutic management.

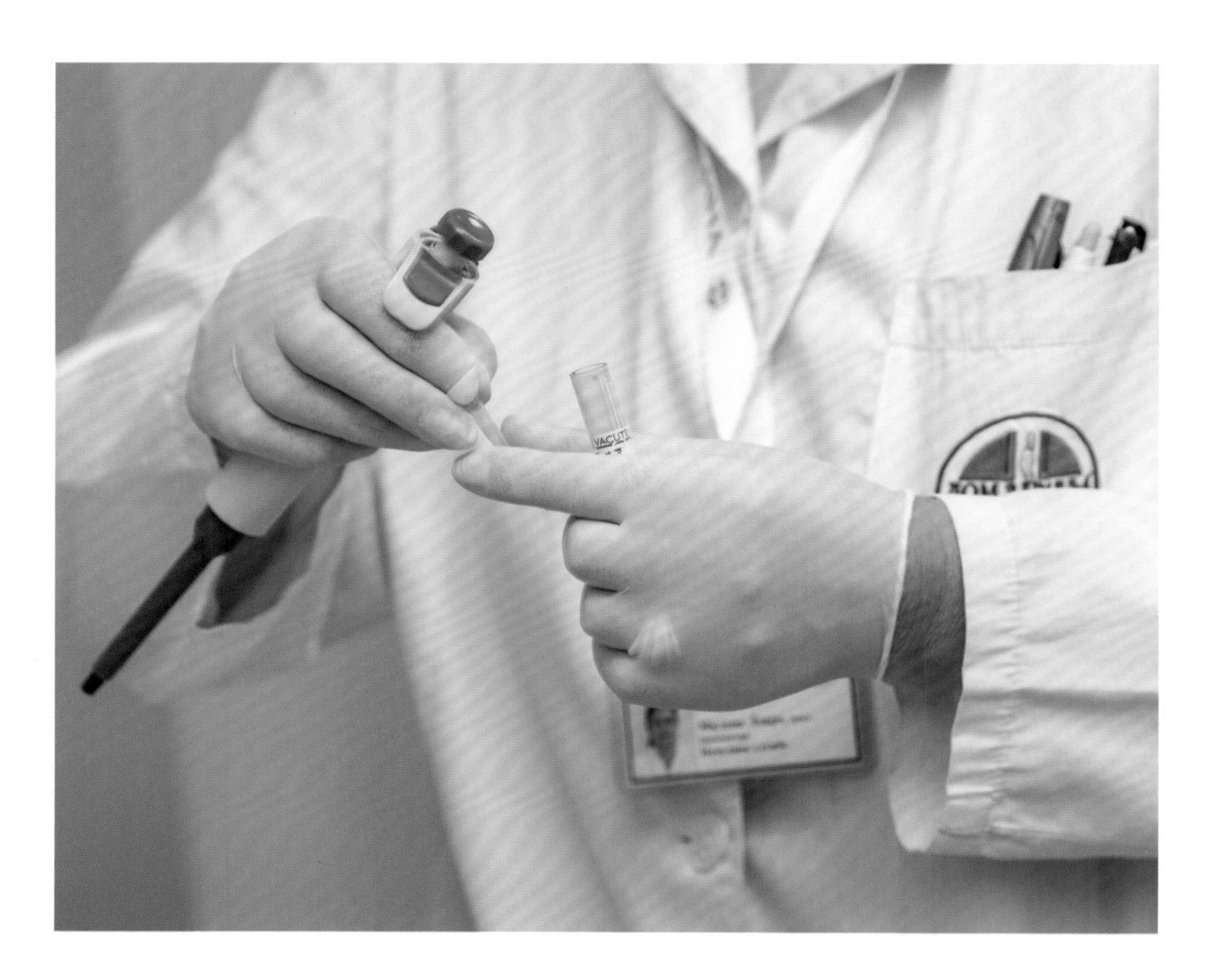

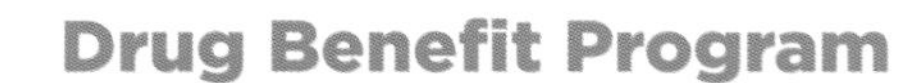

Drug Benefit Program

The **Ontario Drug Benefit** (ODB) Program covers people 65 or older, residents of long-term care facilities, people receiving home care, and Trillium drug program recipients. Recipients may have to pay a deductible and/or co-pay for any required medication. The drug benefit program is explained in detail on the Ontario Ministry of Health website (http://www.health.gov.on.ca/english/public/pub/drugs/odb.html) and covers most of the cost of 3,800 prescription drug products, some nutrition products, and some diabetic testing agents.

Listed under the "Formulary" section are products covered by the ODB program. Under special circumstances, the Exceptional Access Program may cover most of the cost of various drug products not on the formulary list, though a doctor must apply on behalf of the patient. A drug that is not on the formulary list must be granted approval by the ministry before the drug is funded by the program.

In order to qualify for ODB, an Ontario doctor must prescribe the drugs and they must be purchased from either:

- An accredited Ontario pharmacy OR
- An Ontario doctor who is licensed to sell prescription drug products and is linked to the ministry's Health Network System.

After turning 65, a patient must wait until the first of the month following their birthday and inform the pharmacist of their eligibility to access the ODB program. The patient must also present a valid Ontario health card to obtain their prescription. Depending on income, a lower payment per prescription may be arranged through the Seniors Co-Payment Program.

The Seniors Co-Payment Program is available to lower income seniors to have their deductible waived and only have to pay up to $2 each time they fill a prescription for an approved product. Patients have to apply for this program to qualify for the lower ODB or else they have to pay the higher fees. This form is available at local pharmacies, 1-888-405-0405, or online (http://www.forms.ssb.gov.on.ca/mbs/ssb/forms/ssbforms.nsf/GetFileAttach/014-3233-87~1/$File/3233-87E.pdf).

Trillium Drug Program

http://health.gov.on.ca/en/public/programs/drugs/programs/odb/opdp_trillium.aspx[14]

Another option available to patients with high drug costs relative to their income is the **Trillium Drug Program**. In order to apply for this program, a valid Ontario health card is needed and you need to reside in Ontario. There are limitations to who can apply and qualify for this program.

The restrictions are:

- You cannot be covered under the Ontario Drug Benefit Program as a senior over 65 years of age.
- You cannot receive financial help through Ontario Works or the Ontario Disability Support Program while receiving home care services.
- In order to be considered for the Trillium Drug Program, you cannot be a resident of a long-term care home or home for special care.

Limited Use of Drug Programs

Not all drugs are covered by these programs—some drugs are only covered by the Ontario Drug Benefit program under certain circumstances. For example, the program may cover medication if it is prescribed for only certain ailments, or only if other drugs have been tried first with no improvements. In these circumstances, the physician must fill in **a limited use number** on the prescription. If the limited use number is not present, or if the patient does not meet the requirements for the drug to be covered, the pharmacist cannot fill the prescription.

Limited use number:

Offered under the ODB program for specific situations such as for a particular medical condition(s) and/or for a limited period of time.

Prescription Repeats and Renewals

Medical office assistants must handle prescription repeats for the continuation of long-term medications and must pass the message onto a physician to authorize the request. Prescriptions for long-term use medications are usually valid for a limited number of refills before a new doctor prescription is required. Depending on the physician's orders, a repeat of a medication may be denied.

Upon denial, the physician will contact the patient to answer any questions they may have regarding why they were not granted a repeat. A medical assistant may be tasked with the responsibility to answer questions only as directed by the physician, and any information relayed over the phone should be minimal. If the patient has additional questions regarding the denied request, it is the physician's responsibility to answer them when they come in for a follow up appointment.

The patient may not be responding to the medication as well as was intended at the time of prescription. In this case, the physician may ask the patient to schedule another appointment to discuss other options available to control the illness or disease.

If a short-term prescription has run out, a patient may call the medical office to request a renewal or an extension. Policies for handling renewals vary between physicians—some physicians authorize the prescription over the phone, where others require a patient to be present in the office for a renewal. If the physician allows telephone renewals, make sure to record all information about the patient and the medication desired for the physician to review.

Prescriptions for sleeping pills, narcotics, and tranquilizers cannot be renewed without an assessment. This is usually the same for antibiotics as well. For renewing prescription medication, check with the physician before informing the patient of the status of their renewal request.

Phoned or Faxed-in Requests

Physicians rely heavily on prescription medication for treating patients and, as a result, prescription requests made to a medical office involve refilling a previously written prescription. Medical office assistants spend a significant amount of time managing prescription refills, making it essential to have an accurate and efficient system in place. Telephone conversations and faxed-in requests where personal information is collected and exchanged must be recorded in the medical record in the same manner as any other physician-patient encounter.

The documentation of these exchanges should include the date and time of the call or fax received, as well as the physician's advice. When a patient phones or faxes prescription requests, it is crucial to always have a physician approve it before granting the request. The best way to achieve this, is to have written protocols that minimize error rates. All employees should also be aware of the costs associated with refills and renewals that the patient will be responsible for.

When a request has been submitted for the physician's approval it is important to let the patient know, even if they have been on the medication for long-term. Notify the patient regarding the status of their prescription request; i.e. whether it has been granted or denied. Patient satisfaction and efficiency is the responsibility of everyone working in the office.

If a patient requests a refill but is due for an appointment with the physician, they are typically granted a one-month supply. This prescription is faxed or communicated over the phone to the patient's pharmacist. Unless the patient sees the physician, the refill request will be denied. The physician may need the patient to schedule a follow-up appointment to re-assess the medical condition, request tests to screen for any side effects, and monitor the patient's progress.

After receiving a refill request, before submitting the request to the physician, make sure that you have obtained the following information:

- Patient's first and last name
- Patient's address and phone number
- Name of medication
- Prescription number
- Dose and frequency
- Date issued
- Preferred pharmacy (unless the pharmacy is the party calling)
- Pharmacy's location and telephone number

Once prescription requests have been submitted and handled, make sure this physician-patient exchange is properly documented. Where possible, copy all emails for the patient chart, especially those dealing with significant clinical impact. Records should also reflect any prescriptions or repeats authorized over the telephone by the physician.

Managing the volume of prescription requests is a daunting task that medical office assistants may have to handle daily, but protocols ensuring efficiency, accuracy, and patient satisfaction will make the process easier. Some offices have fewer issues with prescriptions because patients are required to have an appointment to be granted renewal for their medication.

The medical record is a legal file that must contain a complete and accurate reflection of the patient's health status. All phoned or faxed-in requests should be handled in a timely fashion and contribute to the office's quality patient care.

my notes

Deterioration of Drugs

Certain drugs require special packaging and handling—exposure to light, moisture, temperature, and/or air may compromise the efficacy of the medication, rendering it defective. It is important to store and handle medication according to the manufacturer's recommendations. Become familiar with these recommendations and educate patients on how to properly handle and store their medication.

In the case of deteriorated and expired drugs, proper disposal should be carried out according to office protocol. Medicine take-back programs are a good way to remove expired, unwanted, or unused medication from the home. Contact your city or county government's household trash and recycling service to see if there are any medicine take-back programs available to your office's patients. You can also speak with your pharmacist to see if they know how to dispose of medications properly.

According to the Government of Canada, there are certain steps to take if a medicine take-back program is not available and you have no choice but to discard your prescription drugs in the garbage.

Tips to Safely Discard Prescription Drugs in the Garbage

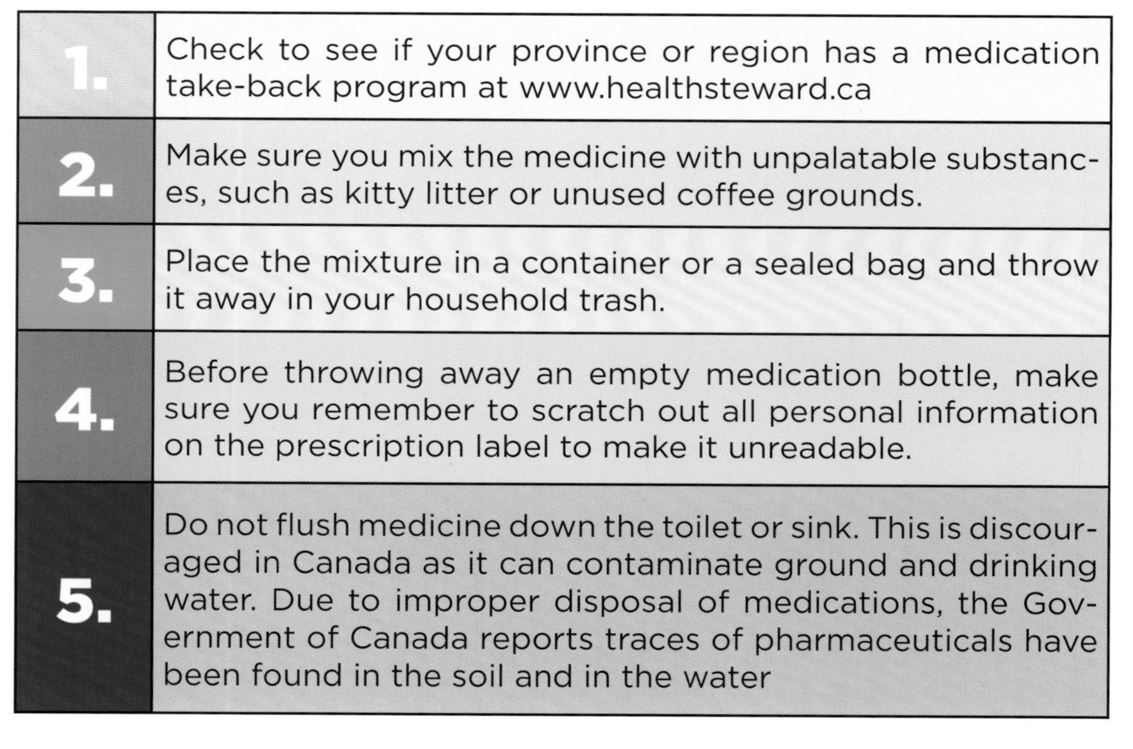

1.	Check to see if your province or region has a medication take-back program at www.healthsteward.ca
2.	Make sure you mix the medicine with unpalatable substances, such as kitty litter or unused coffee grounds.
3.	Place the mixture in a container or a sealed bag and throw it away in your household trash.
4.	Before throwing away an empty medication bottle, make sure you remember to scratch out all personal information on the prescription label to make it unreadable.
5.	Do not flush medicine down the toilet or sink. This is discouraged in Canada as it can contaminate ground and drinking water. Due to improper disposal of medications, the Government of Canada reports traces of pharmaceuticals have been found in the soil and in the water

Even though the potential human health risks associated are minute levels in general, taking preventative actions through proper pharmaceutical disposal will help protect our drinking water source in the long term.

Medications that are past their expiration date may produce adverse effects in the body. You may also receive proper disposal directions for these medications when you pick up your prescription from your pharmacy.

Take the time to return unused or expired prescription medication. Medication that is leftover can be dangerous in several regards. It has the potential to harm water sources if improperly dumped and it poses a risk to those living in the household where leftover medications are kept.

Avoiding Drug Errors

Despite the high volume of medications taken by adults, injuries due to errors in medication prescribing, dispensing, and administration are preventable. Efforts should be made to improve medication safety with a focus on accurate patient information. The following low-cost strategy recommendations are taken from research conducted by the Institute for Safe Medication Practices (ISMP).

Patient Information

Use two patient-specific identifiers to ensure the right patient receives the right medication. When preparing medication or vaccines for the physician, confirm the patient's name and date of birth with a "name alert" process for situations where patients have the same or similar names. Make sure that patient files are accurate so physicians can choose the appropriate medication, dose, route, and frequency.

Verify allergies and reactions in the medication process. Set up a protocol that requires staff members to ask about allergies and reactions to medications, latex, and food before prescriptions or office-administered medications are given to the patient. Include this information on the front of a paper chart, on the top of each progress note page, or on the electronic health record screen. Avoid the use of abbreviated names for medication when documenting allergies or reactions, as these can be easily misread.

Some diagnoses with significant impacts on medication selection, dosing, and frequency are diabetes mellitus, kidney disease, liver disease, and mental diseases. These should be highlighted for easy reference. It is also important to highlight the patient's smoking status and alcohol consumption, as these factors alter the effects of medication, dosing, and frequency. Keep this information for easy reference when prescribing a patient medication.

Keeping a current medication profile in a standard location on each patient's chart is an important safety measure.

This chart should be updated at each visit and should include reminders to ask about prescription drugs, but also any additional medication, supplements, and vitamins taken without a prescription. The medication list should include a record of the drug, dose, route, frequency, and purpose for each medication, herbal supplement, or vitamin.

Communication

Open communication is critical for avoiding drug errors. In order to avoid miscommunication, do not use potentially confusing abbreviations, symbols, and dose designations in various forms of medical communication, as these shortcuts may hinder effective communication. Misinterpreting an abbreviation can result in significant harm to patients.

To check for accuracy, read back any prescription information delivered verbally, either in person or over the phone. Be alert and be mindful for drugs with similar names when transcribing or entering notes. Ask for interpretation if poor handwriting makes it difficult to read a written prescription. Try writing in print rather than cursive, or have the prescription typed to avoid illegible handwriting.

Keep open communication with all medical personnel, and practice an "equal team member" concept that encourages everyone to be vigilant in detecting errors. This prevents any employees from hesitating to speak up or act on any potential error that occurs. Be a model for this behaviour by asking other members for their input and sharing information on a regular basis.

Medication and vials check list	
Ensure that:	
	Single dose vials are not reused. Leftover contents are not combined or pooled.
	A sterile syringe and needle or cannula is used when entering a vial.
	All needles and syringes are single patient use only.
	Multidose vials are not used wherever possible.
When the use of multidose vials cannot be avoided, follow these requirements:	
	Use each vial for a single patient whenever possible and mark the vial with the patient's name, as well as date of entry. Discard the open vial at the appropriate time. If vials are not marked with the patient's name or date, discard immediately.
	Vials are accessed aseptically on a clean surface and away from dirty, used, or potentially contaminated equipment.
	Before inserting a new needle and a new syringe, scrub the diaphragms of vials using friction and 70% alcohol.
	A needle is not left in a vial (to be attached to a new syringe).
	The vials are discarded immediately when sterility is questioned or compromised.
	Opened vials are discarded according to manufacturer's instructions or within 28 days of opening, whichever is shorter unless the vials are used for a single patient.

Controlled Drugs and Drug Information

The lack of drug information, such as outdated or limited references, is one of the most common causes of medication errors[1]. More than half of medication errors occur as a result of lack of drug information at the time of prescribing. The Controlled Drugs and Substances Act (CDSA) governs controlled drugs—the act classifies eight schedules of controlled substances and the regulations to control their use. The different schedules classify drugs and quantities based on legality and potential punishment for possession.

The federal government developed the CDSA in an effort to categorize regulated drugs based on the potential for abuse and benefits they provide from a medical standpoint. It prohibits unauthorized possession of drugs that the government determines to be dangerous, habit-forming, or otherwise not appropriate for use without a prescription. Criminal fines and incarceration can result if these laws are violated. The severity of the penalty is case dependent, determined by the quantity of controlled drugs involved.

In the medical office, pay close attention to high-alert medications that require extra precautions when administered, prescribed, dispensed, or refilled.

Drugs should be scheduled according to:

- Potential for abuse
- Medical usefulness
- Degree of possible physical or psychological dependence

Keep a list of these high-alert medications for easy reference. Decide on a set of core drug information references that you may use, and keep them updated at least annually, or whenever a new edition is available. Establish guidelines and consult national guidelines (http://www.guideline.gov) and other drug resources that will be easy for all office members to follow.

my notes

1) Leape, L.L., et al. (1995) Systems analysis of adverse drug events. JAMA. 274(1): 35-43.

Handling Controlled Drugs

Controlled drugs should be recorded and kept for two years, and records should detail which controlled drugs have been dispensed, administered, or prescribed. Inventories and records of controlled substances must be maintained and updated. All drugs should be stored in a locked, immovable cabinet to ensure that controlled substances are adequately safeguarded.

Be alert to break-ins or misplacements—in either case, the incident must be reported to authorities immediately. The theft or significant loss of any controlled substance must be reported within one business day of the incident. Certain details should be recorded, including the quantity and type of controlled substances lost by the practitioner. It is important to inform authorities about the loss in case diverted drugs are traced back to the practitioner's office.

Promote safe medication use with simple, low-cost system changes. Improved practice protocols and a heightened level of security can help avoid drug errors. Maintain open and effective communication with all members in the medical office to avoid misinterpretation. It is important for both the physician and medical office assistants to keep patient files updated and to avoid using abbreviations.

Safe Drug Handling Protocols
* Keep all medication in their original containers
* Check manufacturer's storage recommendations
* Keep drugs in dark containers or dark rooms
* Refrigerate drugs that must be kept cold
* Do not open bottles unnecessarily
* Do not return unused drugs to the original container
* Keep external use medications away from internal use medications
* Store medications away from cleaning supplies
* Organize drugs on the shelf
* Discard all unused, expired medication
* Never leave drugs out in the exam rooms

Preventing Drug Abuse

A patient's risk for drug addiction and drug abuse increases if they use the medication prescribed outside of the physician's orders. This includes the dosage, the frequency of medication taken, and interaction between drugs.

Drug abuse is not something that should be taken lightly—it can cause serious physical and mental illnesses in patients. Drug abuse can also lead to social dangers such as driving under the influence, violence, stress, and abuse. Drug abuse can lead to homelessness, crime, missed work, or difficulty in keeping a job. It destroys lives, which is why preventing and recognizing the warning signs for drug abuse is important for a medical office assistant.

Ways to Prevent Drug Abuse:

Physician's Written Prescription

Physicians may prescribe only small amounts of drugs with high potential for abuse to protect susceptible patients. The physician may choose to limit the number of refills that a patient can have filled by the pharmacy to avoid the possession of a high quantity of addictive medication.

The physician only prescribes narcotics and controlled substances when clinically appropriate, even if the patient has been prescribed these drugs in the past. It is up to the physician to take careful measures to prevent the theft of drugs, as well as educating patients about their risks. A physician needs to have a balanced approach to managing a patient's pain and relief while minimizing any potential negative consequences.

Prior to any prescription for medication, the patient must disclose every prescription or narcotic that they have obtained within the previous 30 days. Under the CDSA, a person who has been prescribed a narcotic must not seek or receive another prescription for narcotics from a different physician without disclosing this information.

Be Aware of Warning Signs

If patients ask for larger quantities or for a drug to be renewed early, this is a warning sign that they may be abusing the medication. As a medical office assistant, you should bring your concerns to the attention of the physician and ask the patient why they require a prescription renewed early if they are indeed following doctor's orders.

Walk-ins looking for narcotics should be dealt with promptly and efficiently. Politely explain your concerns regarding the patient's well-being and the downfalls of drug abuse. Following the guidelines of CDSA, it will be easy to recognize when a patient is not following the treatment agreement, and unusual drug-related behaviour should be noticeable.

A patient immediately requesting a specific controlled drug by name should also raise a red flag and prompt you to notify the physician before the appointment. Expressing your concerns before the appointment will help prevent the patient's abuse of a drug.

Reviewing Drug Prescriptions

Before the patient leaves the building, ask them if the physician has gone over the instructions for the medication prescribed. Explain the prescription directions once again and ask the patient if they have any questions regarding the medication that they have been prescribed.

Don't let a patient leave the office feeling confused about how they should be taking their medication. Be sure to go over any additional instructions, such as taking a prescription on an empty stomach or if a medication has to be stored in a specific manner to avoid deterioration.

When you are going over the prescription with the client, take the opportunity to double check that the physician has signed the written or printed prescription. If the patient goes to a pharmacy to have their prescription filled without a signed document, the pharmacy will decline the prescription request.

Educate the Patient

Inform the patient that they must speak with a physician before stopping or changing their drug dosage regimen. Go over any side effects and what to look for should an allergy develop to a prescribed medication. Let the patient know that they should contact the office if they have any concerns or questions when they get home. Sometimes the office visit can be overwhelming to a patient, and questions may come to mind once they have had some time to settle.

Explain that the patient must never use another person's prescription, even if the medication is the same as that which a physician has prescribed them. Consuming medication that was not prescribed to a patient can be dangerous and harmful.

The patient must be aware of this as well—they must not give their medication to someone else, as this is also considered a form of drug abuse. Remind the patient to be mindful of where they store their medication, and to keep it out of reach of children.

Educate the patient on what the medication does and how it interacts with the body to help alleviate their symptoms. For example, the medication may not be effective until after a certain amount of time on the drug. The patient must be aware of the signs of side effects or allergic reactions.

Preventing drug abuse and recognizing warning signs of patients are important responsibilities for a medical office assistant. The non-medical use or abuse of prescription drugs is a serious and growing public health concern. In order to control and prevent drug abuse in your practice, the medical office assistant must work with the physician as well as the patient to help meet the latter's needs.

Quiz

CHAPTER 4 QUIZ

1. What is a prescription? ________________________________
____
____
____
____
____
____

2. What kinds of drugs are considered over-the-counter?

____
____
____
____
____
____
____

3. True or false? Long-term prescriptions should be added to the patient's medication profile and kept on their record.

4. To prevent prescription fraud, what should the physician do with the prescription pad?

____
____
____
____
____
____
____

5. True or false? A cubic centimetre is occupied by the same volume of one millimetre, so the two units can be used interchangeably.

6. Rx, an abbreviation that means "Take Thus" or "take," is part of which section in a prescription?

    a. Superscription

    b. Inscription

    c. Subscription

    d. None of the above

7. What do the following abbreviations stand for?

    a. q.i.d.

    b. q.h.

    c. p.r.n.

    d. b.i.d.

    e. q.4h.

8. Metre for distance, second for time, and Kelvin for temperature all fall under which category of measurement? ______________________

9. Fill in the blanks: ______________________ is the only ____________________ unit of measurement used to administer medication, as patients are comfortable measuring medication in drops and teaspoons.

10. Why must a patient follow the physician's exact order when it comes to taking antibiotics?

____

____

____

____

____

____

____

11. What are the five main principles in the Canadian Health Act? List them.

______________________________ ______________________________

______________________________ ______________________________

____

12. What is/are the differences between the Drug Benefit Program and the Trillium Drug Program?

a. The Drug Benefit Program covers residents of long-term care facilities and the Trillium Drug Program is available to those that are not a resident of a long-term care home or home for special care.

b. The Drug Benefit Program covers those that are not a resident of a long-term care home or home for special care and the Trillium Drug Program is available for residents of long-term care facilities.

c. The Drug Benefit Program covers Trillium Drug Program recipients.

d. The Trillium Drug Program helps people who have high drug costs in relation to their income.

13. Which prescriptions require an assessment before the renewal of prescription is approved? ______________________________

____

____

14. Which of the following information should be obtained before submitting a prescription request?

a. Client's first and last name

b. Name of medication

c. Prescription number

d. Dose and frequency

e. All of the above

15. What should you use to ensure the right patient receives the right medication?

____

____

____

16. All are considered to be protocol for safe drug handling, except:

    a. Return all unused drugs to the original container

    b. Do not open bottle unnecessarily

    c. Keep external use medications away from internal use medications

    d. Store medications away from cleaning supplies

17. True or false? Eliminate the use of potentially confusing abbreviations, symbols, and dose designations in various forms of medical communication as it leads to effective communication.

18. How long should controlled drug records be kept for?

    a. 1 year

    b. 2 years

    c. 5 years

    d. 10 years

my notes

Chapter 5

Diagnostic Testing Theory

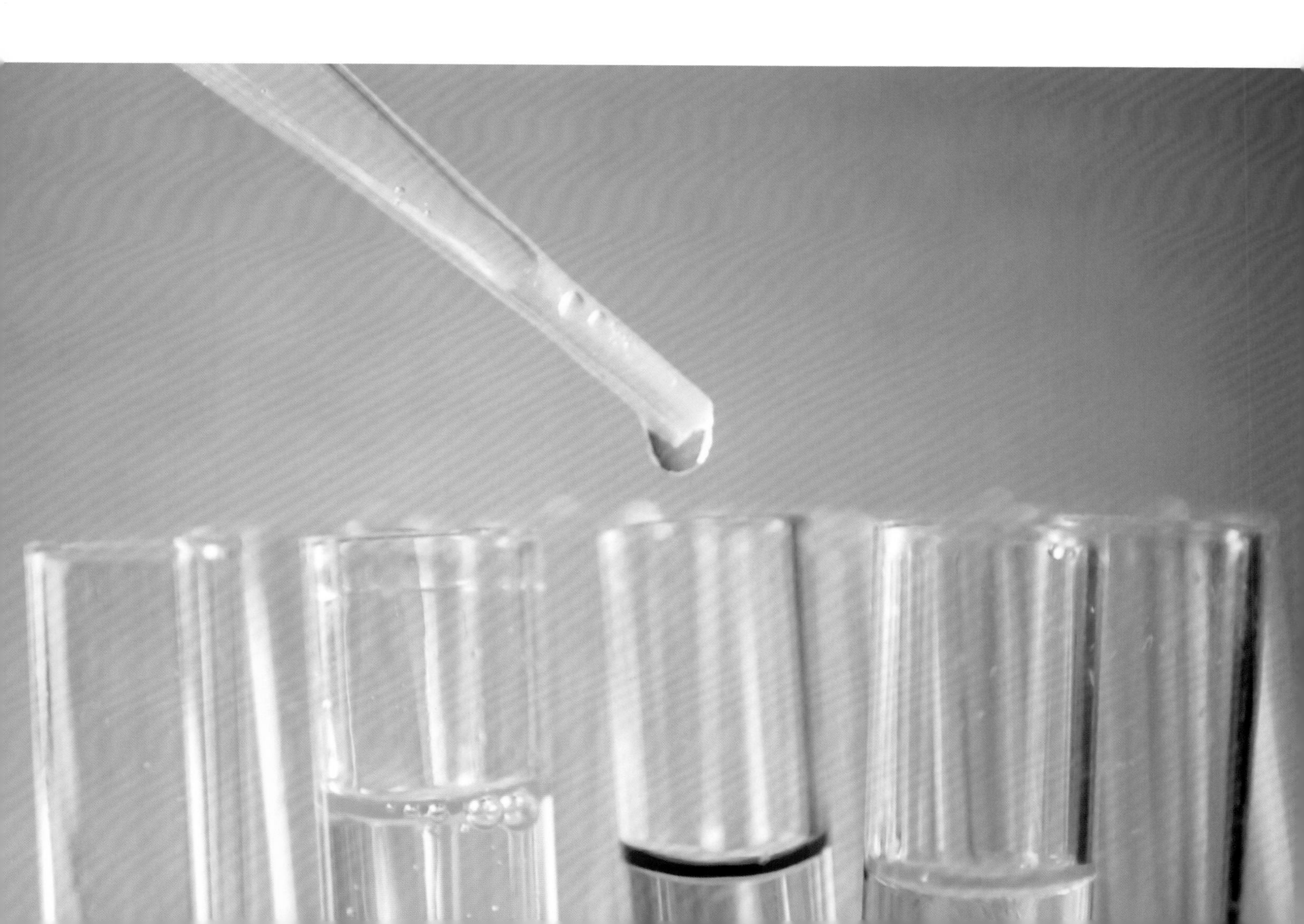

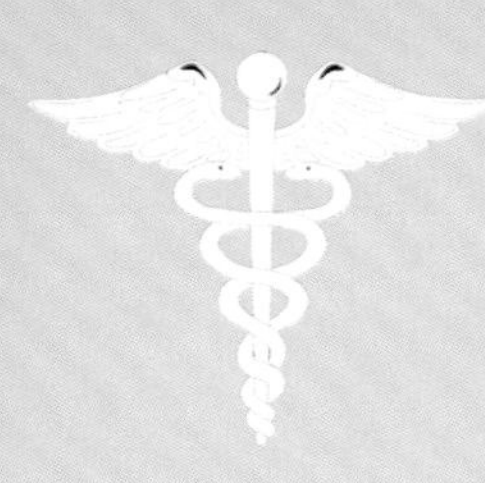

CHAPTER FIVE LEARNING OBJECTIVES

After completing this chapter, you should be able to:

- ❑ **Understand why diagnostic testing is performed**
- ❑ **Define and understand diagnostic imaging terminology**
- ❑ **Identify and understand different professions in the medical field**
- ❑ **Identify and define the term *allied health***
- ❑ **Identify and distinguish medical health care facilities**
- ❑ **Understand and implement how to fill out a lab requisition form**

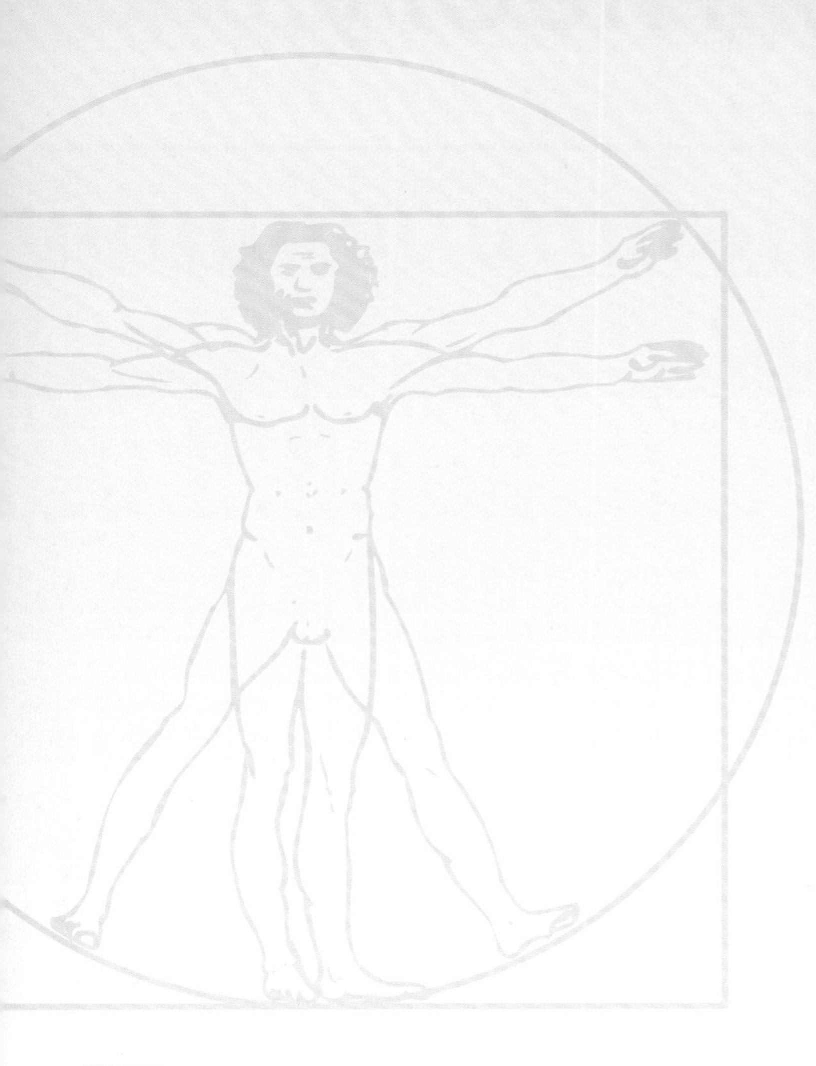

Why Perform Diagnostic Testing?

Diagnostic testing reveals valuable information and is often the most important tool in concluding a medical diagnosis. Testing allows the physician to screen for diseases—it helps visualize and analyze body structures, tissues, and fluids. Early detection of a problem helps physicians to arrive at a diagnosis and allows for prompt treatment. Without physician-ordered diagnostic testing, it is difficult to proceed from the treatment plan to monitoring a patient's progress.

Diagnostic testing can serve many functions in the medical field, and is ordered by physicians to answer a specific question. The physician can use it to monitor therapy by looking for benefits or side effects and make changes accordingly. In asymptomatic patients, a physician can screen for diseases and provide prognosis for individuals with established diseases.

The results from diagnostic testing also provide baseline information for patients undergoing treatment or surgery. It helps the physician determine if the patient has a particular condition or not.

Test results must be reliable and accurate—they usually result in parameters that include the test's sensitivity, specificity, predictive values, and likelihood ratios.

Important Terms for Diagnostic Testing

- **Homeostasis:** the normal state of balance (equilibrium) in the human body. Our physiological state tries to maintain a balanced environment.
- **Reference range:** the range of values normally expected for a particular test.
- **Abnormal value:** results that are above or below the reference range.
    - Note that an abnormal result that is potentially life-threatening and requires immediate action is called a **critical value**.
- **Test Profiles:** tests that are commonly ordered in groups.
    - Examples of test profiles would include, but are not limited to, Complete Blood Count (CBC), Liver Function Tests, Lipid Profile, Comprehensive Metabolic Panel, and T4 (Thyroxine).

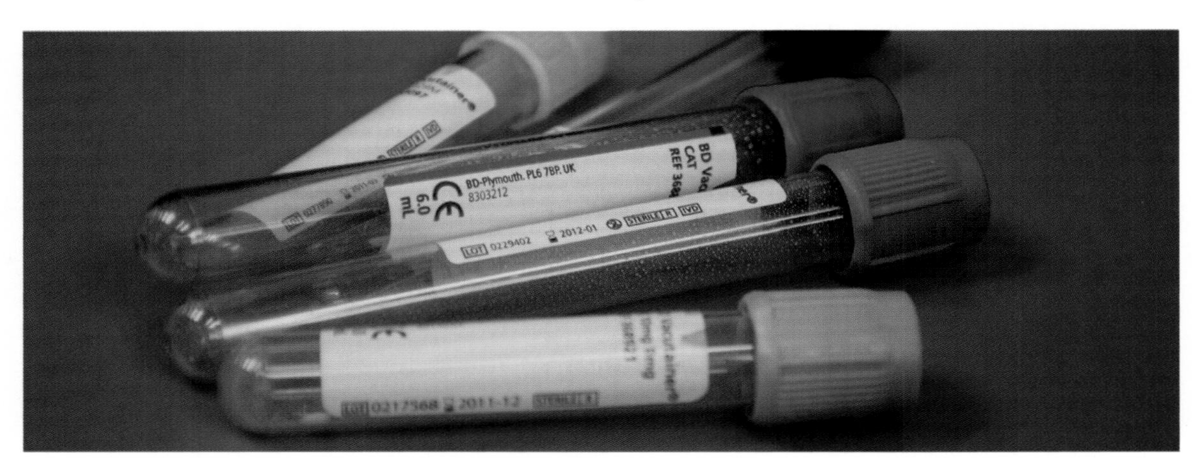

Homeostasis: *The tendency toward a stable equilibrium, as maintained by physiological processes in the body.*

Reference range: *The range of values for a physiologic measurement in healthy persons.*

Abnormal value: *Test results that are above or below the reference range.*

Critical value: *Abnormal results that are potentially life-threatening and require immediate medical action.*

Test Profiles: *A combination of laboratory tests usually conducted by automated methods to evaluate organ systems of patients.*

Professionals in the Medical Field

Allied health professions: *Health care professions that are not in the field of nursing, medicine, or pharmacy.*

Allied health professions are health care professions that are not in the field of nursing, medicine, or pharmacy. These professions work directly, or indirectly, with a patient's health by providing evaluations as well as assessments of patient needs. They also play a role in informing patients of their progress and response to treatment.

Here are a few of the 200 or more careers that fall into the category of allied health professions, and will often work closely with medical assistants:

- **Medical Laboratory Technologist:** Laboratory technologists supervise and carry out all clinical laboratory testing. Training consists of a three-year college and/or university program.
- **Medical Laboratory Technician:** A technician can perform clinical testing under supervision. Training consists of a one-year college course.
- **Phlebotomist:** Phlebotomists collect hematological samples (blood) for clinical or medical testing, transfusion, donations, or research. A trained phlebotomist collects blood through intravenous access or finger pricks. Phlebotomy is a skill often possessed by lab technologists or other specially certified health professionals.

Physicians may choose to specialize in laboratory fields such as:

Cytology

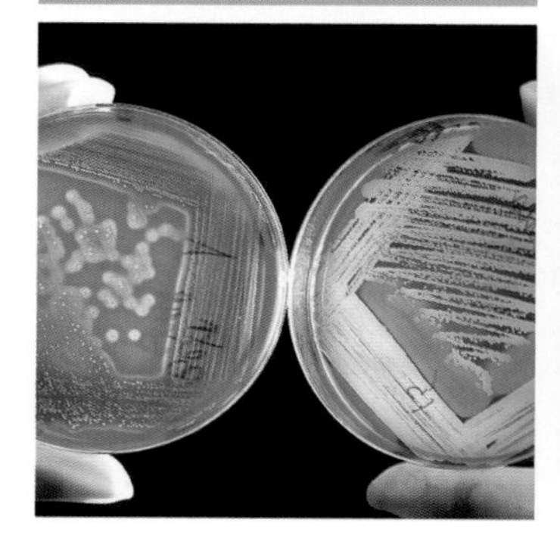

The study of cells on the microscopic level to diagnose any abnormalities and malignancies.

Hematology

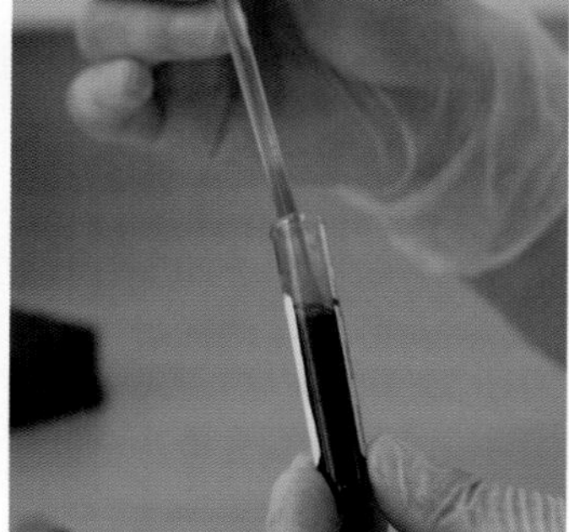

The science and study of blood, blood-forming organs, and blood diseases. The medical aspect of this profession includes the treatment of blood disorders and malignancies such as hemophilia, leukemia, lymphoma, and sickle-cell anemia.

Pathology

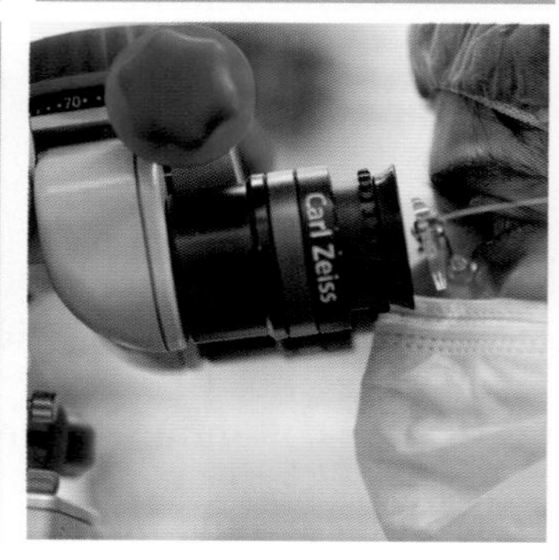

The medical science concerned with examining tissues, diseases, and bodily fluids in order to diagnose a disease.

Radiology

The use of diagnostic imaging technology to examine organs and tissues inside the body. This non-invasive process helps diagnose injuries and illnesses so a treatment plan can be made.

These health professions make up medical health care teams. Together, they help with the assessment, treatment, and recovery process of patients. Allied health professions support a person's medical care and aim to help with diagnosis, recovery, and quality of life.

Medical Health Care Facilities

Many medical facilities are available for people who require medical attention or a particular medical service. A medical assistant should know the locations and contact information of nearby facilities in case they need to direct patients to a different facility. Keep a list of local facilities and phone numbers by the front desk for easy access.

According to the Public Health Agency of Canada, four levels of laboratories form the public health laboratory system. These include: 1) private, local and hospital laboratories, 2) provincial public health laboratories, 3) national laboratories, and 4) international laboratory networks. In this chapter, the focus will be on private, provincial public health, and hospital laboratories.

These different levels of laboratories function as a hierarchy, though there are no formal reporting relationships or requirements between them. The specialization of diagnostic capacity and scientific expertise usually increases at higher levels in the system. In response to an epidemic, the role of each laboratory varies with the disease or stage of the epidemic.

Private Laboratories

Private laboratories may be freestanding, located within clinics, or have satellite locations for specimen collection. They can analyze blood as well as perform imaging and testing of tissues using x-rays, ultrasonography, mammography, and other diagnostic technologies. Many laboratory services for infectious diseases have been privatized for cost-efficiency, but problems may arise due to the reluctance to perform labour-intensive, low-profit-margin tests.

The private laboratory's role is to diagnose infections and this positions them outside of the formal public health system. As such, privatization makes it difficult to monitor proper procedure due to federal privacy legislation.

Notifiable diseases still require reporting due to public health obligations.

Public Health Laboratories

Public health laboratories are operated by the government and provide analyses of specimens for diseases of public concern (for example: HIV, Hepatitis, SARS, and West Nile).

A public health laboratory is made up of one or more professional laboratory scientists and a number of technologists. Public health laboratories provide the following services:

- Clinical and environmental testing
- Clinical consultation
- Technical and customer service support
- Education and training programs for laboratory professionals
- Evaluation of new laboratory technologies and methodologies

Hospital Laboratories

Major teaching hospitals contain larger laboratories and may play a major academic role in training and research. Most hospitals have facilities for:

- Hematology
- Immunohematology
- Chemistry
- Microbiology
- Histology/pathology/cytology
- X-ray and other imaging (CT scan, MRI, Ultrasound)

According to the Public Health Agency of Canada, hospital laboratories are a key component in the response to institutional outbreaks of infection because of their position within the system. The hierarchical system of laboratories creates a slow process as information needs to pass from one level to the next. A hospital laboratory must be well managed to allow quick movement of information through the system.

Hospital laboratories provide surveillance, investigate outbreaks, test for bioterrorism, and support and contribute resources to incident management.

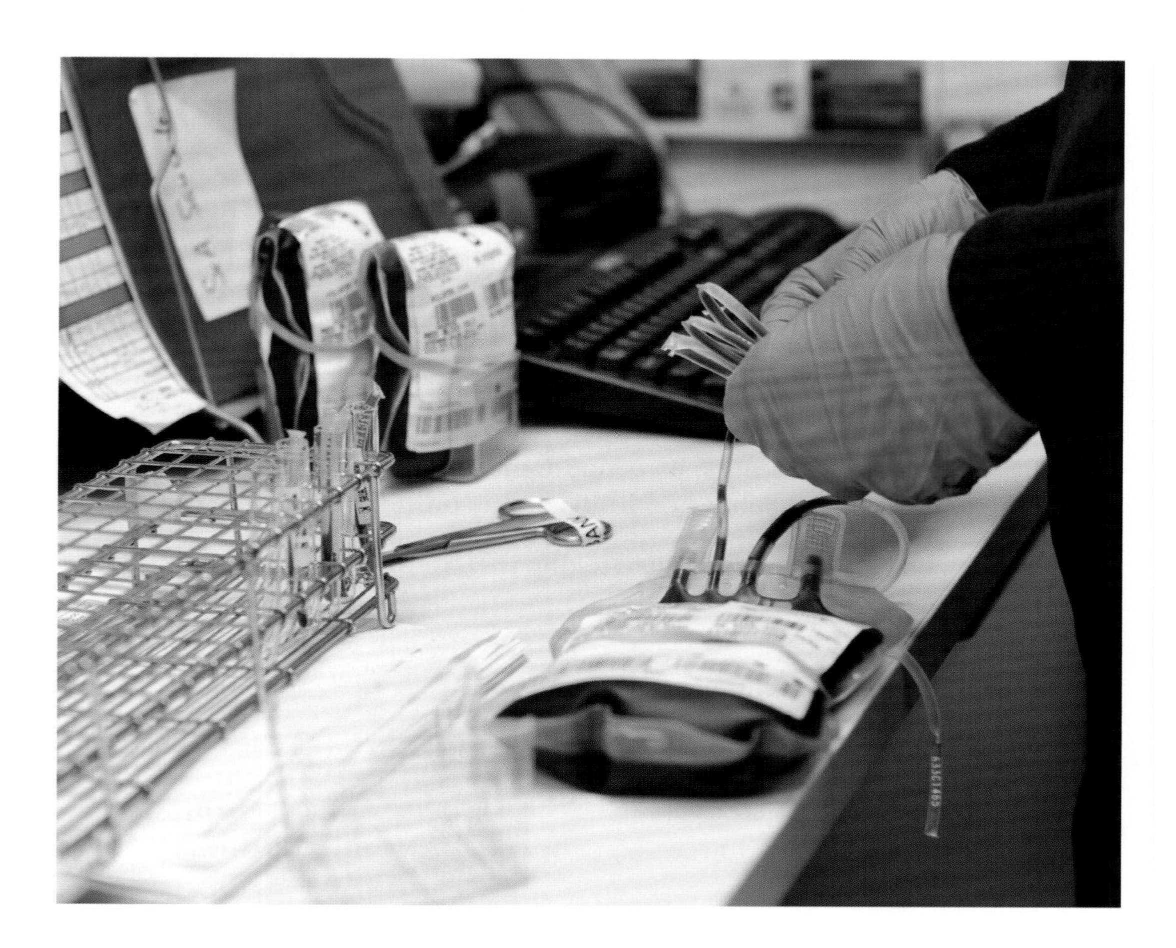

Laboratory Requisition Forms

Lab requisition forms should look something like this:

Public Health Ontario | Santé publique Ontario
PARTNERS FOR HEALTH | PARTENAIRES POUR LA SANTÉ

Date received yyyy / mm / dd — PHOL No.

General Test Requisition

ALL Sections of this Form MUST be Completed

1 - Submitter

Courier Code

Provide Return Address:
Name
Address
City & Province
Postal Code

Clinician Initial / Surname and OHIP / CPSO Number

Tel: ____ Fax: ____

2 - Patient Information

Health No. | Sex | Date of Birth: yyyy / mm / dd

Medical Record No.

Patient's Last Name *(per OHIP card)* | First Name *(per OHIP card)*

Patient Address

Postal Code | Patient Phone No.

Submitter Lab No.

Public Health Unit Outbreak No.

cc Doctor Information

Name: ____ Tel: ____
Lab/Clinic Name: ____ Fax: ____
CPSO #: ____
Address: ____ Postal Code: ____

Public Health Investigator Information

Name: ____
Health Unit: ____
Tel: ____ Fax: ____

3 - Test(s) Requested *(Please see descriptions on reverse)*

Test: Enter test descriptions below

Hepatitis Serology

Reason for test (Check (✓) only one box):
☐ Immune status
☐ Acute infection
☐ Chronic infection

Indicate specific viruses (Check (✓) all that apply):
☐ Hepatitis A
☐ Hepatitis B
☐ Hepatitis C *(testing only available for acute or chronic infection; no test for determining immunity to HCV is currently available)*

4 - Specimen Type and Site

☐ blood / serum ☐ faeces ☐ nasopharyngeal
☐ sputum ☐ urine ☐ vaginal smear
☐ urethral ☐ cervix ☐ BAL
☐ other - *(specify)*

Patient Setting

☐ physician office/clinic ☐ ER (not admitted)
☐ inpatient (ward) ☐ inpatient (ICU) ☐ institution

5 - Reason for Test

☐ diagnostic ☐ immune status
☐ needle stick ☐ follow-up
☐ prenatal ☐ chronic condition
☐ immunocompromised
☐ post-mortem
☐ other - *(specify)*

Date Collected: yyyy / mm / dd

Onset Date: yyyy / mm / dd

Clinical Information

☐ fever ☐ gastroenteritis ☐ respiratory symptoms
☐ STI ☐ headache / stiff neck ☐ vesicular rash
☐ pregnant ☐ encephalitis / meningitis ☐ maculopapular rash
☐ jaundice
☐ other - *(specify)*

☐ influenza high risk - *(specify)*
☐ recent travel - *(specify location)*

For HIV, please use the HIV serology form. - For referred cultures, please use the reference bacteriology form.To re-order this test requisition contact your local Public Health Laboratory and ask for form number F-SD-SCG-1000. Current version of Public Health Laboratory requisitions are available at www.publichealthontario.ca/requisitions

The personal health information is collected under the authority of the Personal Health Information Protection Act, s.36 (1)(c)(iii) for the purpose of clinical laboratory testing. If you have questions about the collection of this personal health information please contact the PHOL Manager of Customer Service at 416-235-6556 or toll free 1-877-604-4567. F-SD-SCG-1000 (08/2013)

Ontario — Agency for Health Protection and Promotion / Agence de protection et de promotion de la santé

The MOA has to fill out the admin portion—this is not the responsibility of the doctor. They need to make sure that the physician has signed and dated the form or the lab will not complete the testing. If the lab calls you, you will need to have the form filled out, signed, and faxed over to the testing facility.

Other generalized lab forms are available at:

www.publichealthontario.ca/en/eRepository/General_test_fillable_requisition.pdf

Quiz

CHAPTER 5 QUIZ

1. A range of values normally expected for a particular test is known as:

    a. Test profiles

    b. Test range

    c. Reference range

    d. Reference profile

2. What's the difference between an abnormal value and a critical value?

____
____
____
____
____
____

3. True or false? The normal state of balance or equilibrium in the human body is called homeostasis.

4. The study of cells on the microscopic level to diagnose any abnormalities and malignancies is the definition of:

    a. Hematology

    b. Pathology

    c. Cytology

    d. Radiology

5. Define what a hematologist specializes in.

____
____
____
____

6. True or false? A medical laboratory technician can supervise and carry out all clinical laboratory testing.

7. Which laboratory technician uses diagnostic imaging technology to examine organs and tissues inside the body to diagnose injuries and illness?

    a. Radiologist

    b. Pathologist

    c. Radiography

    d. Radiograph

Chapter 6

Types of Testing

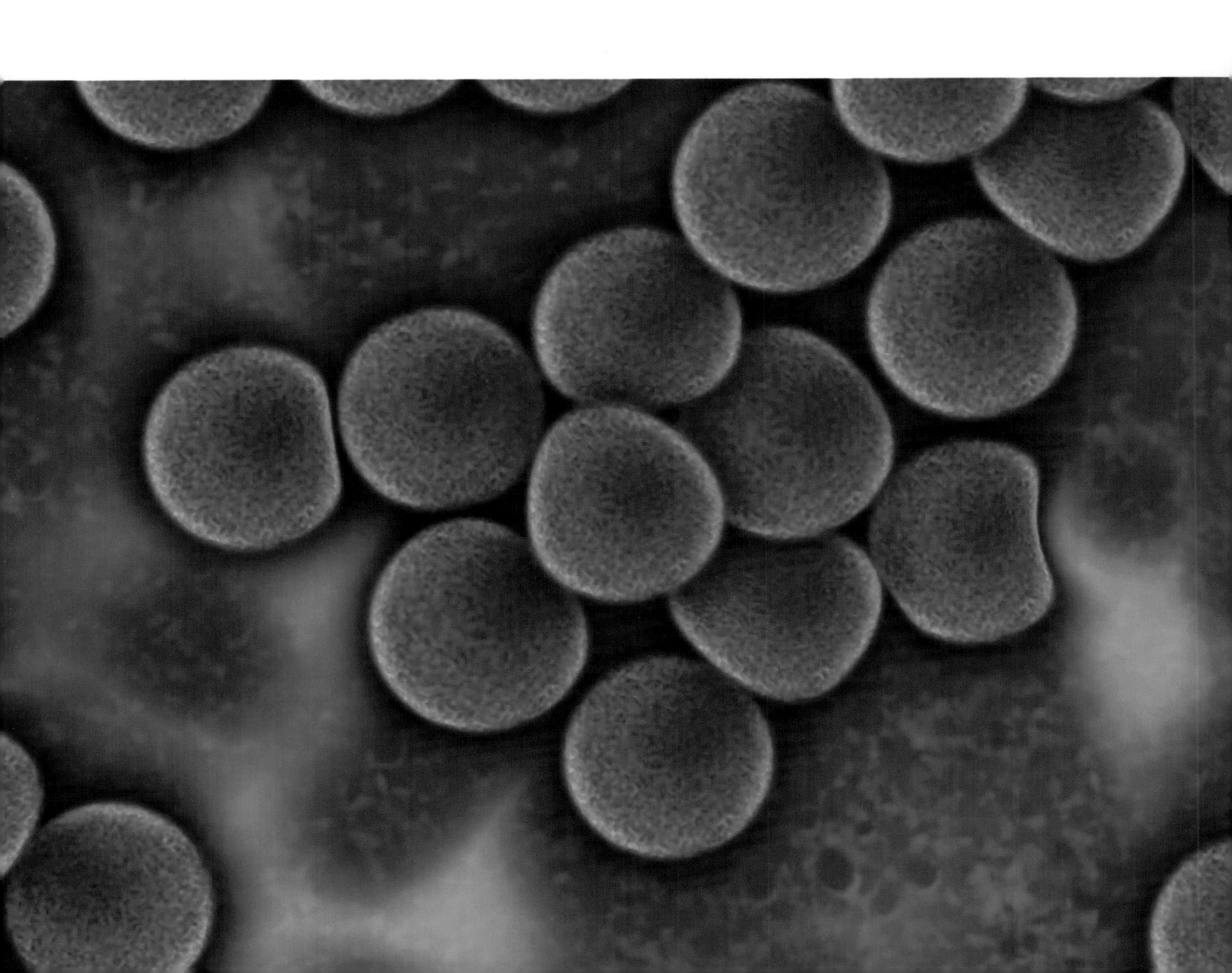

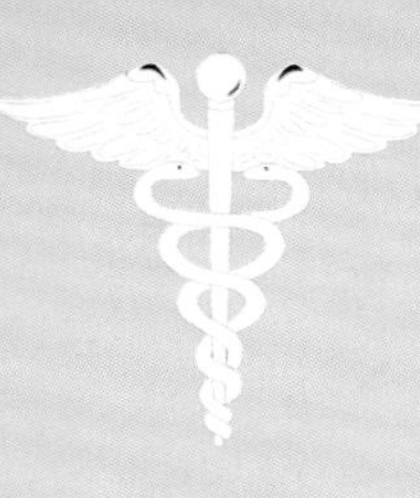

CHAPTER SIX LEARNING OBJECTIVES

After completing this chapter, you should be able to:

- ❑ Define and explain the terms hematology, biochemistry, immunology
- ❑ Define and understand the results from a complete blood count (CBC)
- ❑ Understand and explain microbiology ID and sensitivity
- ❑ Understand how to properly prepare and handle blood specimens
- ❑ Define, distinguish, and know how to implement the four methods of urine collection
- ❑ Understand how to handle urine specimens and prepare a urine sample for microscopic examination
- ❑ Understand how to perform and analyze a urine specimen with the use of reagent strips
- ❑ Understand the Transportation of Dangerous Goods Act

Hematology

Hematology is the study of blood. It includes processing and evaluating blood. This study also looks at blood components, including morphologic appearance, function, blood diseases, and blood-forming tissues. Some common hematologic tests include hemoglobin (Hgb), hematocrit (Hct), white blood cell count (WBC), red blood cell count (RBC), differential white blood cell count (diff), prothrombin time/INR (PT/INR), erythrocyte sedimentation rate (ESR), and platelet count (Plt). Details on these tests and their purposes appear later in this section. Hematological testing is mostly concerned with the cellular components of blood.

***Hematology:** The study of blood, including the processing and evaluation of blood.*

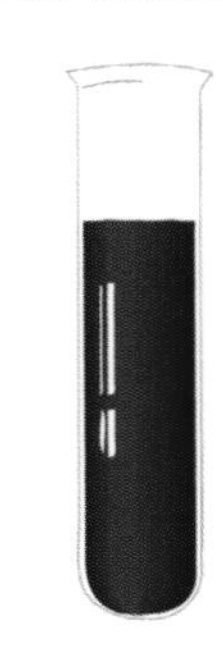

Before moving forward with information on hematological tests, we will review the basics of blood physiology. The human body contains four to five litres of blood. Blood is composed of plasma, red and white blood cells (erythrocytes and leukocytes respectively), platelets (thrombocytes), in addition to various proteins, hormones, antibodies, and nutrients.

Erythrocytes are produced in red bone marrow in various bones of the body. This includes the ribs, skull, sternum, and pelvic bone, as well as in the ends of the long limb bones. A major component of all erythrocytes is hemoglobin. Hemoglobin is responsible for the red colour of erythrocytes. Hemoglobin contains an iron atom, which binds to oxygen, similar to the way free iron oxidizes (or rusts).

***Erythrocytes**: A red blood cell found in humans that are typically the shape of a biconcave disc without a nucleus.*

Hemoglobin can be measured to determine blood's oxygen-carrying capacity. This is a routine test for individuals who are at risk of developing anemia. A decrease in hemoglobin reduces the blood's ability to carry oxygen to the body's tissues. Increased levels of hemoglobin may indicate conditions such as polycythemia (chronic obstructive pulmonary disease), congestive heart failure, or severe burns.

Laboratory analysis in hematology examines blood to detect pathologic conditions, and includes performing blood cell counts, evaluating clotting ability, and identifying cell types. This helps determine if each blood component falls within its reference range.

Prothrombin time, measured in seconds, determines how long it takes an individual's blood to form a clot. Depending on the test used (and the reagents used to stimulate clotting), different laboratory techniques produce different results for clotting time. To account for these differences, the PT results are converted to a standardized ratio known as an international normalized ratio (INR).

***Prothrombin time (PT):** How long it takes for an individual's blood to form a clot, measured in seconds.*

INR allows the comparison of a patient's PT test results regardless of the testing reagent.

Certain hematological laboratory tests take place in the medical office. These are conducted using automated blood analyzers designed specifically for medical office use. They perform laboratory tests with accurate test results in a shorter period than having blood samples sent to an outside laboratory technician for analysis.

Ontario Ministry of Health and Long-Term Care
Laboratory Requisition
Requisitioning Clinician / Practitioner

Name

Address

Laboratory Use Only

Clinician/Practitioner's Contact Number for Urgent Results ( )

Service Date yyyy mm dd

Clinician/Practitioner Number | CPSO / Registration No.

Health Number | Version | Sex ☐M ☐F | Date of Birth yyyy mm dd

Check (✓) one: ☐ **OHIP/Insured** ☐ **Third Party / Uninsured** ☐ **WSIB**

Province | Other Provincial Registration Number | Patient's Telephone Contact Number ( )

Additional Clinical Information *(e.g. diagnosis)*

Patient's Last Name *(as per OHIP Card)*

Patient's First & Middle Names *(as per OHIP Card)*

☐ Copy to: Clinician/Practitioner
Last Name First Name

Address

Patient's Address *(including Postal Code)*

Note: Separate requisitions are required for cytology, histology / pathology and tests performed by Public Health Laboratory

x	Biochemistry
	Glucose ☐Random ☐Fasting
	HbA1C
	Creatinine (eGFR)
	Uric Acid
	Sodium
	Potassium
	ALT
	Alk. Phosphatase
	Bilirubin
	Albumin
	Lipid Assessment (includes Cholesterol, HDL-C, Triglycerides, calculated LDL-C & Chol/HDL-C ratio; individual lipid tests may be ordered in the "Other Tests" section of this form)
	Albumin / Creatinine Ratio, Urine
	Urinalysis (Chemical)
	Neonatal Bilirubin:
	Child's Age: days hours
	Clinician/Practitioner's tel. no. ( )
	Patient's 24 hr telephone no. ( )
	Therapeutic Drug Monitoring:
	Name of Drug #1
	Name of Drug #2
	Time Collected #1 hr. #2 hr.
	Time of Last Dose #1 hr. #2 hr.
	Time of Next Dose #1 hr. #2 hr.

I hereby certify the tests ordered are not for registered in or out patients of a hospital.

X
Clinician/Practitioner Signature Date

x	Hematology
	CBC
	Prothrombin Time (INR)
	Immunology
	Pregnancy Test (Urine)
	Mononucleosis Screen
	Rubella
	Prenatal: ABO, RhD, Antibody Screen (titre and ident. if positive)
	Repeat Prenatal Antibodies
	Microbiology ID & Sensitivities (if warranted)
	Cervical
	Vaginal
	Vaginal / Rectal – Group B Strep
	Chlamydia *(specify source)*:
	GC *(specify source)*:
	Sputum
	Throat
	Wound *(specify source)*:
	Urine
	Stool Culture
	Stool Ova & Parasites
	Other Swabs / Pus *(specify source)*:

Specimen Collection
Time 24 hour clock Date yyyy/mm/dd

x	Viral Hepatitis *(check one only)*
	Acute Hepatitis
	Chronic Hepatitis
	Immune Status / Previous Exposure *Specify*: ☐ Hepatitis A ☐ Hepatitis B ☐ Hepatitis C or order individual hepatitis tests in the "Other Tests" section below

Prostate Specific Antigen (PSA)
☐ Total PSA ☐ Free PSA
Specify one below:
☐ Insured – Meets OHIP eligibility criteria
☐ Uninsured – Screening: Patient responsible for payment

Vitamin D (25-Hydroxy)
☐ Insured - Meets OHIP eligibility criteria: osteopenia; osteoporosis; rickets; renal disease; malabsorption syndromes; medications affecting vitamin D metabolism
☐ Uninsured - Patient responsible for payment

Other Tests - one test per line

Fecal Occult Blood Test (FOBT) *(check one)*
☐ FOBT (non CCC) ☐ ColonCancerCheck FOBT (CCC) no other test can be ordered on this form

Laboratory Use Only

4422-84 (2013/01) © Queen's Printer for Ontario, 2013 7530-4581

The most common test performed in a hematologic laboratory test is the **complete blood count** (CBC). Physicians will routinely request this test for new patients as well as patients with a pathologic condition. Running a CBC provides:

White blood cell count	Assists in diagnosis and prognosis of disease including meningitis, diphtheria, and viral infections.
Red blood cell count	Assists in diagnosing conditions such as anemia, polycythemia, dehydration, and leukemia.
Platelet count	Assists in evaluating bleeding disorders occurring in liver disease, thrombocytopenia, uremia, and anticoagulant therapies
Hemoglobin	Screens for anemia, determines its severity, and monitors the patient's response to treatment
Hematocrit	Assists in the diagnosis and evaluation of anemia
Differential white blood cell count	Assists in the diagnosis and prognosis of diseases
Red blood cell indices	Provides information about the size and hemoglobin content of a patient's red blood cells
	Assists in the diagnosis and evaluation of the type of anemia
	Determines the cause of this anemia

Hematology results provide information to the physician to make the proper diagnosis while evaluating the patient's progress and treatment. The study of a patient's blood can reveal abnormalities in blood formation and other blood disorders. Using laboratory tests and work ups, a medical professional can diagnose various blood-related disorders and cancers.

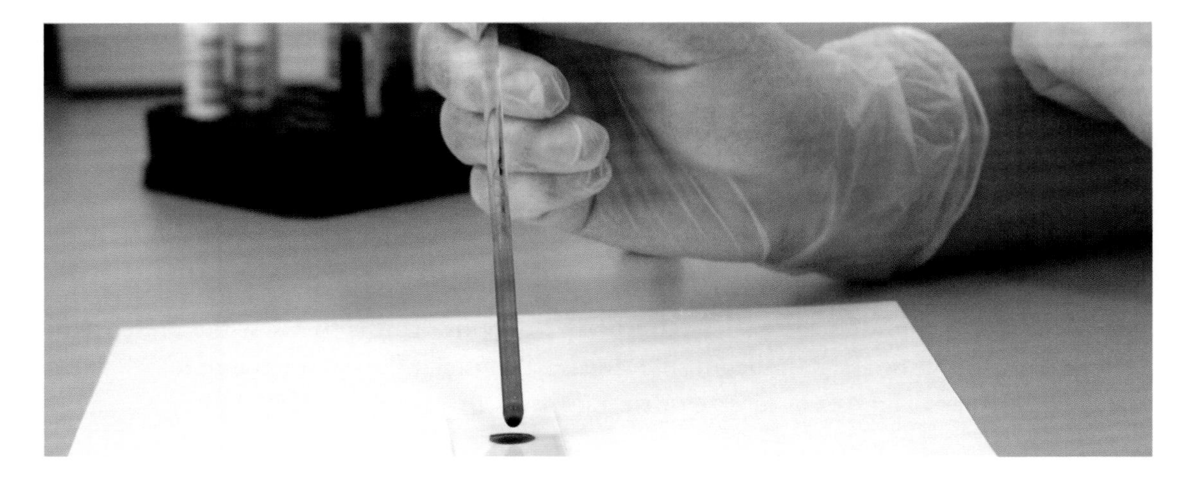

Biochemistry

Biochemistry testing: *The chemical analysis of bodily fluids for diagnostics and/or therapeutic monitoring.*

Biochemistry testing is the chemical analysis of bodily fluids for diagnostics and/or therapeutic monitoring. Fluids mainly include urine and blood plasma or serum. A physician will order a biochemistry test for a patient if a specific part of the body appears to function abnormally. The medical biochemist will quickly inform the physician of any abnormalities.

Biochemistry involves the knowledge of normal and abnormal biochemistry as well as physiology. This knowledge is applied to the understanding of human disease, which will help with the consultation and interpretation of results and how to apply this information to monitor a patient's treatment.

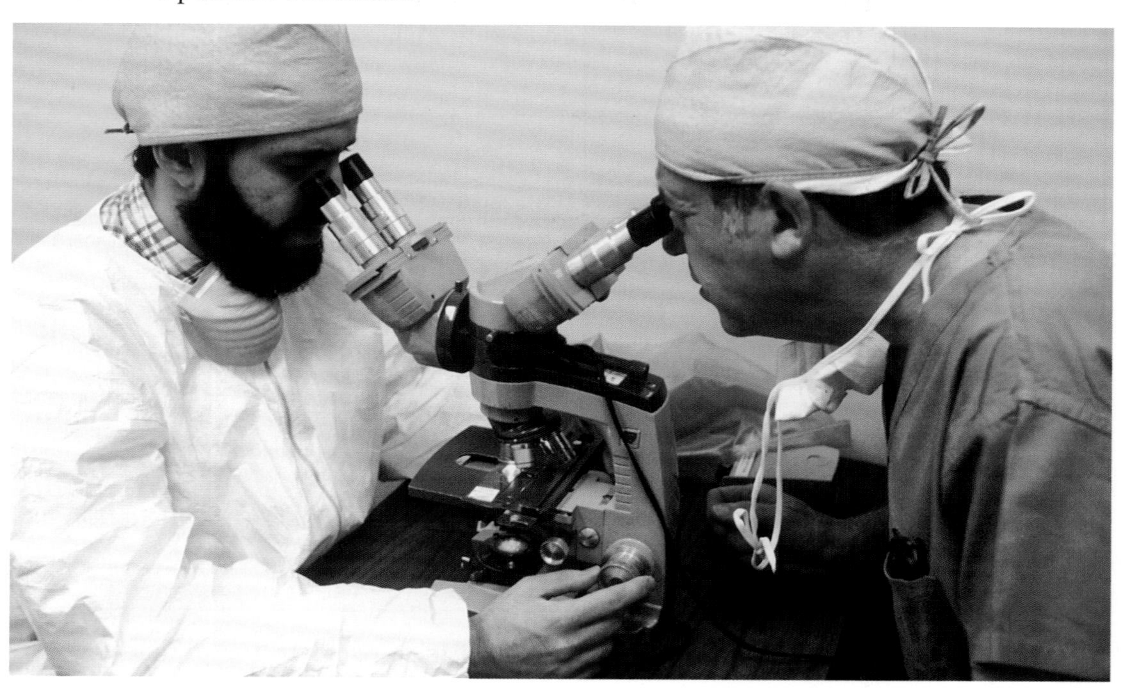

Immunology: *A scientific study of antigen and antibody reactions.*

Immunology

Antigen: *A chemical marker that stimulates an immune reaction and induce the formation of antibodies.*

Antibody: *A protein with the ability to combine with an antigen, resulting in an antigen-antibody reaction.*

Immunology is the scientific study of the reactions of antigens and antibodies. Immunological tests assess the action of the immune system by identifying antibodies present in the blood. **Antigens** are chemical markers—including protein, glycoprotein, complex polysaccharides, and nucleic acid—that stimulate an immune reaction and induce the formation of antibodies in a person. Specific sources of antigens include bacteria, viruses, bacterial toxins, allergens, and blood antigens.

Antibodies are proteins with the ability to combine with antigens. This results in an antigen-antibody reaction

Laboratory testing studies the antigen-antibody reactions. This is to assess the presence of an antigenic source or assist in diagnosing diseases. Physicians often use the results of these tests for the early diagnosis of disease or to track its course.

Microbiology Identification and Sensitivity

Sensitivity test: *A test to determine the bacterial source of infection and the most appropriate treatment.*

A physician may request a **sensitivity test** to locate a source of bacterial infection and determine the most appropriate treatment. The results of this test allow the physician to prescribe the best antibiotic to treat the condition. Not all antibiotics are effective in destroying all pathogens—some pathogens may have developed a resistance, or are unaffected by antibiotics.

The most common form of sensitivity testing is the **disc-diffusion method**, in which commercially prepared discs with known concentrations of various antibiotics are dropped on the surface of a solid culture medium. The laboratory will incubate the culture in a Petri plate inoculated with the pathogen in question to allow the antibiotics time to diffuse. A clear zone without bacterial growth will surround the disc if the pathogen is sensitive to the antibiotic.

Another method to identify which pathogens are present is cytology. Cytology tests evaluate cells in fluids, or cells that have been aspirated, scraped, or washed away from a body surface. These tests may be requested to aid the physician in diagnosing diseases and conditions through examining tissue samples from the body.

Samples collected from the body are examined under a microscope after being spread onto glass slides and stained accordingly. A laboratory technician determines the abnormalities, forms, and functions of cells. This test differs from a biopsy, as it only examines cells and not complete pieces of tissue. An example of cytology a physician might request is a Pap smear, in which they examine cells from the cervix.

Specimens are cultured to diagnose infectious organisms and may be treated with various antibiotics to determine which mediations can stop the infection. The additional sensitivity testing is requested on behalf of the physician to decide the correct antibiotics to prescribe to the patient. Without the clear zone present, it is evident that a given antibiotic will not effectively destroy the pathogen.

my notes

Preparing and Handling Blood Specimens

Many physicians send patients directly to a lab to have blood work done. A minimum of four (4) mL of blood should be collected and placed in appropriate blood collection tubes. Depending on the type of blood test to be done, some patients should not eat or drink 12 to 14 hours prior to collection. Samples that are rejected for testing include non-fasted samples, improper labeling of the tube, and hemolysis.

If the physician collects his or her own specimens:

- Physicians will place all specimens in appropriate vials and label them.
- A requisition form should be printed (or obtained from physician) and checked to make sure all information is filled in.
- Place vials in refrigerator (if appropriate) until ready to prepare shipment.
- Before the lab courier arrives, double check requisition forms against vials and place the forms in the cooler bag.

Blood specimens for biochemistry serum testing have to be centrifuged before being sent, and should not be placed in the fridge until the centrifugal process is complete. Blood that must be centrifuged should be placed in SST tubes (gold or red grey tops) and spun within two hours of blood collection, after letting the SST tube stand for 30 minutes. This separates the serum from cells with a gel barrier. Many centrifuges require that they be balanced, so wait until you have several tubes to centrifuge or balance the centrifuge with a tube of water.

www.who/int/csr/emc97_3.pdf

When handling blood samples, carriers must follow the guidelines set by the **Transportation of Dangerous Goods Act with Respect to Diagnostic Specimens** document. The lab courier is responsible for ensuring proper transport and provides any necessary containers that meet the requirements for safe transfer of biohazardous samples.

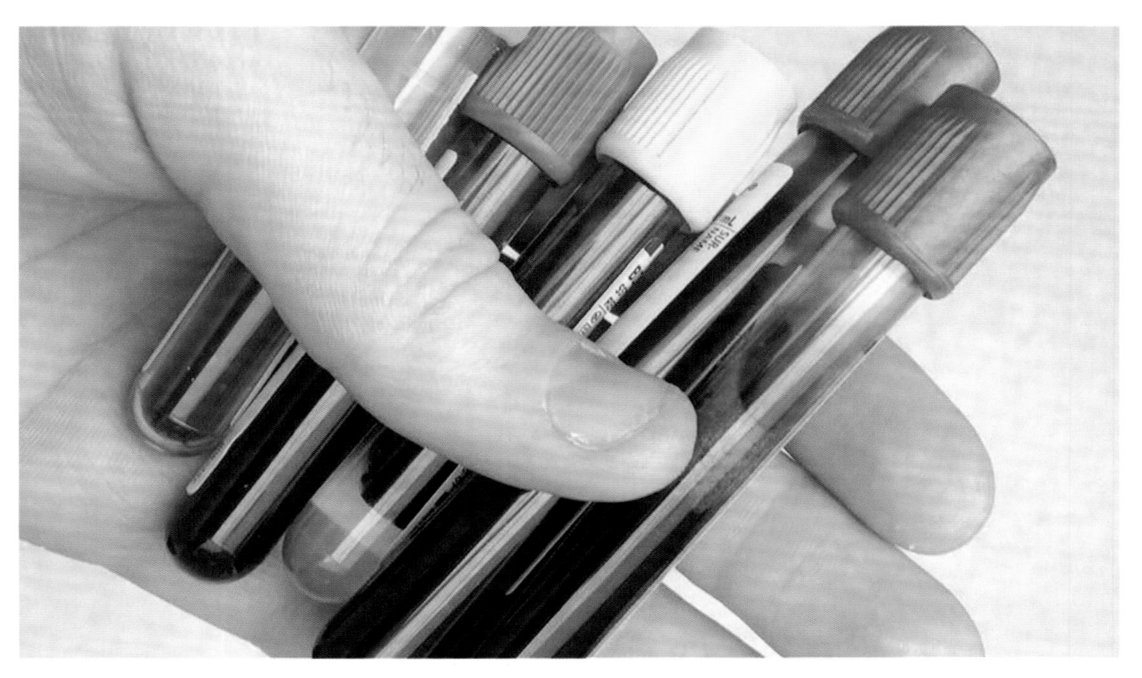

Photo by Tom Mallinson

https://commons.wikimedia.org

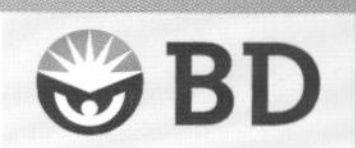

Helping all people live healthy lives

BD Vacutainer® Venous Blood Collection

Tube Guide

For the full array of BD Vacutainer® Blood Collection Tubes, visit www.bd.com/vacutainer.
Many are available in a variety of sizes and draw volumes (for pediatric applications). Refer to our website for full descriptions.

BD Vacutainer® Tubes with BD Hemogard™ Closure	BD Vacutainer® Tubes with Conventional Stopper	Additive	Inversions at Blood Collection*	Laboratory Use	Your Lab's Draw Volume/Remarks
Gold	Red/ Gray	• Clot activator and gel for serum separation	5	For serum determinations in chemistry. May be used for routine blood donor screening and diagnostic testing of serum for infectious disease.** Tube inversions ensure mixing of clot activator with blood. Blood clotting time: 30 minutes.	
Light Green	Green/ Gray	• Lithium heparin and gel for plasma separation	8	For plasma determinations in chemistry. Tube inversions ensure mixing of anticoagulant (heparin) with blood to prevent clotting.	
Red	Red	• Silicone coated (glass) • Clot activator, Silicone coated (plastic)	0 5	For serum determinations in chemistry. May be used for routine blood donor screening and diagnostic testing of serum for infectious disease.** Tube inversions ensure mixing of clot activator with blood. Blood clotting time: 60 minutes.	
Orange		• Thrombin-based clot activator with gel for serum separation	5 to 6	For stat serum determinations in chemistry. Tube inversions ensure mixing of clot activator with blood. Blood clotting time: 5 minutes.	
Orange		• Thrombin-based clot activator	8	For stat serum determinations in chemistry. Tube inversions ensure mixing of clot activator with blood. Blood clotting time: 5 minutes.	
Royal Blue		• Clot activator (plastic serum) • K_2EDTA (plastic)	8 8	For trace-element, toxicology, and nutritional-chemistry determinations. Special stopper formulation provides low levels of trace elements (see package insert). Tube inversions ensure mixing of either clot activator or anticoagulant (EDTA) with blood.	
Green	Green	• Sodium heparin • Lithium heparin	8 8	For plasma determinations in chemistry. Tube inversions ensure mixing of anticoagulant (heparin) with blood to prevent clotting.	
Gray	Gray	• Potassium oxalate/ sodium fluoride • Sodium fluoride/Na_2 EDTA • Sodium fluoride (serum tube)	8 8 8	For glucose determinations. Oxalate and EDTA anticoagulants will give plasma samples. Sodium fluoride is the antiglycolytic agent. Tube inversions ensure proper mixing of additive with blood.	
Tan		• K_2EDTA (plastic)	8	For lead determinations. This tube is certified to contain less than .01 µg/mL(ppm) lead. Tube inversions prevent clotting.	
	Yellow	• Sodium polyanethol sulfonate (SPS) • Acid citrate dextrose additives (ACD): **Solution A -** 22.0 g/L trisodium citrate, 8.0 g/L citric acid, 24.5 g/L dextrose **Solution B -** 13.2 g/L trisodium citrate, 4.8 g/L citric acid, 14.7 g/L dextrose	8 8 8	SPS for blood culture specimen collections in microbiology. ACD for use in blood bank studies, HLA phenotyping, and DNA and paternity testing. Tube inversions ensure mixing of anticoagulant with blood to prevent clotting.	
Lavender	Lavender	• Liquid K_3EDTA (glass) • Spray-coated K_2EDTA (plastic)	8 8	K_2EDTA and K_3EDTA for whole blood hematology determinations. K_2EDTA may be used for routine immunohematology testing, and blood donor screening.*** Tube inversions ensure mixing of anticoagulant (EDTA) with blood to prevent clotting.	
White		• K_2EDTA and gel for plasma separation	8	For use in molecular diagnostic test methods (such as, but not limited to, polymerase chain reaction [PCR] and/or branched DNA [bDNA] amplification techniques.) Tube inversions ensure mixing of anticoagulant (EDTA) with blood to prevent clotting.	
Pink	Pink	• Spray-coated K_2EDTA (plastic)	8	For whole blood hematology determinations. May be used for routine immunohematology testing and blood donor screening.*** Designed with special cross-match label for patient information required by the AABB. Tube inversions prevent clotting.	
Light Blue Clear	Light Blue	• Buffered sodium citrate 0.105 M (≈3.2%) glass 0.109 M (3.2%) plastic • Citrate, theophylline, adenosine, dipyridamole (CTAD)	3-4 3-4	For coagulation determinations. CTAD for selected platelet function assays and routine coagulation determination. Tube inversions ensure mixing of anticoagulant (citrate) to prevent clotting.	
Clear	New Red/ Light Gray	• None (plastic)	0	For use as a discard tube or secondary specimen tube.	

Urine Collection Methods

Patient urine samples are often required for **urinalysis** testing. Commonly performed in medical offices, this type of testing consists of physical, chemical, and microscopic examination of a urine specimen. Results from a urinalysis assist the physician in the diagnosis and treatment of pathologic conditions. It can be performed as a screening measure during a physical exam, the diagnosis of a pathologic condition, or evaluation of the effectiveness of therapy after the start of treatment.

Fresh or preserved samples are considered suitable for testing, but anything left standing at room temperature for more than an hour renders any tests void. Chemical additives can be used to preserve a urine specimen, but these are generally used for specimens that require longer storage and have to be shipped long distances.

The medical assistant must obtain an adequate volume of urine to perform the necessary type of urinalysis. This volume is typically 30 to 50 mL. Properly label each specimen with the patient's name, date of birth, and type of specimen, plus the collection date and time. Document any medication the patient is taking, particularly if the specimen requires further testing in a lab. Some medication may interfere with the accuracy of test results. If possible, women should avoid providing a urine sample during menstruation and for several days afterwards. This will help avoid a false positive measure of blood in the urine.

As a health care provider, it is important to know the different methods of collection in order to address any questions or concerns that patients may have related to their medical problems.

Here are four different methods of collecting urine in a sterile and clear plastic container:

Method One: Timed Urine Collections (24-hour)

The patient must collect all urine for a 24-hour period in a large bottle to see cumulative elements in the urine. In order to collect a timed urine sample, patients should perform the first **void** of the morning into the toilet, and then collect for 24 hours thereafter, including the first void the next day.

***Void:** emptying the bladder*

Remind the patient to note the exact time of the first emptying of the bladder. Every drop of urine during the day and night is to be collected in an empty collection bottle. This can be stored at room temperature or in the refrigerator.

It doesn't matter how much urine the patient passes each time, as they must still collect every drop. If the patient has a bowel movement, they should collect any urine passed with the bowel movement. The patient should avoid including any feces with the urine collection. If fecal matter does mix with the urine, do not try to remove it from the collection bottle.

Send samples to the lab as soon as possible and educate the patient on how to store their urine properly.

Activity

TIMED URINE COLLECTIONS (24-HOUR)

In groups of two, use the below flowchart (or create your own) to explain to your partner ("patient") how they will complete a timed urine collection over 24 hours.

1	**Void**	Perform the first void of the morning into the toilet and record the time on the container's label.
2	**Collect**	Start collecting for the 24 hours thereafter, including the first void the next day in a given large container (approximately one gallon), labelled with the patient's name and date.
3	**Record**	All urine must be collected in the container until the next morning. The patient should be instructed to avoid fecal contamination. Record the exact time when the test ended.
4	**Storage**	Store the urine sample either at room temperature or in the refrigerator, depending on the preservative requirements provided by the laboratory specimen collection manual.
5	**Return**	After the collection process, return the sample to the medical office as soon as possible.

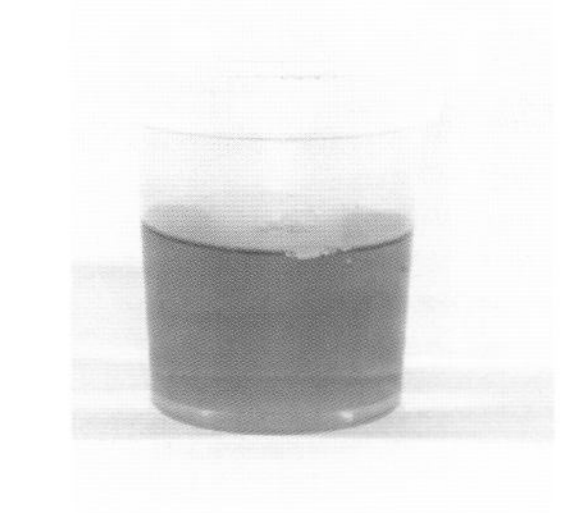

my notes

Activity

Method Two: Random Urine Collection

A random urine collection can be obtained anytime and usually takes place at the doctor's office, primarily for screening purposes. This type of specimen is not used for a culture and sensitivity test. Provide the patient with a sterile and clear urine collection container for the preliminary screening. Instruct the patient to void into the container provided and obtain a midstream specimen in the container. Instruct the patient to return the urine sample immediately so that it can be tested at the medical office.

RANDOM URINE COLLECTION

Read the scenario and discuss what needs to change in order to achieve a valid random urine sample.

Patty's physician ordered a random urine collection. She receives the urine collection kit from the medical office assistant. Entering into the washroom, she untwists lid of the sterile container and places the lid on the counter. Holding the cup tightly by the rim, Patty prepares for collection.

Voiding the first part of the urine into the toilet, Patty quickly places the sterile container in the path of the stream and collects a sample midstream. Filling the container nearly up to the rim, she stops urinating and twists the cap back on tightly. After she finishes urinating in the toilet, she washes her hands, returns an email on her phone, then returns the sample back to the medical assistant.

my notes

Method Three: Early First-Voided Morning Specimens

The first void in the morning contains the greatest concentration of dissolved substances. Any abnormal substance is easily detected because the volume and composition is more uniform. The pH is also lower, so formed elements are preserved for easy detection.

Inform the patient they need to collect the first urine sample after they wake up in the morning. Instruct them to preserve the sample in their refrigerator until they bring it into the medical office. Always provide the patient with a specimen container for the collection process. A container from the patient's home is not sterile and, as a result, has the potential to change the results of the urinalysis, rendering it inaccurate. A physician often uses early first-void morning specimens to monitor pregnancy. Physicians will request these specimens during the patient's visit to the medical office.

EARLY FIRST-VOIDED MORNING SPECIMENS

Number the following steps to obtain an accurate early first-voided morning specimen. (1-first step, 9-last step)

	Return the sample to the medical office within one hour of collection OR place the specimen in the refrigerator until it can be returned.
	Patient performs proper hand washing technique.
	Lid is firmly re-secured, and sample cup is carefully set aside.
	Place the sterile empty container in the path of the stream.
	Finish urinating into the toilet.
	Urinate into the toilet for a few seconds, then stop.
	Patient prepares and remove lid of urine container, taking care not to touch the inside of the container to preserve sterility.
	Patient wakes up and readies themselves for collection.
	Restart the urine stream into the container and stop when the container is approximately half-full.

Method Four: Clean Catch Midstream Urine (CCMSU)

Urine that needs to be cultured and screened for the presence of bacteria requires a urine sample caught midstream. This ensures the sample is sterile or near-sterile. The urinary bladder and most of the urethra are normally free of microorganisms, whereas the distal urethra and urinary meatus often harbour microorganisms. A physician may request a CCMSU to detect a urinary tract infection (UTI) or for treatment evaluation.

For CCMSU, strict sterility practices need to be adhered to, similar to the other collection methods. This includes proper hand washing, as well as careful handling of the collection container. The patient must cleanse the urinary opening, and they must void a small amount of urine to flush out microorganisms present in the distal urethra. Careful attention must be taken to ensure that no contaminants make it into the sample.

Many offices will provide the patient with a collection kit to use for CCMSU specimens. These kits include a sterile container, wipes for cleansing, and instructions on how to collect a urine sample properly. These instructions help to clarify the process for a patient who is unsure about what they need to do. Medical office assistants should be able to answer any questions that the patient has regarding the CCMSU method.

Bladder catheterization: *the passing of a sterile tube through the urethra and into the bladder to obtain a sample of urine.*

A properly collected sample can prevent other, more invasive collections techniques such as **bladder catheterization**, which is the passing of a sterile tube through the urethra and into the bladder to obtain a sample of urine.

Suprapubic aspiration: *the passing of a sterile needle through the abdominal wall into the bladder to remove urine.*

Another process that can collect a sample for this particular screening is **suprapubic aspiration**, which involves passing a sterile needle through the abdominal wall into the bladder to remove urine. All of these processes are performed using sterile techniques, but CCMSU is easiest and the least invasive.

The type of test performed often dictates the method used to collect the urine sample. As part of the medical office's inventory, the office assistant should have a supply of disposable plastic urine specimen containers to provide to patients when a urine sample is requested. These containers come in different sizes and include a lid to prevent spillage and reduce bacterial and transferable contamination.

Handling Urine Specimens

With any type of laboratory specimen, there are certain criteria that need to be met for proper collection and transportation of urine specimens. In order to ensure accurate test results, all urine collection and transport containers must be clean and free of particles or interfering substances. Do not reuse specimen containers. Always ensure each container is labelled properly. Collect the sample from patients following standard precautions.

If reagent strip testing is performed in the office:

- Mix the urine before testing
- Make sure the sample does not spill
- Wear proper safety gear (gloves, glasses, mask, etc.)
- Hold the test strip horizontally after removing it from the container and do not touch the container with the contaminated stick

If the specimen is being sent to the lab:

- Either label the container prior to giving to a patient, or paste an adhesive label on the container after the patient submits their sample
- Refrigerate all samples that will not be tested within 30 minutes of collection to preserve pH and prevent bacterial growth
    - Refrigerated samples should warm up to room temperature before tests are performed and should spend no longer than one hour at room temperature before being returned to the refrigerator.
- Make sure all specimens required by the tests selected on the requisition are sent

Proper handling and storage of urine samples is important when performing urinalysis for clinical diagnosis. The labelling, collection method, preservation, can alter test results if guidelines are not followed. Factors such as temperature, and even exposure to light, can affect the sample.

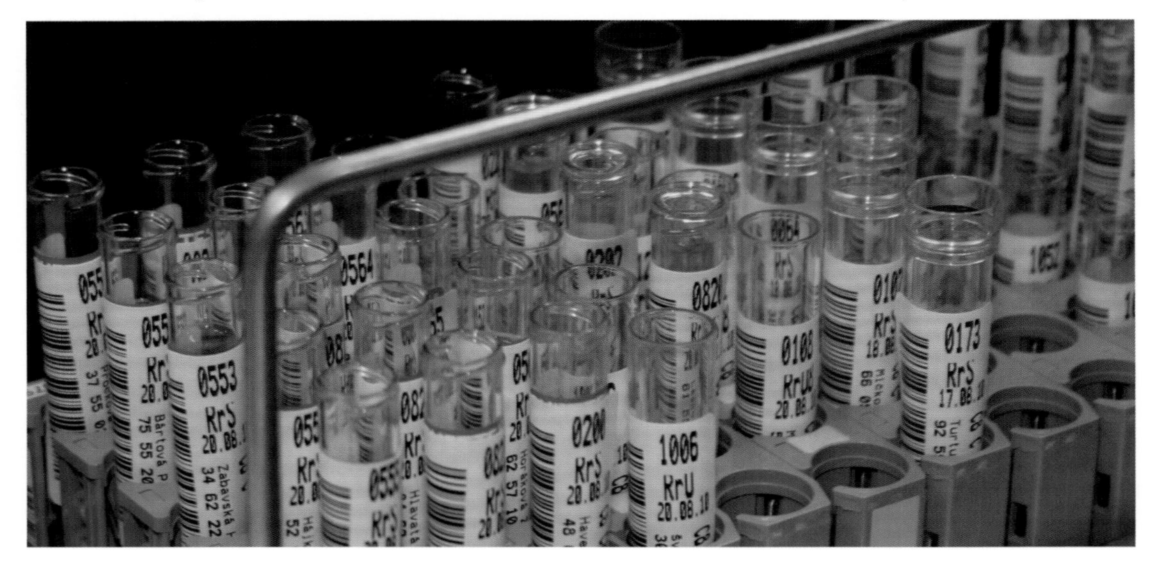

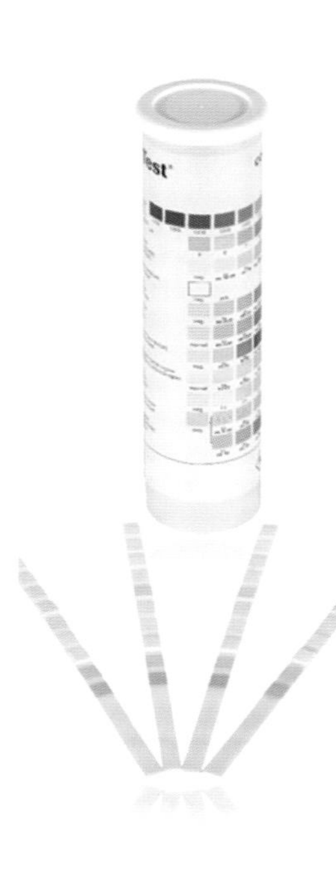

Reagent Strips

Commonly used as a part of the diagnostic urine testing kit, reagent strips are disposable plastic strips with multiple reagent areas. Each reagent square tests for specific chemical constituents that may indicate pathological conditions. It is important to read the manufacturer's instructions before performing a urinalysis.

The results of the reagent strips provide the physician with information to assist in diagnosing:

- Conditions affecting kidney or liver function (e.g. kidney stones or hepatitis)
- Urinary tract infections
- Conditions affecting carbohydrate metabolism (e.g. diabetes mellitus)
- Urine acid-base imbalance and urine concentration

Results from reagent strips are considered a qualitative test. This means if there is a positive result, further testing needs to be done for confirmation.

The plastic strip typically contains 10 reagent areas for testing pH, protein, glucose, ketone, bilirubin, blood, urobilinogen, nitrite, specific gravity, and leukocytes. Fill in the form accurately so the results can be entered into the patient file.

It is fairly easy to perform reagent strip testing, but there are certain guidelines that need to be followed to obtain accurate results.

Quality of Specimen

The best results are obtained with freshly voided and thoroughly mixed urine specimens. The urine specimen needs to be tested within one hour of collection, otherwise it must be refrigerated immediately. Allow the specimen to return to room temperature prior to testing with a reagent stick.

Type of Collection

Most reagent strips are designed for random specimen collection. For specific tests, however, clean catch midstream and first-void morning specimens are suggested. Examples of specific tests include testing for nitrite, for which first-voided morning midstream collection is best suited. The testing recommendation for the presence of leukocytes is clean catch midstream collection.

Specimen Container

Ideally, the container should be sterile. Avoid leaving any traces of cleansing agents such as detergent, as they contain oxidants that can cause a reaction with the sample. If such a reaction occurs, the test results are inaccurate.

Time Intervals

Read results at the exact time intervals the colour chart specifies.

Interpretation of Results

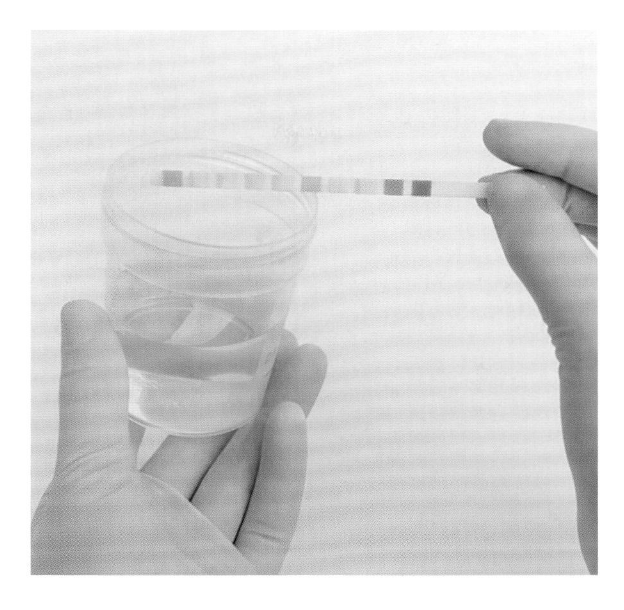

Compare the reagent strip with the provided colour chart in a well-lit area. This helps obtain a good visual match of the colour reactions with the test kit's colour chart.

Storage of Reagent Strips

Ensure reagent strips are stored in a cool, dry area, away from direct sunlight, as they are sensitive to light, heat, and moisture. Tightly seal the cap after each use. This helps maintain the reactivity of the reagent strips. Store the bottle of strips between 15°C and 30° C, and keep the desiccant in the bottle. Doing so keeps the internal moisture level in the bottle low as the desiccant draws in surrounding moisture. Never store reagent strips in a refrigerator or freezer. This causes the strips to deteriorate, which renders any test results inaccurate.

The accuracy of these reagent strips is important, as they play a crucial part in the physician reaching a proper diagnosis. Quality control testing ensures the tests results are accurate and reliable. Testing includes determining if the strips are reacting properly and if the individual conducting the reagent strip test is doing so properly, including the interpretation of the results.

In order to run a quality control test, the manufacturer should have a control allowing you to determine if the reagent sticks are providing accurate results. A quality control test should be done every time a new bottle of reagent strips is opened and when the accuracy of the reagent strips is questioned.

my notes

How to

PREPARING A URINE SAMPLE FOR MICROSCOPIC EXAMINATION

You will need the following:

- **Disposable gloves**
- **Urine specimen**
- **Urine centrifuge**
- **Urine centrifuge tube**
- **Pipette**
- **Glass slide**
- **Coverslip**
- **Stain**
- **Test tube rack**
- **Mechanical stage microscope**

Follow the steps to prepare a urine specimen for microscopic analysis by the physician.

1. Wash your hands and collect the equipment.

2. Put on gloves and use the pipette to mix the urine specimen. Transfer a standardized volume into a centrifuge tube according to laboratory procedures. This will often be to approximately the 12 mL graduation mark.

3. Cap the tube and place it into the urine centrifuge. Spin the centrifuge for five minutes at approximately 1500 revolutions per minute (RPM) to allow heavier components to settle at the bottom of the tube.

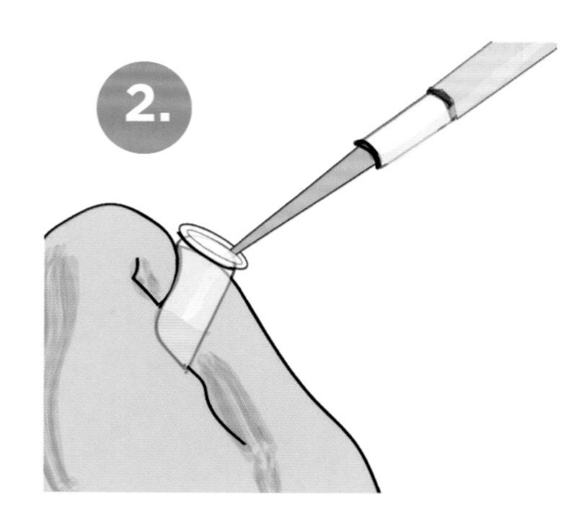

4. Remove the tube from the centrifuge. Avoid dislodging or otherwise disturbing the sediment. Pour out the supernatant fluid in the sample by inverting the tube, which will leave approximately 1 mL of sediment in the bottom.

5. Add a drop of stain into the sediment and use the pipette to mix the sediment with the stain vigourously. Place the urine tube back on the test tube rack after confirming the sediment and stain are well mixed.

6. Transfer a sample of the stained sediment on the glass slide.

7. Place a coverslip over the drop of sample on the glass slide carefully. Avoid bubbles and ensure the specimen does not overflow.

8. Place the microscopic slide on the stage of the microscope.

9. Focus the specimen under the microscope.

10. Once the physician is done examining the urine slide, discard the slide into the sharps container and the pipette into a regular waste container.

11. Rinse the remaining urine sample down the sink or toilet.

12. Dispose of all other waste, including the gloves, into a regular waste container.

13. Wash and sanitize hands.

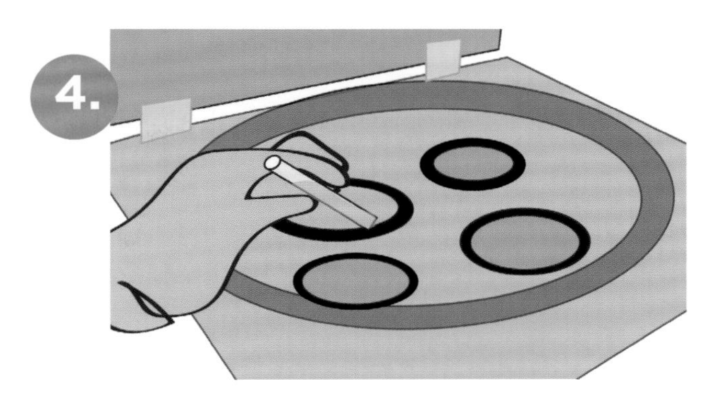

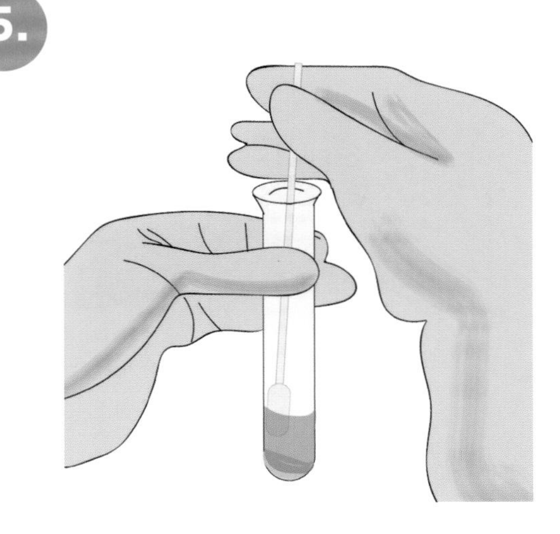

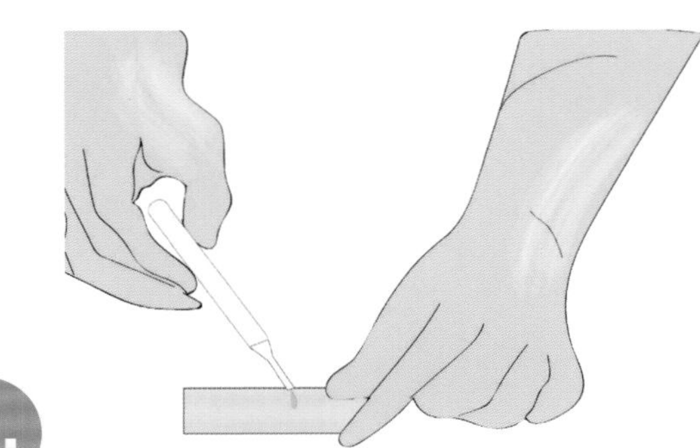

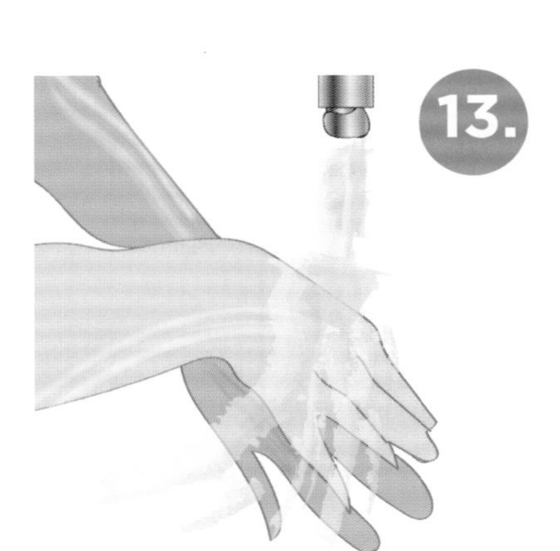

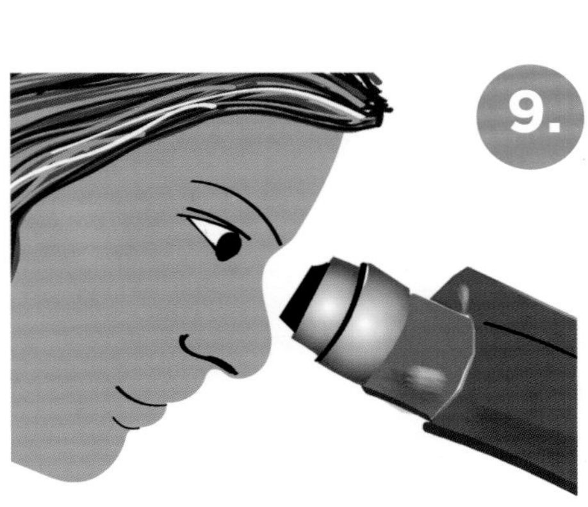

Transportation of Specimens

All specimens, whether blood or other bodily samples, must be transported in accordance with the **Transportation of Dangerous Goods Act** (TDG). Anyone handling, transporting, or offering the transport of dangerous goods must use containers that are in accordance with safety standards. Along with the TDG regulations, the standards indicate what containers are permitted for particular dangerous goods, the requirements for the container use, and maintenance.

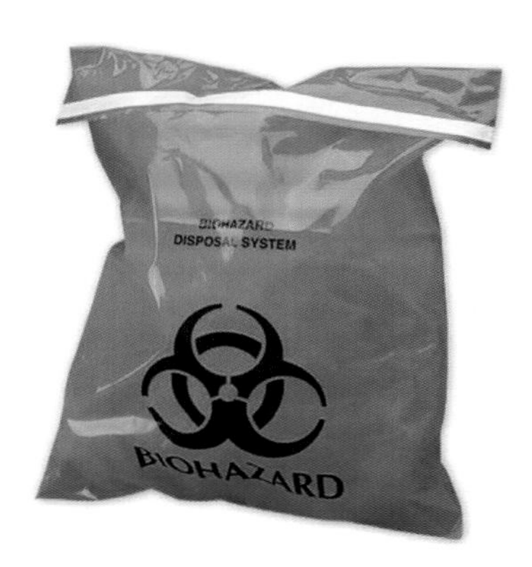

Biohazard transport bags should be used for specimens and are to be sealed tightly to avoid any spillage. There should be a separate pouch where the requisition can be placed on the outside of the bag. Proper handling and the disposal of biohazardous waste will limit exposure to potentially infectious microorganisms. Check for updates on rules and regulations regarding the proper disposal of biohazardous waste material in your area.

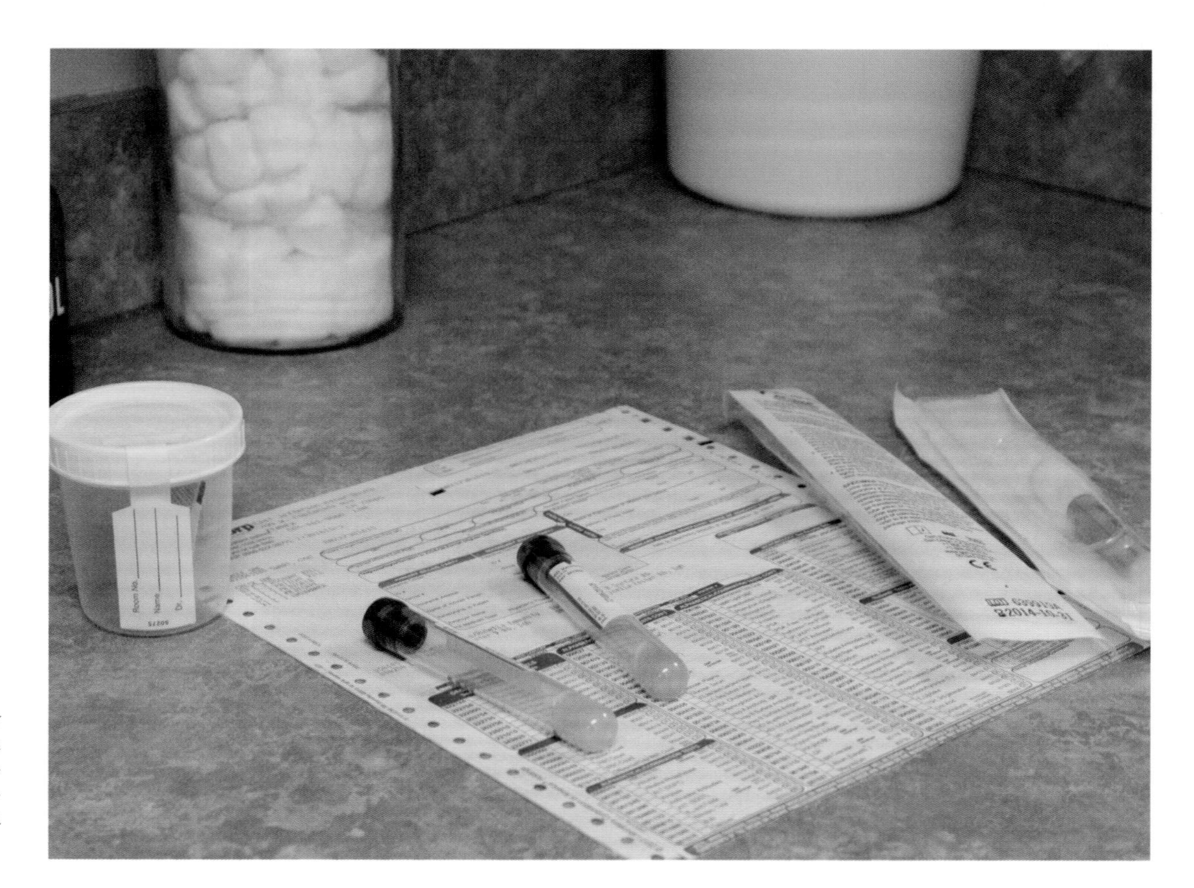

Photo by Community Emergency Response Team (CERT) (http://www.citizencorps.gov/cert/IS317/medops/) [Public domain], via Wikimedia Commons

Activity

TESTS AND SPECIMEN COLLECTION

Identify and match the purpose of the test with the specimen that is required for a physician to reach a diagnosis. Use an online search to help, if needed.

	Specimen		Purpose of Test
1	Urine	a	Spinal fluid pressure
2	Stool	b	Cystic fibrosis
3	Blood	c	Adrenal/hormone levels
4	Cerebrospinal fluid	d	Urinary tract infection
5	Synovial fluid (fluid within a joint)	e	Leukemia and/or lymphoma
6	Sweat	f	Level of acidity in the stomach
7	Saliva	g	Colon cancer or polyps
8	Gastric juices	h	Gout and other types of arthritis

my notes

Quiz

CHAPTER 6 QUIZ

1. True or false? Hematology is the study of blood, including the processing and evaluation of blood.

2. What is Prothrombin time (PT)?

____

____

____

3. What does INR stand for?

    a. International National Range

    b. International Normalized Ratio

    c. Internship Normalized Range

    d. Internship National Ratio

4. What information does a platelet count provide to the physician?

____

____

____

____

____

5. Define immunology.

____

____

____

____

____

____

6. When might a physician request a sensitivity test?

____

____

____

____

____

7. How much blood needs to be collected and placed in collection tubes to run a test?

a. 2 mL

b. 4 mL

c. 6 mL

d. 8 mL

8. How much urine should be collected to perform a urinalysis?

a. 10 to 15 mL

b. 15 to 25 mL

c. 30 to 50 mL

d. 70 to 100 mL

9. What are the other two methods to collect a sterile urine sample aside from clean catch midstream urine (CCMSU)?

____

10. If a urine specimen is being sent to the lab, what should you not do?

a. Refrigerate samples not tested within 30 minutes of collection

b. Label the container prior to giving to a patient

c. Refrigerate after a minimum of one hour at room temperature

d. Allow refrigerated samples to come up to room temperature before testing

11. List five out of the 10 reagent areas on a reagent strip for urinalysis.

____

____

____

____

____

12. True or false? All specimens must be transported in accordance with the Transport of Dangerously Good Act.

13. True or false? Biohazard bags should be sealed, labeled accordingly, and used only for specimens to limit exposure to possible infectious microorganisms and to avoid any spillage.

14. If urinalysis is performed in the office, which of the following should you not do?

a. Mix urine before testing

b. Hold test strip horizontally after removal from container

c. Label the container prior to giving to a patient

d. Hold the stick horizontally to read results after carefully dipping it into the container

my notes

Chapter 7

Diagnostic Imaging

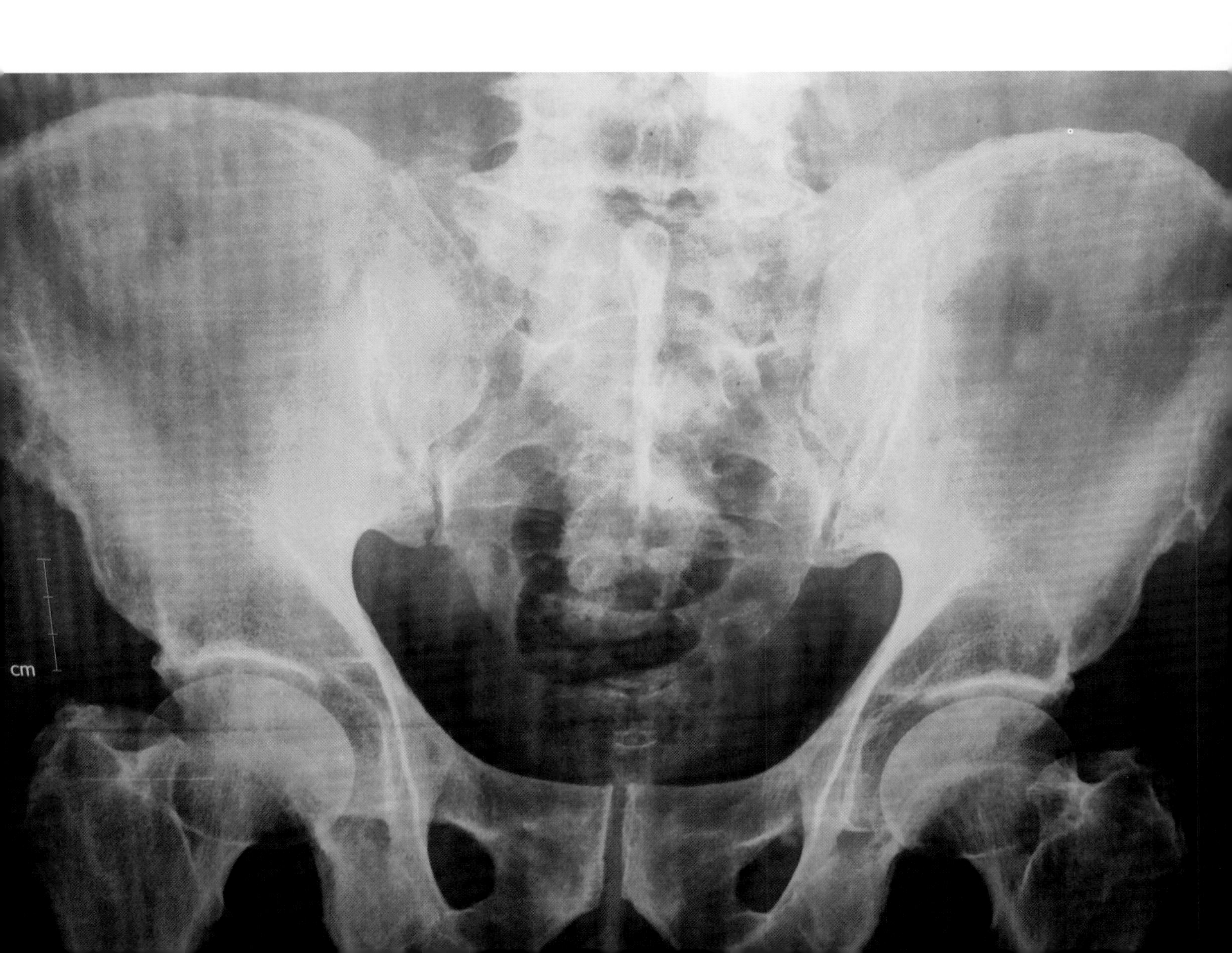

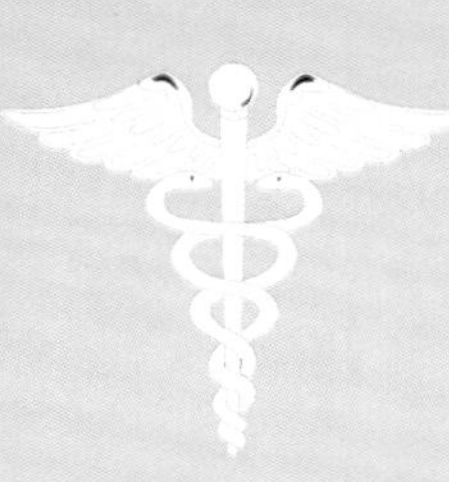

CHAPTER SEVEN LEARNING OBJECTIVES

After completing this chapter, you should be able to:

- ❑ Define the term diagnostic imaging
- ❑ Understand the importance of radiography
- ❑ Understand and explain the difference between upper gastrointestinal series and lower gastrointestinal series
- ❑ Understand other examples of fluoroscopy
- ❑ Understand the importance and methods of cardiovascular radiography
- ❑ Understand the importance and methods of CT or CAT scanning
- ❑ Explain the importance and methods of Magnetic Resonance Imaging (MRI)
- ❑ Understand the importance and methods of ultrasonography
- ❑ Understand the importance and methods of mammography
- ❑ Comprehend the importance and methods of bone densitometry (DEXA) along with its relation to osteoporosis
- ❑ Understand and distinguish the importance between colonoscopy and gastroscopy (endoscopy)
- ❑ Identify and understand the reason for patient positioning
- ❑ Understand how to receive and record test results

What is Diagnostic Imaging?

Diagnostic imaging is any visual display of structural or functional patterns of organs or tissues for diagnostic evaluation. It includes measuring physiologic and metabolic responses to physical and chemical stimuli.

***Diagnostic imaging:** any visual display of structural or functional patterns of organs or tissues for diagnostic evaluation.*

While medical office assistants are only rarely part of the actual imaging process, it is important that the MOA has a general idea of the processes so they can help instruct patients and answer questions. Many of these tests are done in hospitals or specialized facilities and have dedicated staff who assist the patients and prepare the images.

Radiography

Radiology is a branch of medicine that uses imaging to diagnose internal injuries or diseases. A **radiograph** is an x-ray image that images solid internal structures with the use of radiation. A **radiologist** is a physician who contributes to the diagnosis and treatment of disease using radiation and other imaging techniques.

***Radiology:** the use of radiation to diagnose and treat diseases.*

A variety of machines and techniques can create images of the structures inside the body. The type of imaging requested by a physician depends on the ailments and part of the body examined. Many imaging tests are painless and easy. Some may be uncomfortable and involve exposure to a small amount of radiation.

***Radiograph:** the making of an x-ray image that helps visualize internal structures with the use of radiation and other imaging techniques.*

***Radiologist:** a physician who contributes to the diagnosis and treatment of disease using radiation and other imaging techniques.*

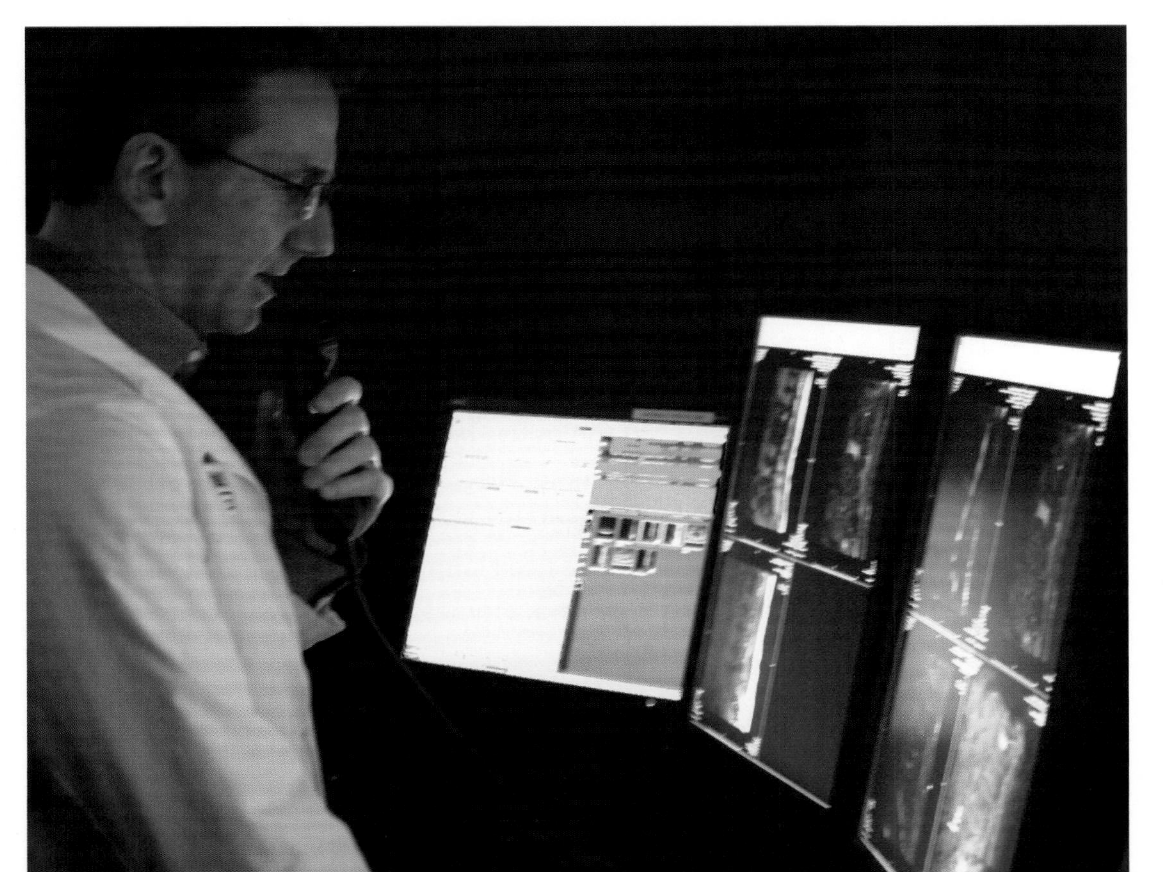

By w:User:Zackstarr - w:File:Radiologist in San Diego CA 2010.jpg, https://commons.wikimedia.org/w/index.php?curid=11834258

Imaging technologies include, but are not limited to, the following:

- Fluoroscopy
- Cardiovascular radiography
- CT Scans
- Magnetic Resonance Imaging
- Ultrasound
- Mammography
- DEXA
- Colonoscopy
- Gastroscopy

Wilhelm Konrad Röentgen, a German physicist, discovered x-rays in 1895, while working on the cathode ray tube. Since then, these radiation rays have been renamed roentgen rays, but are still commonly known as "x-rays." X-rays are helpful in identifying abnormal conditions of skeletal structures and some soft tissues. Radiotherapy is also used in the treatment of cancer, in which high doses of radiation are delivered to cancerous tumours in the body.

Radiotherapy

A beam of radiation passes through the skin to target a specific location of where the tumour is located. Radiation damages the DNA of the cancer cells, causing tumour cells to die and the tumour to shrink. The process of radiotherapy is painless and the side effects are often limited to the areas of the body that receive the treatment. For example, clinical trials[1,2] have shown the use of radiotherapy on patients with limited-stage small cell lung cancer has presented favourable outcomes of remission.

1) Wang, P., Liu, W., and Wang, P. (2015) Does the response to induction chemotherapy impact the timing of thoracic radiotherapy for limited-stage small-cell lung cancer? Thoracic Cancer (5): 605-612. Accessed on the 8th of October, 2015.

2) Haas, M.L. (2008) Advances in radiation therapy for lung cancer. Semin Oncol Nurs. (1):34-40. Accessed on the 8th of October, 2015.

Photo by By Michael Anderson (Photographer) [Public domain], via Wikimedia Commons

When traditional x-ray film is exposed to x-rays, it darkens. X-rays pass through materials based on their density. Dense objects such as metal and bone will appear clearer or brighter than less dense materials such as liquids or soft tissues, which will appear darker as they are able to let more x-rays pass through.

Many facilities now use digital radiography that does not require film, but uses the same principle. The x-rays strike a plate that relays a digital image instantly to the radiographer's computer.

Various parts of the human body have different capabilities of obstructing x-rays. Bone is the densest, so it will appear white on the film (radiopaque). Air, gas, and soft tissues cause less disruption of the x-rays' path and these will display as varying shades of black and grey (radiolucent).

X-ray Example

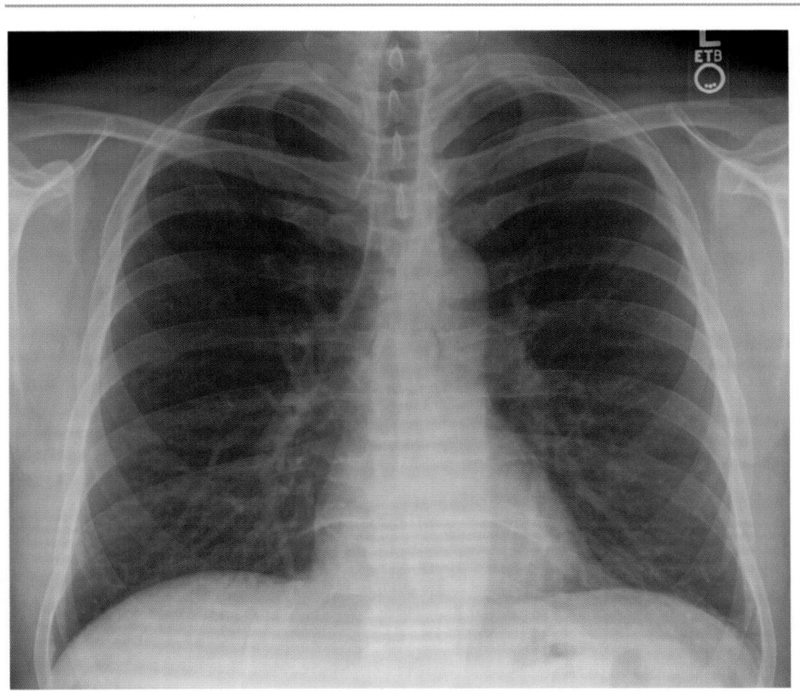

X-rays can be used to diagnose various conditions, such as pneumonia, blockages, fractures, enlargements, etc.

Contrast media are used in x-ray studies so that hollow organs can become visible on x-ray images. Chemicals and substances, such as barium sulphate or iodine compounds, can make soft organs appear radiopaque and visible for diagnosis. Patients ingest these substances before the imaging.

When scheduling a radiograph appointment, medical office assistants should inform the patient of any required preparation needed prior to imaging and also provide a reminder the day before the procedure takes place.

X-Ray Fluoroscopy

***Fluoroscopy**: with the use of x-rays, this special technique allows the radiologist to see x-ray images in real time.*

***Fluoroscope:** an instrument used to view internal organs and structures of the body directly on a display screen.*

X-rays are also used in **fluoroscopy**, which is a procedure that allows a radiologist to see x-ray images in real time. This technique uses a **fluoroscope**, which is a medical instrument capable of displaying a view of internal organs and body structures on a screen.

When conducting this test, a physician will place the patient between a radiographic tube and fluorescent screen. The screen is comprised of zinc cadmium sulfide crystals.

During this test, the x-rays from the radiographic tube pass through the patient's body and hit the fluorescent screen, specifically the crystals, on the other side. This process emits a light onto the screen so the radiologist is able to view and examine the patient's body organs and structures.

It can also be used to aid in catheterization or for "spot" images. Radiograph images may be taken to permit the study of the structure in detail. The radiograph serves as a permanent record and the findings are entered into the patient file.

X-ray radiation, like other forms of radiation, has the potential to damage living cells. X-rays are specifically harmful because of their ability to pass through and expose tissues to damaging radiation. Typically, the only tissues that are accustomed to dealing with the effects of radiation, are those that are exposed to the outside environment, like skin.

A small amount of x-ray radiation exposure is fine for the average patient, but continued exposure can increase the risk of diseases such as cancer. Risks and benefits need to be weighed and patient exposure to radiation should be minimal. With proper shielding in place, radiography is an effective way to help physicians make a proper diagnosis.

Upper Gastrointestinal (GI) Series Test

A physician will often order an upper gastrointestinal series test if the patient complains of difficulty swallowing, severe indigestion, vomit, abdominal pain, or if they find blood in their stool. This is an x-ray diagnostic imaging test also known as a barium swallow.

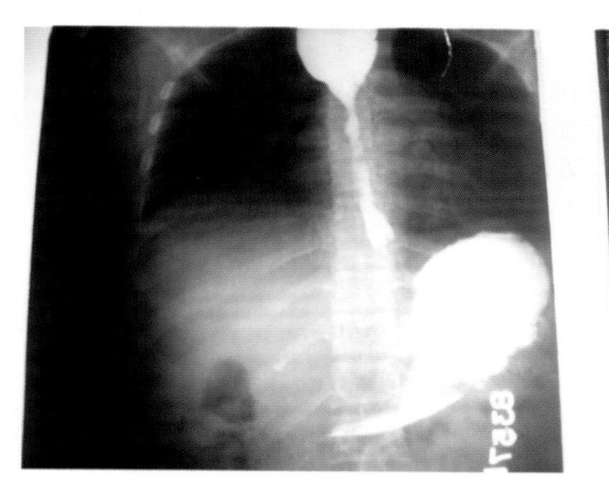

Photo by Netha Hussain (Own work) [CC BY-SA 3.0 (http://creativecommons.org/licenses/by-sa/3.0)], via Wikimedia Commons

This type of diagnostic imaging uses fluoroscopy and radiography to examine the upper digestive tract to identify ulcers, tumours, and other abnormalities of the esophagus, stomach, and duodenum. It can diagnose gastroesophageal reflux disease (GERD), hiatal hernia (when the stomach bulges up into the chest through an opening in the diaphragm), peptic ulcers, and benign or malignant tumours.

Food and drink can obscure the radiographic image, which is why the patient's stomach must be empty at the beginning of the test. The patient must refrain from eating or drinking anything after midnight on the day prior to the test. This includes water and medications. However, the patient can consume a light evening meal the day before.

The patient should fast for at least eight hours before the test.

It is important to review any test instructions with the patient before the procedure and any tests that are to be done. Having an instruction sheet to hand out is ideal to reinforce the instructions and serve as a reminder for the patient.

The procedure itself will begin with the patient ingesting a carbonated beverage with baking soda granules. The solution expands the patient's stomach with gas. Then, the patient must also drink barium sulphate. This is a chalky mixture of barium, water, and flavouring that resembles the consistency of a milkshake. The expanded stomach, along with the barium mixture, allows the radiologist to view the stomach in detail.

After the patient swallows the barium solution, the radiologist will observe its passage down the esophagus into the stomach and duodenum. The barium will make the tract visible on the fluoroscopy screen as it coats the lining of the gastrointestinal tract. The radiologist monitors the passage of the contrast medium with fluoroscopy for 30 to 60 minutes.

The radiologist will take periodic radiographs to allow a detailed study of the upper gastrointestinal tract and provide permanent records. The patient will be repositioned various times so the radiologist can observe the upper GI tract from different angles. If the procedure is to observe the small and large intestines, the radiologist may require the patient to return for additional radiographs after enough time has passed for the solution to make its way through the system.

After the radiologist prepares the upper GI tract report, they will send the results to the referring physician. The medical office assistant should explain to the patient that after the barium series is done, the barium suspension will appear in the stool for up to three days. This means their stool will often be whitish in colour. The use of laxatives might be necessary, as a common side effect of ingesting barium is constipation. It is recommended that the patient increase their fluid and fibre intake following the procedure.

Lower Gastrointestinal (GI) Series Test

Known as barium enema, this diagnostic imaging procedure involves the insertion of a catheter into the rectum through the anus where the colon in the lower GI is filled with barium sulphate. Permanent pictures of the colon and rectum are obtained through examination using fluoroscopy and radiography.

Lower GI images may be requested by the physician to assist in diagnosing disorders of the colon, such as polyps, cancerous tumours, diverticulosis. It can also determine the extent of irritable bowel diseases like ulcerative colitis and Crohn's disease. This procedure often follows if the patient has chronic diarrhea, blood in their stool, irritable bowel syndrome, and/or other disorders of the lower GI.

As with any medical procedure, the instructions the patient must follow prior to the lower GI series test are important. The medical office assistant should instruct the patient to limit their consumption to clear liquid the day prior to the exam. This includes water, plain coffee or tea, clear broth, and strained juice. Gas and fecal material must be voided in advance because gas can show up as confusing shadows on radiographs. Fecal matter can obscure the colon image. To avoid this, the patient should take a laxative the day before the procedure.

Other instructions for proper pre-procedure preparation include refraining from drinking anything but water after midnight on the day before the procedure. An enema, which requires an injection of fluid into the rectum, will help to eliminate any feces present in the colon. This may be required before the procedure begins.

At the beginning of the procedure, the radiologist will instruct the patient to relax on their side while they insert a rectal catheter. As the barium enters the colon, the inner lining of the large intestine will display. The radiologist will watch the movement of barium on a fluoroscopic screen and periodically take radiographs.

The patient will experience fullness and may feel the need to defecate while the barium enters the colon. The catheter usually has a balloon on the tip that expands for a tight seal in order to avoid leakage.

During this procedure, the radiologist will instruct the patient to move into various positions. This will allow the barium to fill the colon completely, which will give the radiologist a better image. At the end of the procedure, the patient will evacuate the barium. The radiologist will take the final radiographs at this point. Once the radiologist prepares a lower GI report, they will send it to the patient's physician.

While a double-contrast barium enema radiographic study is similar to a lower GI study, it uses air to distend the wall of the colon. This is how the radiologist views the colon in detail, to make it easier to detect small tumours and polyps.

Other Examples of Fluoroscopy

- **Intravenous urogram (IVU):** Used to identify kidney stones, tumours, abnormalities of the urinary tract
- **Arthrogram:** Iodine compounds are injected into a joint capsule to view the soft tissues of the joint.
- **Myelogram:** Iodine compounds injected into the spinal column to diagnose tumours, herniated disks, etc.

Cardiovascular Radiography

Angiography is a diagnostic radiology that can identify any narrowing or blockages in the cardiovascular system. This procedure involves the taking of x-ray images of the coronary arteries and the vessels that supply blood to the heart. In order to obtain clear images, a contrast medium is injected through a catheter into the desired location. The dye makes the blood vessels visible when a radiograph is taken and allows the physician to clearly see how the blood flows into the heart.

Angiography: *Diagnostic radiology to identify any narrowing or blockages in a cardiovascular system.*

Coronary Angiography

An angiograph is recommended for patients with chest pain, or patients suspected to have coronary artery disease (CAD). Angiography allows the physician to gather important information about the coronary arteries. Valve malfunction, blood flowing backwards through the heart valves, and atherosclerosis are all health conditions that can be detected through cardiovascular radiology. This is a common procedure and is generally considered safe.

Photo by Maria A Pantaleo, Anna Mandrioli, Maristella Saponara, Margherita Nannini, Giovanna Erente, Cristian Lolli and Guido Biasco : Development of coronary artery stenosis in a patient with metastatic renal cell carcinoma treated with sorafenib. BMC Cancer, 2012, 12:231 doi:10.1186/1471-2407-12-231 Published: 11 June 2012 - http://www.biomedcentral.com/1471-2407/12/231/abstract, CC BY 2.0, https://commons.wikimedia.org/w/index.php?curid=19874515

Cardiovascular radiography is performed in a hospital or clinic and is also used when a patient is being evaluated for surgery, or having angioplasty or stent placement. It is advised that patients check with the hospital or clinic regarding how long an angiography procedure may take, as this may vary upon location. Generally, the procedure takes one to two hours.

Patients will be expected to lie down on a table while the site where a catheter is to be inserted—usually the groin or an arm—will be cleaned. A local anesthetic will be given to numb the skin so that no pain is felt. A series of x-rays is taken and shown on a monitor to be evaluated. The catheter is guided carefully through a vein or artery so that it is positioned near the heart. With the catheter in place, a special iodine dye is released into the bloodstream. Patients might experience a warm sensation that quickly passes.

Patient Preparation for Cardiovascular Radiography

When an office assistant confirms or reminds patients about their scheduled appointment, it is important to recap the following with them before they come in:

- Patients should wear comfortable, loose-fitting clothing to the procedure. A gown will be given to wear during the procedure.
- The day before the angiogram procedure, patients should not eat or drink anything after midnight (or six to eight hours before the procedure).
- Take all medications to the hospital in their original bottles. Ask the physician about whether or not to take usual morning medications.
- Patients with diabetes must ask the physician if insulin or other oral medications should be taken before the procedure.
- Before the procedure starts, medical history and vital signs will be taken and a physical exam will be performed.
- The patient should empty their bladder and remove contact lenses, eyeglasses, jewellery, and hairpins.
- The patient will have the opportunity to present any concerns or questions before the procedure.

After Procedure

Inform the patient that they may experience the following after the procedure. Encourage any questions or concerns they may have at this time. Provide them with the office's phone number and emergency contact information in case any questions, concerns, or complications occur after the office is closed.

- The catheter is removed and the incision is closed with manual pressure, a clamp, or a small plug to prevent bleeding and promote healing. The puncture site is likely to be tender for a few days with slight bruising. This is normal.
- The patient will be monitored in a recovery area until their condition is stable.
- While in the recovery area, the patient needs to lie flat for several hours to avoid bleeding.
- The patient may be able to go home on the same day or they may have to remain in the hospital for a day or longer.
- Instructions will be given for when they should resume taking medications, bathing, showering, returning to work, and other normal activities.

At-Home Care

Once the patient has returned home, they should rest and recover for a few days. They should drink plenty of fluids to help flush the dye from their system. Naturally, they should also avoid strenuous activities and heavy lifting for several days.

While it is a routine procedure, the patient should be made aware of the warning signs that something isn't right. They should call their physician if there is/are:

- bleeding, new bruising, or swelling at the catheter site
- increasing pain or discomfort
- signs of infections, such as redness, drainage or fever
- a change in temperature or colour of the extremity that was used for the procedure
- a feeling of weakness or fainting
- development of chest pain or shortness of breath

Early detection of any cardiovascular defects or blockages will give the patient a better prognosis. The use of cardiovascular radiography allows the physician to obtain accurate results of what is happening inside the heart. Test results of x-ray images give the radiographer the ability to see the cause of any blockage or narrowing of blood vessels in the heart.

ANGIOGRAPH

Jason Ryder was sent to a radiologist by his physician to receive an angiograph after complaining about ongoing chest pain. What does the physician hope to obtain from the results? Is there anything that Jason has to prepare before the procedure? Discuss three at home care steps that Jason should follow after the angiograph is done.

Answer:

Case Study

CT or CAT Scanning

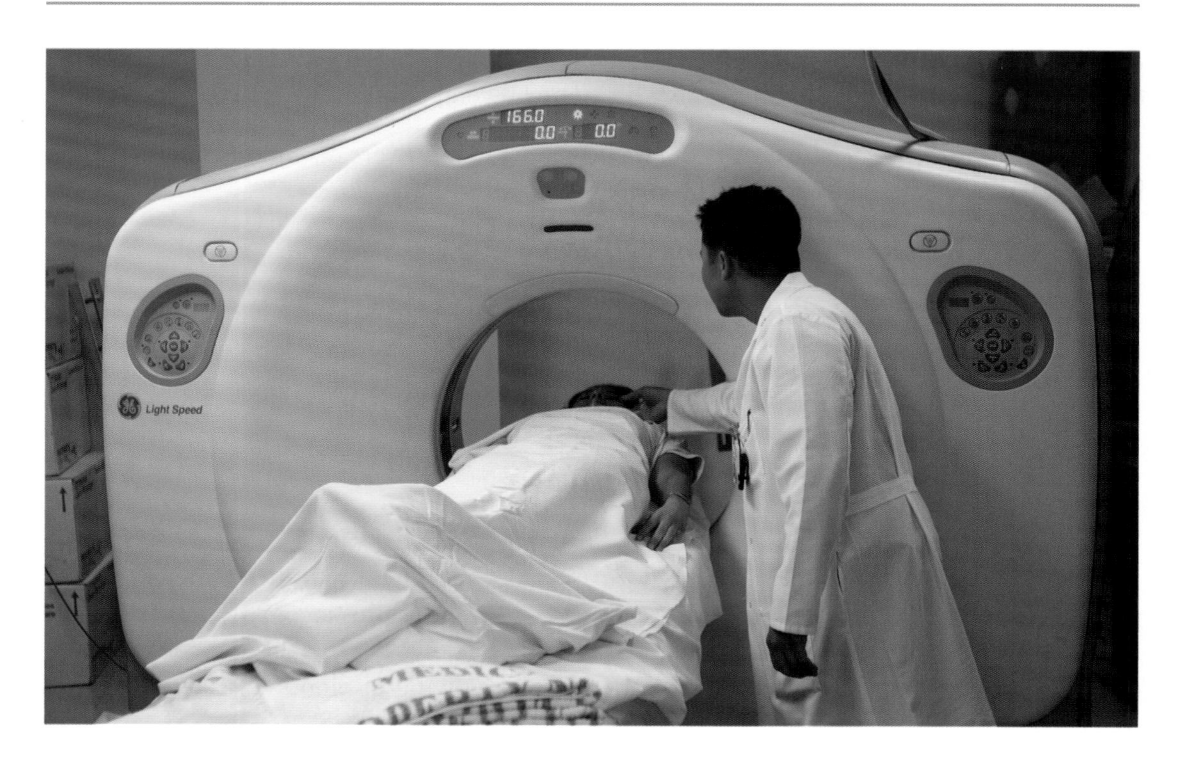

***Computed Tomography (CT):** An imaging procedure that allows a detailed view inside the body with minimal radiation exposure.*

Computed Tomography—also referred to as Computerized Axial Tomography, and CT or CAT scanning—is an advanced radiograph examination carried out by a skilled diagnostic imaging technician. It allows the technician to view bones and organs in fine detail with minimal use of radiation

Using a computer and a specialized x-ray machine to produce cross-sectional images of the body, CT scans allow the imaging of structures that cannot be visualized with conventional radiographic procedures.

The x-ray unit rotates around the body to get a 3D view. The images produced by the x-ray are stitched together by the computer to generate cross-sectional images. This unique perspective has been used successfully in diagnostic studies of the brain, abdomen, and pelvis.

For this procedure, the patient will lie on a motorized table. The technician will remotely move this table from an adjoining room. The table moves the patient or body part through the opening of the CT scanner.

CT scans are used to:

- Diagnose muscle and bone disorders, such as osteoporosis
- Pinpoint the location of a tumour, infection, or blood clot
- Guide procedures, such as surgery, biopsy and radiation therapy
- Detect and monitor diseases, such as cancer or heart disease, and monitor the progression of a disease
- Detect internal injuries and internal bleeding

Patient Preparation for CT Scan

The medical office assistant is responsible for informing the patient about what they can expect during the CT scan, as well as the instructions they must follow before and after the procedure. This ensures the results are as accurate as possible and the patient recovers appropriately afterwards.

Outline the following to a patient before a scheduled CT scan:

- The patient should wear comfortable, loose-fitting clothing to the procedure. They will be given a gown.
- Metal objects, including jewellery, eyeglasses, dentures, and hairpins may affect the CT images—they must be removed prior to the procedure. Patients may be asked to remove piercings, if possible.
- If a contrast medium is used, the patient must not eat or drink anything for several hours beforehand.
- The patient must inform the physician of all medications currently being taken and if there are any known allergies to contrast material or dye (if so, the physician will prescribe a steroid medication to reduce the risk of an allergic reaction). This medication is generally taken 12 hours prior to the contrast material being administered.
- Tell the patient to inform the physician if they have any recent illnesses or medical conditions that may increase the risk of an adverse effect, such as a history of heart disease, asthma, diabetes, kidney disease, or thyroid problems. This is especially important for pregnant women.
- The patient should lie motionless during the procedure and breathe normally. When a radiograph is being taken, the patient is usually instructed to hold their breath for a clearer image.
- The patient will hear mechanical clicking and whirring sounds from the scanner as the images are taken.
- Inform the patient that the procedure takes anywhere from 10 minutes to an hour to complete, depending on the part of the body they are imaging.

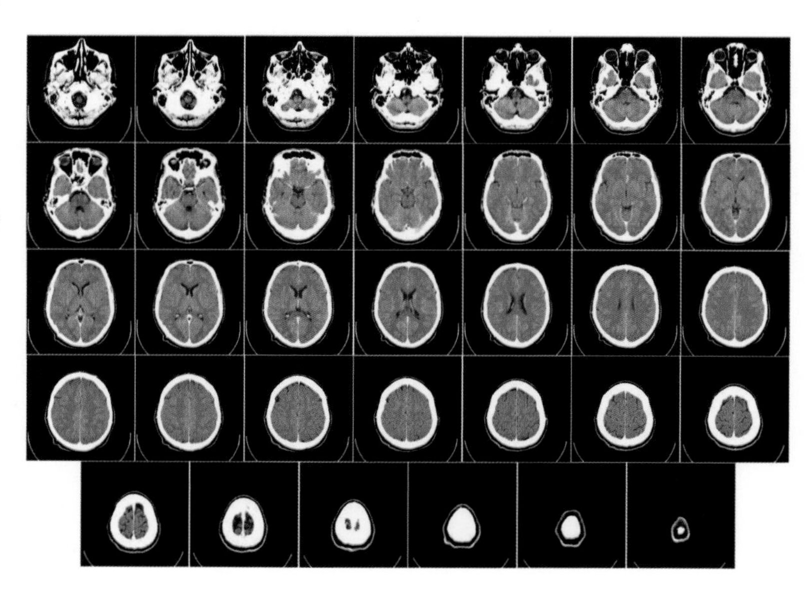

A diagnosis and understanding of diseases and injuries are determined for certain medical procedures through the results of a CT scan. The clear images from this non-invasive procedure provide the physician with a better view of almost every part of the body. Images from a CT scan are a great tool to use when planning medical, surgical, or radiation treatments.

Case Study

CT SCAN

Geoff was sent to have a CT scan by his physician because of symptoms that presented during a physical exam. He is currently taking insulin to control his diabetes and was wondering if he should stop taking it before the procedure. He is also worried that the procedure will be painful and scary because he is claustrophobic. Before going in for his CT scan, what instructions would you advise?

Answer:

my notes

Magnetic Resonance Imaging (MRI)

MRI is able to see through bone and gives detail to fluid-filled soft tissue. It is used for viewing tissue high in fat or water where other radiographic techniques cannot obtain the appropriate detail required for diagnosis. MRI is also quite useful for viewing images of the brain, central nervous system, and joints.

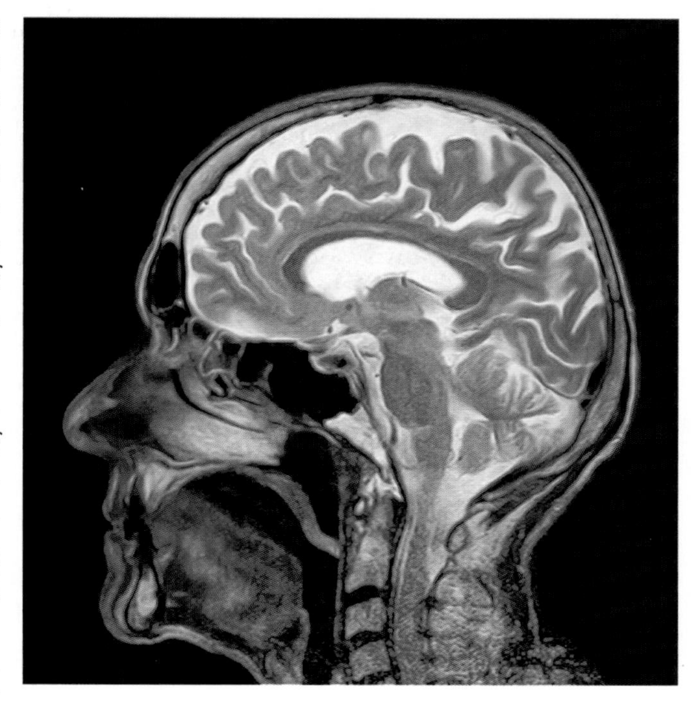

Magnetic resonance imaging assists physicians with diagnosis of intracranial and spinal lesions, cardiovascular and soft tissue abnormalities (e.g. joint disease), brain tumours, multiple sclerosis, and other nervous system diseases.

Magnetic Resonance Imaging: *An imaging technique that takes images of tissues with high fat and water content that cannot be seen with other radiographic techniques.*

The procedure is safe, painless, and non-invasive, because it does not require radiation. The device uses a strong magnetic field and radiofrequency pulses to image various systems, producing computer-processed images. However, despite its safety and non-invasive nature, an MRI is unsuitable for patients who are claustrophobic or have metal in their body. The magnets are extremely powerful and metallic objects can cause damage if they are forced through tissues.

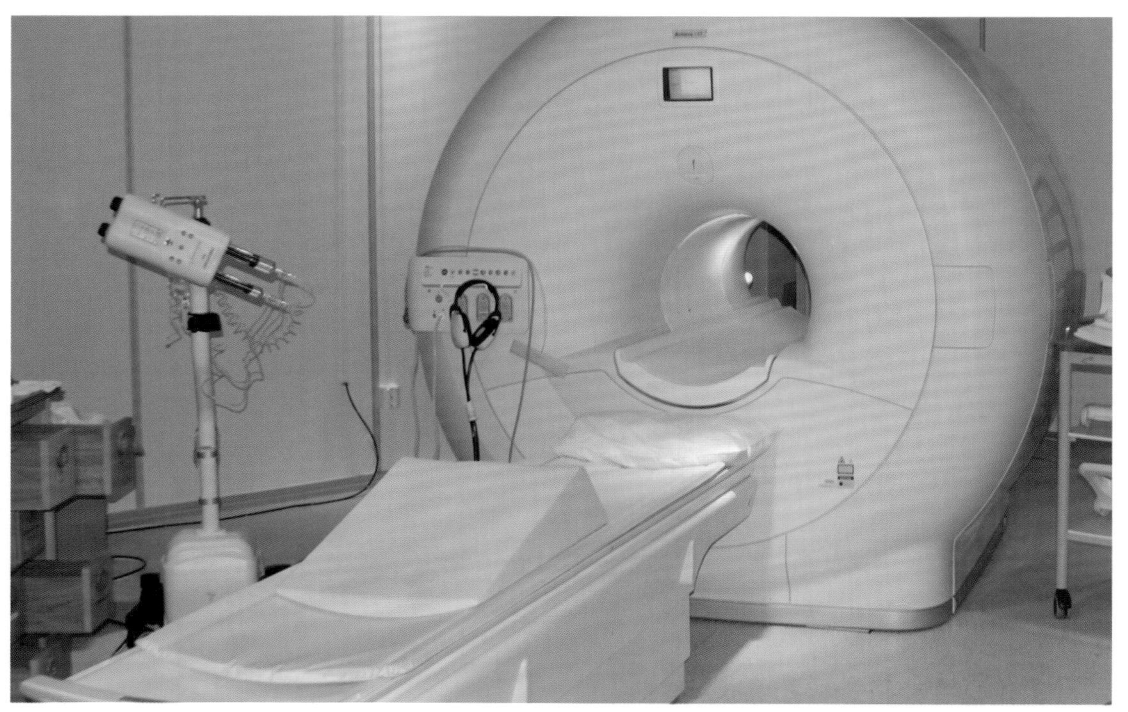

Photo by Jan Ainali (Own work) [CC BY 3.0 (http://creativecommons.org/licenses/by/3.0)], via Wikimedia Commons

During an MRI, the patient lies on a table within the hollow section of the cylindrical machine. A diagnostic technician monitors from an adjoining room. Claustrophobic patients may require a sedative before an MRI as the procedure occurs in an enclosed space.

A potential alternative is an open MRI machine, which is less confining. However, these may not always be available as they are a newer technology.

Depending on the specific model of an open scanner, patients may be able to sit in the machine rather than lie down. These machines can also accommodate larger patients who cannot fit into the conventional machine.

High-resolution, three-dimensional images obtained with MRI are permanently recorded on film or stored digitally on computers for evaluation by a radiologist. Once these images are evaluated, the radiologist will write a report and send it to the patient's physician.

Patient Preparation for MRI

- Let the patient know that the length of the procedure can range from 20 to 90 minutes.
- No special preparation is necessary for the examination, unless they require a sedative. Patients are allowed to eat and drink before the procedure and take any prescribed medication.
- Loose and comfortable clothing should be worn, but tell the patient to avoid wearing cosmetics as certain products contain small amounts of metal.
- With the involvement of a strong magnet, any metal or magnetic-sensitive objects should be removed. These include hairpins, eyeglasses, hearing aids, watches, jewelry, and credit cards.
- Once inside the MRI machine, the patient must remain completely still for 15 to 20 minute intervals during the procedure. The sound of metallic clacking can be heard during the process, but earplugs or headphones are available for use if the patient requests them.

Patients with any of the following cannot undergo an MRI scan:
• A pacemaker or have had heart valves replaced
• Metal plates, pins, metal implants, surgical staples, or aneurysm clips
• Are pregnant or may be pregnant
• Body piercings
• Are wearing a medicine patch
• Permanent eye liner or tattoos
• Have ever had a bullet wound
• Worked with metal (for example, a metal grinder or welder)
• Metallic fragments anywhere in the body
• Inner ear implant
• Cannot lie down for 30 to 60 minutes

Case Study

MRI

What would you do and what would you not do in the following situation?

Sharon Wendl is an 18-year-old high school varsity Jiu Jitsu competitor. For the past 2 months, she has had pain and swelling in her left shoulder. The physician schedules an MRI to determine the cause of the problem. Sharon has had several radiographs done over the past year and is worried about the radiation exposure to her body. She wants to know how much radiation is involved with the procedure and if she needs to fast the night before. She is also claustrophobic and wants to know what options are available to her.
Answer:

my notes

Ultrasonography

Ultrasound Imaging: *A diagnostic procedure that uses sound waves or other vibrations with an ultrasonic frequency to produce images of soft tissue.*

Ultrasonography, better known as **ultrasound imaging**, is non-invasive and safe for patients as it uses sound waves to produce images of soft tissue. Often used for fetal monitoring, ultrasound scans can be 3D and 4D. A 4 dimensional ultrasound still takes a 3D image, but will show the fetus moving in real time (time is the fourth dimension).

Physicians use ultrasound to diagnose conditions of the abdominal and pelvic organs, particularly the liver, gallbladder, spleen, pancreas, kidneys, uterus, ovaries, and abdominal aorta. Specific medical conditions ultrasounds can detect include breast cysts, gallstones, and kidney stones.

Echocardiogram: *An ultrasound examination of the heart to determine its size, shape, and position.*

An **echocardiogram**, which is an ultrasound of the heart, helps to determine the heart's size, shape, and position in the patient. It also allows the ultrasonographer to observe movement in the heart valves and chambers and identify if anything is abnormal.

Other uses for ultrasounds include guiding devices during minimally invasive procedures. Potential procedures include a needle biopsy, cortisone injection, or amniocentesis.

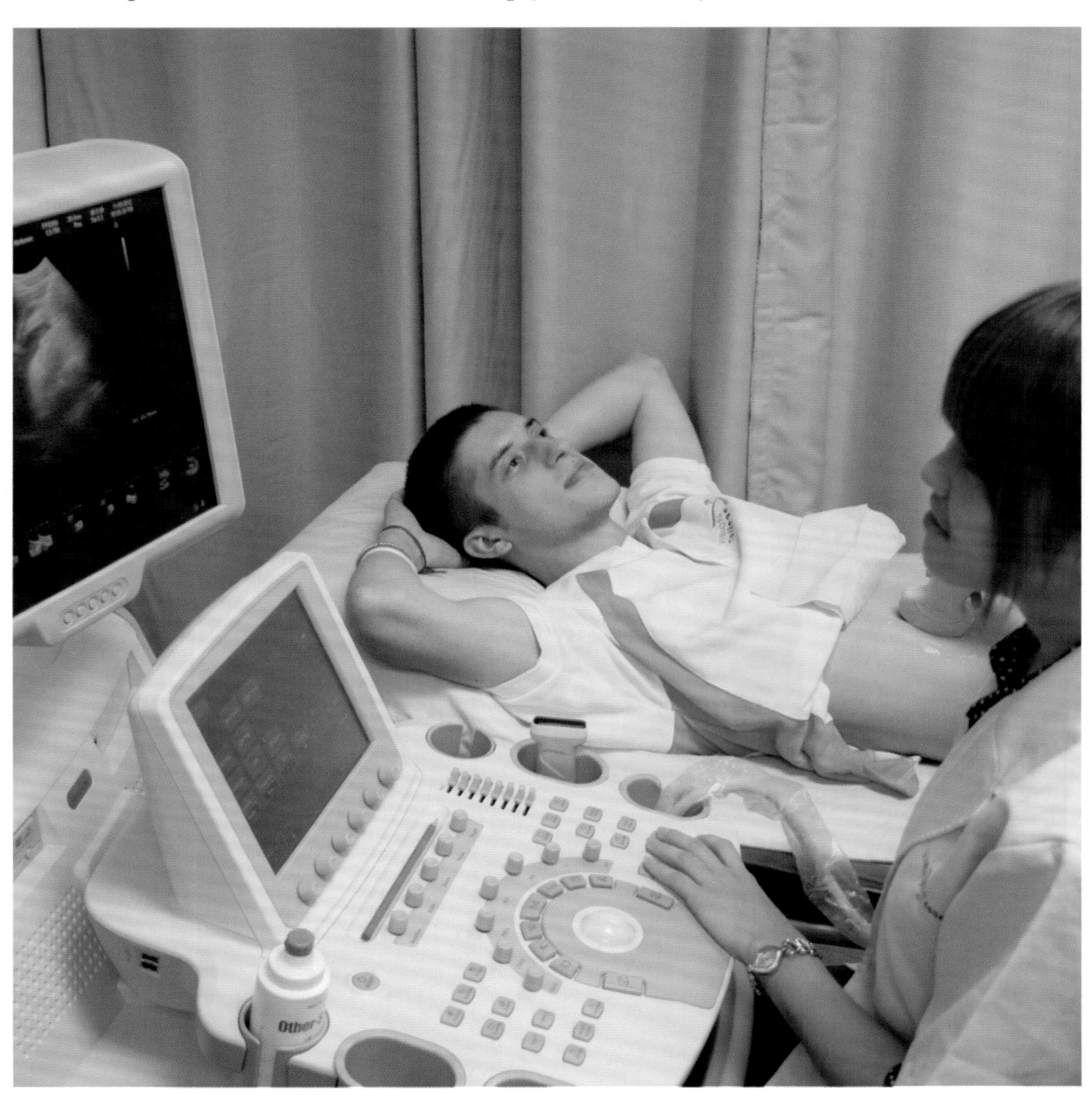

Photo by Aseev artem (Own work) [CC BY-SA 3.0 (http://creativecommons.org/licenses/by-sa/3.0)], via Wikimedia Commons

Ultrasound advantages:

- Shows movement
- Allows continuous viewing of a structure
- Uses sound waves vs. radiation
- Less expensive

Ultrasound disadvantages:

- Sound waves cannot penetrate bone and air or gas-filled cavities
- Difficult to use on obese patients because adipose tissue can interfere with sound wave transmission

Before conducting the examination, the ultrasonographer must spread ultrasound gel on the part of the body to be examined. This increases the conductivity of sound waves between the patient's skin and the transducer. After applying the gel, the ultrasonographer will place the probe on the patient's skin. They will move it around the examination area.

How does the transducer produce an image?

- It generates sound waves directed into patient's skin
- The sound waves reflect back to the transducer, from internal organs and soft tissue.
- The ultrasound machine interprets the sound waves into an image known as a **sonogram** which displays the image's size, shape, and consistency

Sonogram: *a visual image produced from an ultrasound examination.*

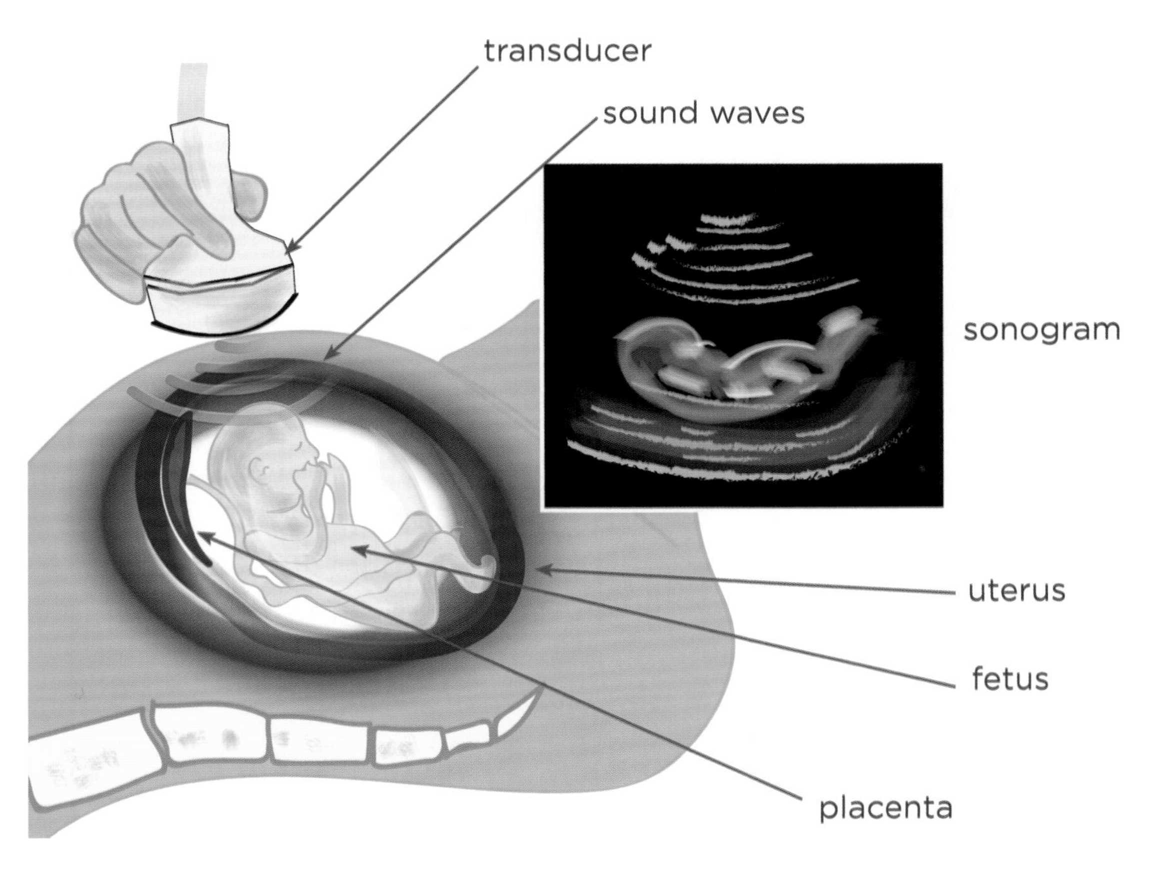

Obstetric ultrasound: *the use of medical ultrasound where sound waves are used to create real-time visual images of the developing embryo or fetus in the mother's uterus.*

The patient can also view the screen while the procedure is performed and selected images are permanently recorded on paper, film, videotape, or a computerized storage medium. Once the radiologist reviews the radiographs and writes up the ultrasound report with the findings, it is sent to the patient's physician.

Most people think of **obstetric ultrasound** when they hear the term ultrasound. Obstetric ultrasound is the method physicians will use to determine a fetus' gestational age, which can confirm the expected due date, along with the fetus' size and position. Additionally, an obstetric ultrasound can help in identifying potential issues such as ectopic pregnancy or conditions like osteogenesis imperfecta (brittle bone syndrome). Based on these images, the obstetric ultrasound helps determine:

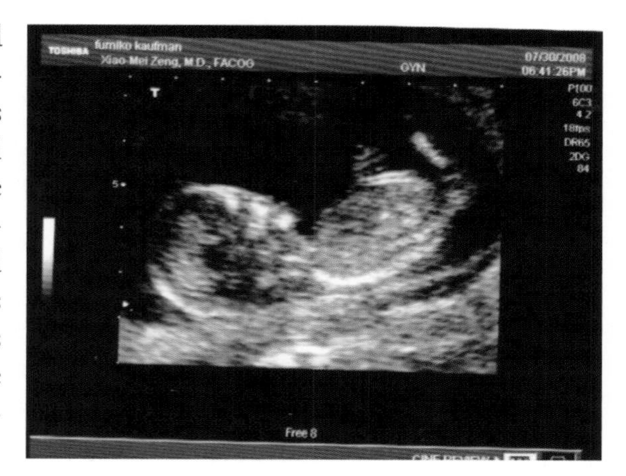

- If the fetus is growing accordingly to the gestation or trimester stage
- If the fetus is positioned correctly
- The fetus' gender, if the fetus is old enough and positioned appropriately

A gynecologist may also use ultrasounds to evaluate and treat infertility issues prior to pregnancy.

Doppler Ultrasound: *a non-invasive test that can be used to assess blood flow through blood vessels by the use of bouncing high-frequency sound waves off circulating red blood cells.*

Another use of ultrasounds is the **doppler ultrasound**, which measures direction and speed of blood flowing through major arteries and veins in the abdomen, arms, legs, and neck. This type of ultrasound can help diagnose issues such as blood flow blockages, narrowing of blood vessels due to atherosclerosis, and congenital malformations.

Patient Preparation for Ultrasound

The patient should be aware that the procedure will take approximately 15 to 45 minutes to complete, depending on the area that is being examined.

- Depending on the area in need of examination, the patient may need to fast.
- Fast for 8 to 12 hours for ultrasounds examining the gallbladder, liver, spleen, or pancreas.
- Obstetric ultrasounds require a full bladder. Consume approximately 32 ounces of fluid one hour before the procedure.
- The patient must remain still during the procedure. Movement can interfere with accurate results. The ultrasonographer may ask the patient to change and hold positions so they can get an alternate view of their organs.

Case Study

ULTRASONOGRAPHY

What would you say and do to ease the concern of the patient in each scenario?

Scenario One: Nicholas Hawk was sent for an echocardiogram after presenting with chest pain. He is worried that the echocardiogram will worsen the pain and wants to know how long the procedure will take, as he has to take time off work. Nicholas also wonders if there are any additional preparations before he comes in for his procedure.
Scenario Two: Sandy Lanesworth is going for an obstetric ultrasound to determine the gestational age of her fetus. She is worried that her baby will be exposed to too much radiation and was wondering if the ultrasound can determine the gender of her baby. Sandy also wonders if she should stop taking her prenatal vitamins and whether or not she should have a full bladder prior to her procedure.
Answer

Mammography

__Mammography:__ a safe and diagnostic imaging procedure that uses low-dose-radiation for the examination of breasts to diagnose and locate breast tumours.

Mammography is a safe and specific type of imaging that uses a low-dose x-ray for the examination of breasts to detect breast diseases. A mammogram can help detect a tumour that is less than one centimetre in diameter before it is even clinically palpable by the physician. Mammography helps monitor the effects of surgery and radiation therapy on breast tumours. On radiographs, abnormal areas appear noticeably different from normal breast tissue. Mammography can detect benign breast masses, breast calcification, fibrocystic breast disease, and, most notably, breast cancer.

According to the Canadian Cancer Society, women who are 40 to 49 should discuss breast cancer and mammography with their physician. Depending on the provincial program, a patient may be able to schedule an appointment without a referral. There is a chance that certain provincial screening programs do not accept women aged 40 to 49—if this is the case, a physician should be consulted.

All provinces have breast cancer screening programs for women age 50 to 69 and do not require a doctor's referral. According to Cancer Care Ontario, the Ontario Breast Screening Program (OBSP) is a province-wide service that provides high-quality breast screening to two groups of women:

- Women aged 50 to 74 who are at average risk for breast cancer with mammography every two years.
- Women aged 30 to 69 years who are identified as being in high risk for breast cancer with annual mammography and breast MRI screening.

Women with a family history of breast cancer should follow the advice of their physician regarding mammography, as age guidelines do not apply—they are at higher risk of breast cancer and need to be monitored more frequently. If abnormality is discovered during a clinical examination, the physician will send the patient for a diagnostic mammogram.

There is no preparation needed when going to a mammogram, except that the patient should avoid applying lotion, powders, or deodorant. These may contain traces of metals that can interfere with the radiograph.

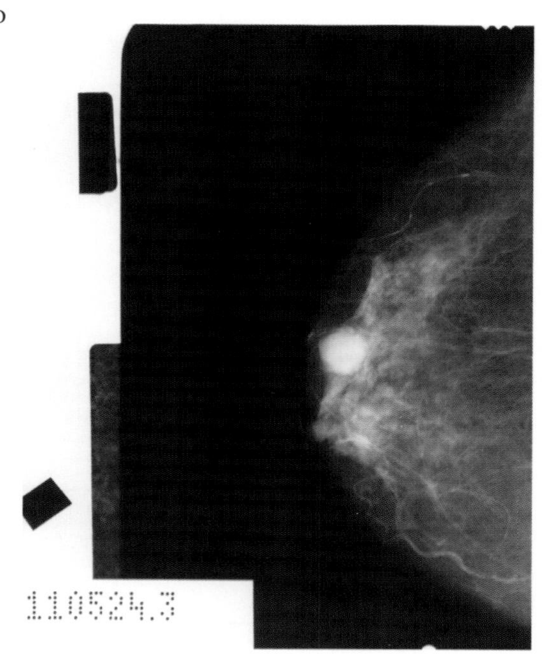

In order to make the procedure easier and more comfortable, the patient should wear two-piece clothing on the day of the mammogram. Before the procedure, the patient must remove clothing from the waist up. A radiology technician will position the patient's breasts on the mammography machine. The plastic compression paddles will apply pressure and flatten the breast. This helps the technician obtain a clearer image and lowers the dosage of radiation. Some patients may experience discomfort or pain during this process.

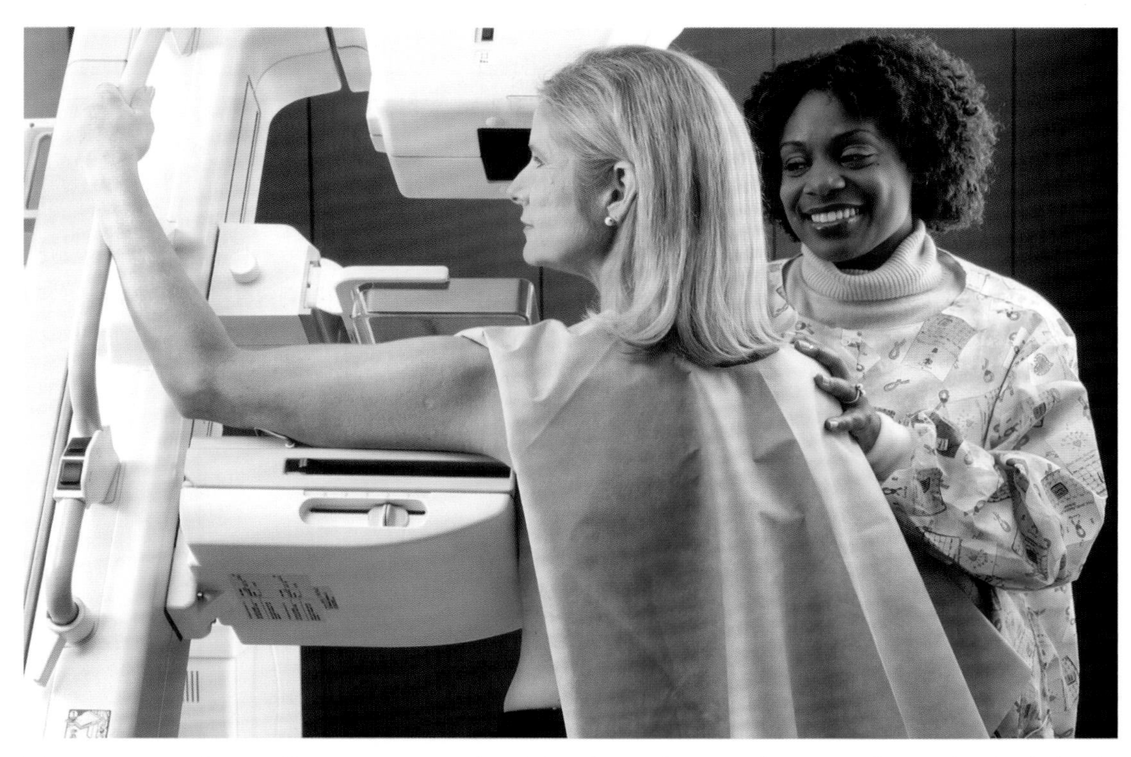

Photo by Rhoda Baer via Wikimedia Commons

To minimize discomfort, a patient should reduce their caffeine intake and schedule the mammogram a week after their menstrual period finishes. The breasts are less tender during this period.

The patient must hold their breath and remain motionless to obtain a clear image. Should the image be unclear or obscured, the image will need to be taken a second time. Slight movements—even as small as breathing creates enough shift to blur the image. From here, two radiographic views are taken from each breast: one side view and one view from top.

The radiologist then checks the mammogram for abnormalities. However, they may also order additional images to increase the accuracy of their findings. Once the radiologist records the results, they will send the report to the patient's physician.

With early diagnosis and treatment, breast cancer survival rates for women can be as high as 93%. Removing a malignant lump due to early detection through mammography can result in conservative treatment followed by less disfigurement and a high survival rate.

my notes

Case Study

MAMMOGRAPHY

Sally Smith was sent by her physician to get a mammogram even though she does regular self-examinations. With this being her first time, Sally is afraid that the procedure will be extremely painful and leave her with a lot of bruising. She asks why she still needs to go for a screening when there were no abnormal findings from self-examination and physical examination with her physician. Her grandmother had breast cancer, but her mother does not, so why is it in her best interest to get a mammogram done? Explain what you would say to ease her worries.

Answer:

my notes

Bone Densitometry (DEXA)

Bone densitometry measures bone mineral density of the human skeleton to detect bone loss. With age, bones may become less dense, resulting in brittle and weak bones leading to possible fractures. Dual energy x-ray absorptiometry (DEXA) is widely used for testing bone density in the human skeleton. Density measures are taken at different parts of the body, including the hip, spine, and peripherals (wrist, fingers, heel, etc.)

Bone densitometry: *A measurement of mineral matter per square centimetre of bone.*

Osteoporosis is the gradual loss of calcium in bones. It causes bones to become thinner, more fragile, and more likely to break. Thyroid and parathyroid conditions, and certain medications are all factors that can cause bone density loss. Physicians recommend post-menopausal women above the age of 65 have a bone density scan every two years as they are at particular risk for osteoporosis.

Osteoporosis: *The gradual loss of calcium that causes bones to become fragile and therefore, more likely to break or fracture.*

Patient Preparation for DEXA

- Instruct the patient to avoid taking a calcium supplement or osteoporosis medication the morning of the procedure. These medications will interfere with the accuracy of the bone density measure.
- Position the patient on an x-ray table and instruct them to remain as still as possible during the procedure.
- The radiologic technician will perform scans on one or more areas of the bone with DEXA on different parts of the body as mentioned previously.

This test will reveal results as either a T-score, which is a comparison against peak bone density, or a Z-score, which compares the results against other individuals who are the same age as the patient. This will help indicate if the patient has experienced a loss in bone density, predict the risk of bone fracture, and the presence of osteoporosis. A normal score is above -1. If the patient has low bone mass, often termed osteopenia, the score will be between -1 and -2.5. Patients who have osteoporosis will have scores below -2.5.

A physician may send patients in for additional testing if they have an unusually high or low Z-score.

A physician may request DEXA to be performed on patients who are genetically prone to osteoporosis, or women who are menopausal. This non-invasive procedure provides valuable information to prevent or delay the weakening of bones.

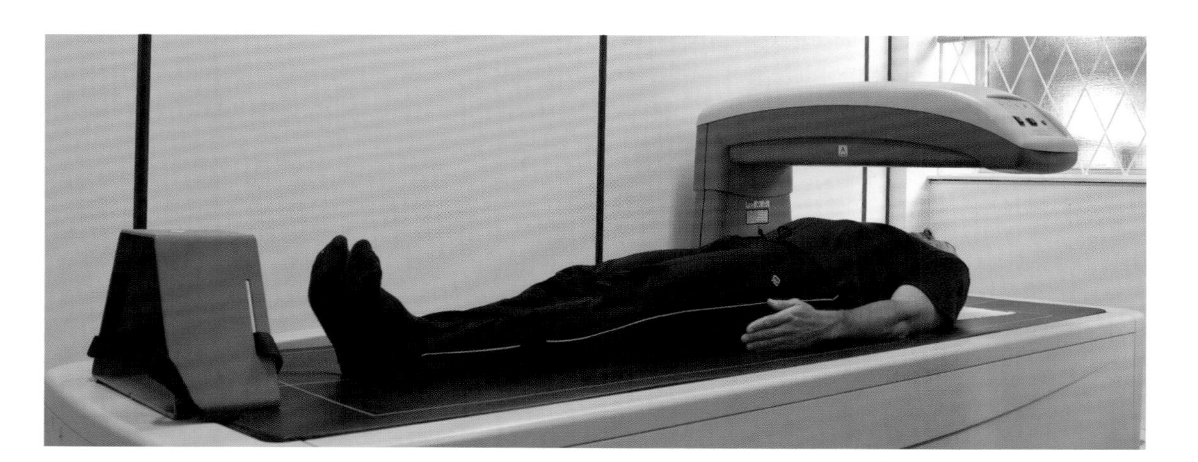

Photo by Nick Smith photography - ALSPAC web site, CC BY-SA 3.0, https://commons.wikimedia.org/w/index.php?curid=26389366

Scopes

Colonoscopy

With the use of a small camera attached to a flexible tube called a colonoscope, this procedure internally examines the mucosa of the rectum and entire length of the colon. The colon consists of the sigmoid colon, descending colon, transverse colon, and ascending colon.

The camera at the end of the insertion tube transmits images back to a video screen for the physician. Before this procedure, the physician will explain the process along with any risks that may be involved. After all questions are answered, the medical office assistant may be responsible for obtaining the patient's signature on treatment forms.

Colonoscope: *A flexible tube with a small camera attached to the end that is inserted through the anus to examine the colon.*

A physician will normally request the patient undergo a colonoscopy when they have tested positive in a fecal occult blood test. This is so the physician can determine the source and cause of the bleeding. It also helps to evaluate colon-related symptoms including lower abdominal pain.

A colonoscopy can detect and assess the following conditions:

- Lesions of the colon or rectum (e.g. benign or malignant growths)
- Colorectal polyps
- Fissures
- Hemorrhoids
- Infection and inflammation

Colonoscopies also help with early detection of colorectal cancer. This early diagnosis and treatment increases the patient's chance of survival.

Patient Preparation for Colonoscopy

Often performed in a hospital on an outpatient basis, a colonoscopy requires the patient's rectum and entire colon flushed out, leaving it completely empty.

Also known as full bowel preparation, the patient needs to be free of fecal material as it can interfere with views of the colon wall. That makes it difficult for the physician to detect abnormalities.

The medical office assistant may need to provide proper instructions on preparing the colon because if patients have not prepared properly, the colonoscopy is usually cancelled and rescheduled for another time. Note that patient preparation procedure for a colonoscopy may vary from one facility to another.

Five days before the procedure, the patient should begin the following instructions:

- Stop taking iron supplements, as they may alter the colour of the colon wall.
- Stop taking aspirin and aspirin products—these will cause more bleeding if a polyp is removed from the colon.

Two days before the procedure, the patient should begin the following instructions:

- Stop taking non-steroid anti-inflammatory drugs, such as ibuprofen and naproxen. This will minimize bleeding if a colon polyp is removed.
- Any other medication restrictions will be advised by the physician and must be followed.

The day before the procedure and continuing until the examination is completed the patient should:

- Not consume any solid food or milk products (including any milk or cream with coffee or tea)
- Consume only gelatin or popsicles (avoid purple or red which could be mistaken for blood in the colon)
- Drink only clear liquids such as water, apple juice, sport drinks, soft drinks, and clear broth.
- Avoid drinking alcohol.

Bowel Preparation:

- The patient must take a laxative, usually in powdered form, in the afternoon the day before the procedure (between 2 p.m. and 4 p.m.). The package will come attached to a plastic gallon container. Make sure the patient reads the instructions before they prepare the laxative solution.
- Fill the gallon container with drinking water and mix in the powdered laxative. Store the laxative solution in the refrigerator after preparing. Many patients find it easier to drink when the solution is chilled.
  - The patient will begin preparing their bowels by drinking one eight-ounce glass of the liquid laxative solution every 10 to 15 minutes until they have consume two quarts (eight 8-ounce glasses).
  - The patient may experience nausea and bloating after drinking the first few glasses. This feeling will disappear once bowel movements begin. If the patient continues to feel nauseous, they should slow down the drinking process or stop for 30 minutes before resuming at the recommended pace.
  - The patient's first bowel movement should start about one hour after they have begun drinking the solution and will have 10 to 15 more bowel movements after that.

- The patient can stop drinking the solution if the first bowel movement appears pale yellow or clear. However, if the bowel movement is neither, the patient must continue drinking the laxative solution every 15 minutes until their bowel movements appear clear.

After midnight the night before the examination:

- Do not eat or drink anything, including water.
- Only take medications if approved by the physician, and only with a small sip of water.

Transportation:

- Notify the patient to arrange for a ride with someone after the procedure as they will be sedated and cannot drive themselves or take public transportation.

Following the procedure:

- Instances of bloating, abdominal cramping, and flatulence may occur after a colonoscopy.
- If the physician removed a polyp or took a biopsy during the procedure, the patient may notice traces of blood in the stool for one to two days.
- If the patient experiences significant rectal bleeding, faintness, dizziness, shortness of breath, or heart palpitations, they must contact the office immediately.

Colonoscopy Procedure

Before the physician begins the colonoscopy, they will administer a sedative to the patient intravenously. This will relax the patient, making them sleepy and less aware of their surroundings. In many cases, the patient will not remember anything about the procedure.

Position the patient on his or her left side in the Sims position. The patient's left thigh should be slightly flexed and the right thigh acutely flexed on the abdomen. The physician will perform a digital rectal exam prior to inserting the colonoscope. A digital rectal exam means the physician will insert a lubricated, gloved finger into the patient's rectum to check for abnormalities. After this, the physician will insert the colonoscope through the entire colon until it reaches the cecum.

For better viewing, the physician will inject air into the colon and use suction to remove any secretions present that might obstruct the visual field. The physician will observe the colon's mucosa while withdrawing the colonoscope slowly and check for any abnormalities.

If the physician detects any abnormalities or lesions in the colon, they will insert a long, thin instrument through the insertion tube in order to remove a specimen for biopsy. They will send this specimen to the laboratory for analysis.

Removing a precancerous polyp prevents it from developing into colon cancer in the future.

After a colonoscopy, the medical office assistant must inform the patient they may experience the following:

- Bloating
- Abdominal cramping
- Flatulence

If the physician did remove a polyp or took a specimen for biopsy, inform the patient they may notice traces of blood in their stool for a couple of days after the procedure. Reassure them that this is completely normal.

COLONOSCOPY

Case Study

Kristen Musson was admitted with abdominal pain, and later tested positive in a fecal occult blood test. Her physician requested a colonoscopy to assess if there were any abnormalities in the colon. Kristen is concerned about the amount of pain that she might experience during this procedure, and was wondering if she should fast the night before her colonoscopy is scheduled. She has asked if there are any specific instructions that she should follow before her procedure and whether she can drive home afterward. What would you do? What would you say?
Answer:

Gastroscopy (Endoscopy)

Gastroscopy: *Uses a gastroscope to examine the upper digestive tract to diagnose abnormalities.*

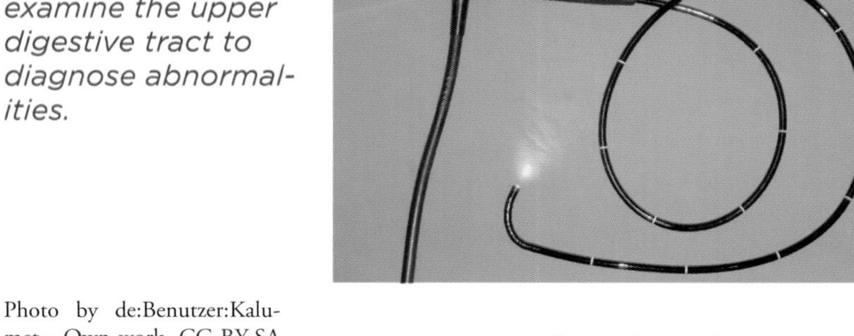

Photo by de:Benutzer:Kalumet - Own work, CC BY-SA 3.0, https://commons.wikimedia.org/w/index.php?curid=958735

Gastroscopy uses a gastroscope to view the lining of the esophagus, stomach, and the first part of the small intestine (or the duodenum) to diagnose abnormalities in the upper part of the gastrointestinal tract. This procedure can control bleeding by injecting medications through the gastroscope, which allows the physician to carefully view inflamed areas that need to be further explored. A laboratory technician may take a biopsy sample for analysis.

A gastroscopy allows for cultures, stretching of narrowed areas and the proper diagnosis of inflammation or gastrointestinal bleeding. Before the procedure, the physician will explain the process and answer any questions the patient may have. The medical office assistant should obtain a signature on a written treatment form that provides consent for the gastroscopy.

Patient Preparation

Before the procedure, advise the patient of the following rules and guidelines. If they are not followed, the gastroscopy will have to be rescheduled.

1. The patient's stomach must be completely empty.
    - If gastroscopy is scheduled for the morning, fast from midnight with no food or liquid intake.
    - If gastroscopy is scheduled for the afternoon, the patient is allowed to have clear fluids such as water, coffee and tea without milk or cream, soft drinks, and gelatin. Breakfast must be eaten before 9 am.
2. Remove all jewellery before the procedure, including any hair accessories, earrings, rings, necklaces, and eyewear.
3. The patient needs to inform the physician in advance of any of the following medical conditions:
    - If the patient is taking Coumadin, Aspirin, Plavix, or diuretics, it is usually necessary to stop taking these medications. It is best for the patient to discuss any medications they are taking with their physician well in advance, so they can prepare properly for a gastroscopy.
    - If the patient has diabetes, the diabetic medication will need to be adjusted prior to starting the procedure for the gastroscopy. It is advised that the patient does not take their diabetic pills on the morning of the procedure. If the patient is on insulin, it is strongly encouraged for them to discuss with the physician what they should do prior to the procedure.
    - If the patient is allergic to any medications or has other allergies, bring this to the attention of a nurse or physician.

Gastroscopy Procedure

A sedative will be administered to the patient intravenously to help relax them and a local anesthetic may be sprayed down the throat to prevent gagging. Oxygen may be provided during the procedure through the nose, and patients usually fall asleep during gastroscopy.

It is best to advise the patient that little to no discomfort is experienced, but due to the use of sedatives, it is strongly recommended to have someone accompany the patient on the day of the gastroscopy procedure. For 24 hours after the procedure, the patient is not allowed to drive or take public transit, so a ride home must be arranged beforehand.

The patient's throat may be sore for a few hours after the gastroscopy and the patient may feel bloated for a few minutes—this is normal. After the effects of the medication have sufficiently worn off, the patient can resume a normal diet.

Bleeding may occur from the site of biopsy and polyp removal. This is usually minor and will stop on its own. If the bleeding does not stop on its own, it can be controlled by cauterization or injecting medication into the bleeding site with a needle through the gastroscope.

Bruising or local irritation may occur at the site of injection of the medication, but this will resolve in a few days. If there are any extreme side effects, such as continual bleeding for many days, pain, or other symptoms, the patient is encouraged to contact the practice and speak with the physician.

Gastroscopy is a low-risk procedure when performed by specialized physicians. It collects valuable information for detailed study of suspicious or inflamed areas that require further investigation. A physician may request a gastroscopy when problems in the upper digestive tract cannot be diagnosed properly by x-ray. A gastroscopic procedure can accurately detect ulcers and cancers.

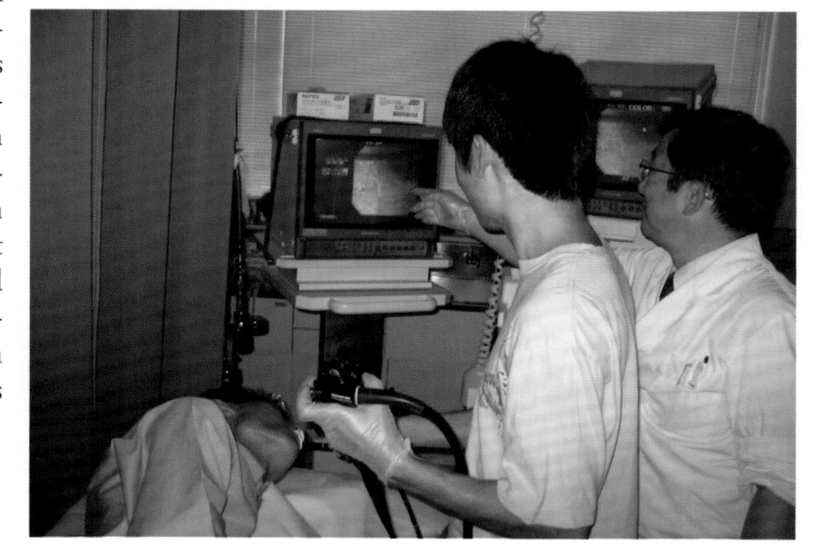

Photo by Yuya Tamai, Flickr.com

Positioning of Patient for Imaging Examinations

How and where the patient is positioned is determined by the purpose of the examination and the area being examined. Ideally, the patient is positioned in such a way that several different views can gather a complete three-dimensional picture of the site of injury. More than one position may be used to examine the same body part during a physical examination. Remind patients to remove any jewellery or hairpins to avoid radiograph obscurity.

Once you have placed the patient in a particular position, let them know that they are to remain completely still until the image is taken so that it isn't blurry. A blurry image will need to be retaken.

There are different types of radiographic views and methods to position your patient. The following are relative positions of body part, film, and x-ray:

1. **Antero-Posterior (AP) view**: The x-ray is directed at the front and the beam passes through to the back of the body. The anterior (directed towards the front) aspect of the body is closest to the radiograph tube and the posterior (directed towards the back) aspect of the body is closest to the radiographic film.

2. **Postero-Anterior (PA) view:** The patient is positioned so that the x-ray beams travel from the back towards the front of the body. Position the patient so that the posterior aspect of the body is facing the radiograph tube and the anterior aspect is facing the radiographic film.

3. **Lateral view:** The patient is positioned so the x-ray beam passes from one side of the body to the opposite side.

    4. **Right lateral (RL) view:** The right side of the body is next to the radiographic film and the x-rays pass through the body from left to right side.

    5. **Left lateral (LL) view:** The left side of the body is positioned next to the radiographic film and the x-rays pass through the body from right to left side—the opposite of right lateral.

6. **Oblique view:** The body is positioned at an angle or semi lateral position.

7. **Supine position:** The patient is positioned on their back with their face upward.

8. **Prone position:** The patient is positioned on their abdomen with their head turned to one side. They are not facing down.

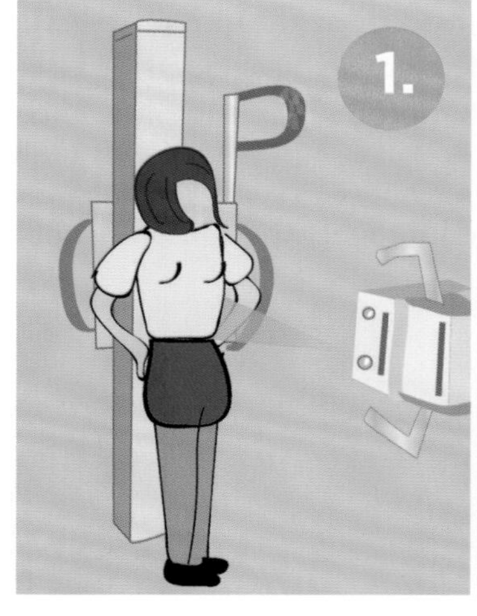

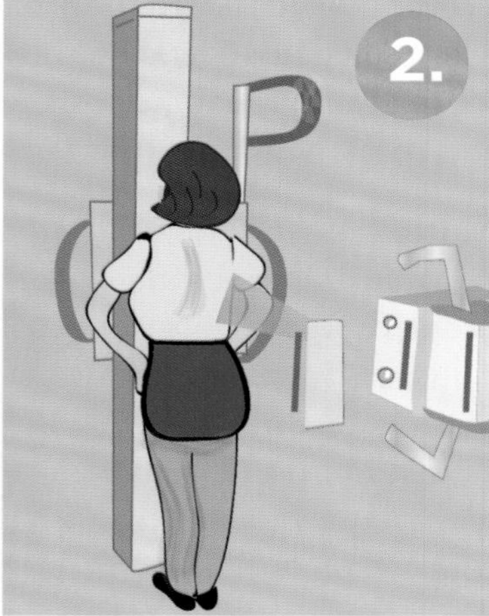

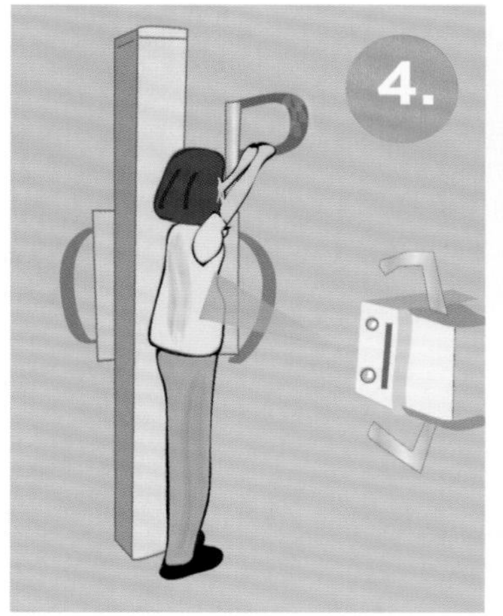

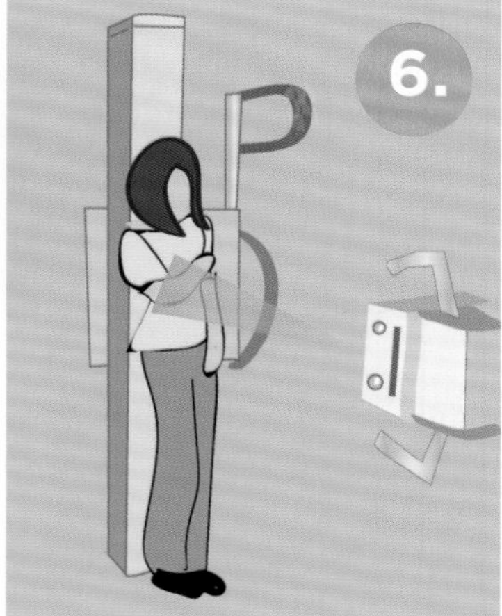

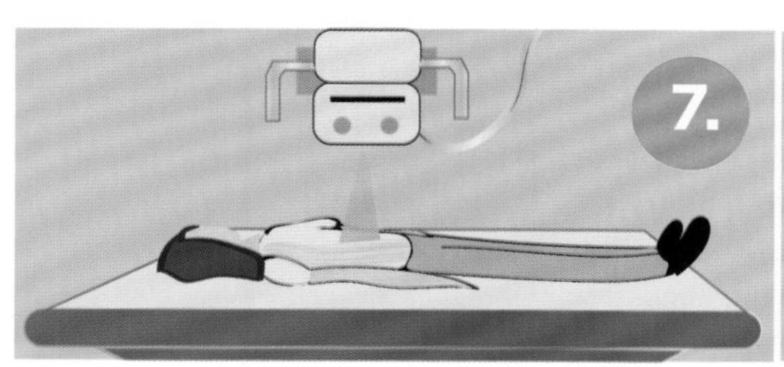

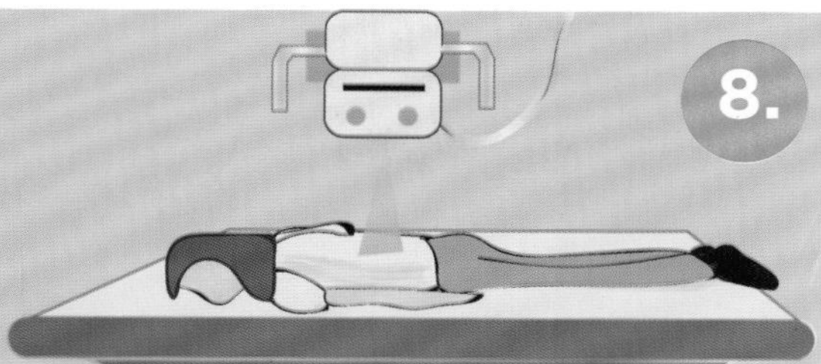

As a medical office assistant, you may need to instruct the patient into the correct position to help the physician during the radiograph imaging process. The patient is usually directed through several positions so that multiple views can be examined. The patient must remain in the position that you have placed them in order to prevent blurring images. Medical assistants should understand the purpose of commonly performed radiographic examinations and should instruct patients into correct positioning for the necessary radiographic view.

Receiving and Recording Test Results

Part of a medical office assistant's responsibilities might also be to organize and maintain a location for receiving test results from labs. Test results can arrive as telephone calls, faxes, email, or by mail. When receiving results over the phone, it is best to request a hardcopy for the patient's file. Office assistants should repeat and confirm the test results to avoid miscommunication. For paperless files, an electronic copy should be obtained and attached to the patient's file with the physician's notes or comments documented.

Reports received by fax, email, or mail should be brought to the physician's attention in a timely manner. For critical cases with clinically significant results, notify the physician immediately that results have been received. Physicians are expected to follow up with appropriate urgency and are encouraged to document any follow-ups in the patient's file. Normal results should be left for the physician to review. When the physician gives back the reports, file the patient's charts accordingly.

Ensure that you match the name on the report to the chart and make sure to check for further instructions, such as calling the patient in for a follow-up appointment. Make note in the file that a physician has seen the test results and that the results have been relayed to the patient. Mark down the date the results were received and when the physician has seen them. All health information collected and exchanged about a patient must be recorded with the same accuracy and care as any other physician-patient encounter.

Medical records are legal documents and should be handled appropriately to avoid losing test results in patient files. At any point, these medical records may provide significant evidence in regulatory, civil, criminal, or administrative matters if the patient care by the physician is questioned.

When converting paper records into an electronic format, destroy the original paper record when the document has been successfully saved in "read-only" format.

The medical record is a tool that provides physicians with the ability to track a patient's medical history, and to identify problems or patterns that may help determine the course of health care. Complete and accurate medical records should meet all legal, regulatory, and auditing requirements. It is a "living document" that tells the story of the patient and the encounters they had with health professionals in facilities involved in their care.

Quiz

CHAPTER 7 QUIZ

1. Define diagnostic imaging.

____
____
____
____
____

2. True or false? Fluoroscopy is a special technique using an endoscope that allows lab technicians to see internal organs and structures of the body in real time on a display screen.

3. Which of the following diagnostic imaging requires the use of strong magnetic field and radiofrequency pulses to image various systems producing computer-processed images?

   a.) CT scan

   b.) MRI

   c.) Ultrasonography

   d.) Mammography

4. Which of the following describes the branch of medicine that uses radiation to diagnose and treat diseases?

   a.) Radiology

   b.) Fluoroscopy

   c.) Angiography

   d.) Geography

5. True or false? A radiograph is an image that shows internal structures with the use of radiation and other imaging techniques.

6. Describe the duties of a radiologist.

____
____
____
____

7. True or false? Radiopaque are radioactive elements in the body that obstruct the x-rays from forming a clear image for the radiologist to make a confirmed diagnosis.

8. This type of diagnostic imaging uses both fluoroscopy and radiography to examine the upper digestive tract. It helps to diagnose ulcers, tumours, and other abnormalities of the esophagus, stomach, and duodenum.

    a.) Upper GI Series

    b.) Lower GI Series

    c.) Intravenous urogram

    d.) Fluoroscopy

9. What does CT stand for?

    a.) Computerized Tomography

    b.) Computerized Axial Tomography

    c.) Computed Tomography

    d.) Computed Telegraphy

10. True or false? CAT scans are used to diagnose muscle and bone disorders, or to pinpoint the location of a tumour, infection, or blood clot. CAT scans are also used to guide procedures such as surgeries, biopsies, and radiation therapies.

11. What does the Doppler Ultrasound measure?

____

____

____

12. What's DEXA? Why is DEXA considered a useful tool for diagnosing osteoporosis?

____

____

____

13. This procedure internally examines the mucosa of the rectum and entire length of the colon with the use of a small camera attached to a flexible tube. This procedure is better known as:

    a.) Colonoscopy

    b.) Endoscopy

    c.) Radiology

    d.) Gastroscopy

14. A physician may order which type of test to view the lining of the esophagus, stomach, and the first part of the small intestine?

    a.) Colonoscopy

    b.) Endoscopy

    c.) Radiology

    d.) Angiography

15. Define postero-anterior and provide an example of when this position would be used.

____

____

____

____

____

____

16. True or false? A right lateral scan is when the right side of the body is positioned next to the radiographic film, and x-rays are directed through the body from the left to right side.

17. Define prone position.

____

____

____

18. When the body is positioned at an angle or semi-lateral position, this is known as which position?

    a.) Lateral view

    b.) Oblique

    c.) Supine position

    d.) Prone position

19. Fill in the blank: With their face upward, this patient is positioned on their back in the ____________________ position.

20. When reports are received by fax, email, or mail, how should a medical office assistant handle critical cases with significant results?

____

____

____

____

____

21. Why is the medical record such an important legal document?

____

____

____

____

____

22. True or false? Original paper records must be destroyed when converting paper records into electronic format and should be saved successfully into the patient's file in "read-only" format.

my notes

my notes

Chapter 8

Assisting with Physical Examinations and Assessment Procedures

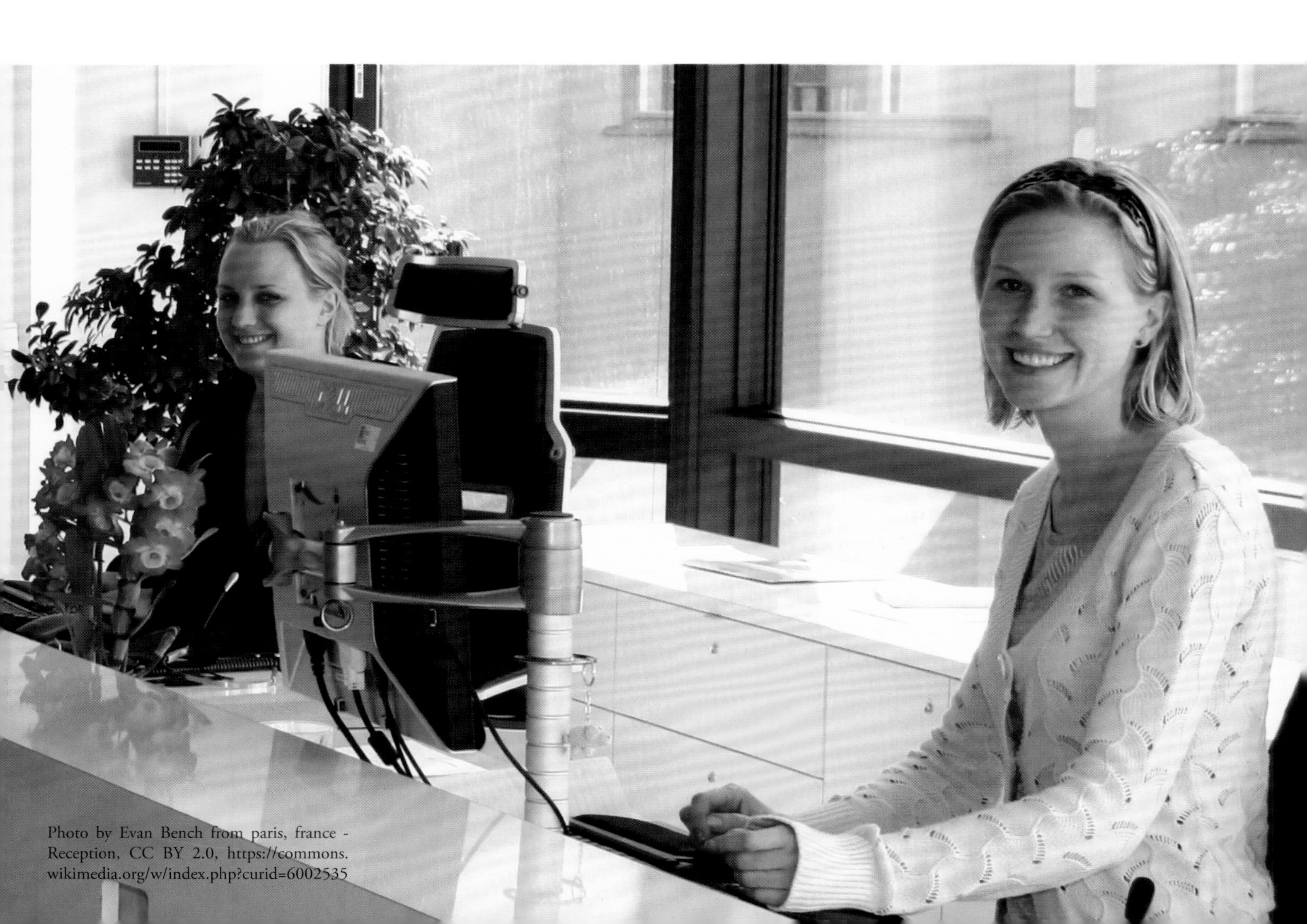

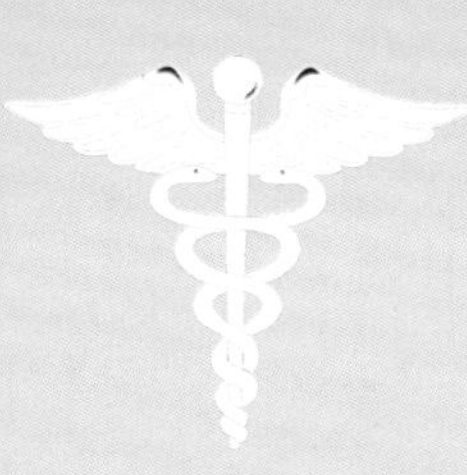

CHAPTER 8 LEARNING OBJECTIVES

After completing this chapter, you should be able to:

- ❑ Define and understand the term physical examination along with terms associated with physical examinations
- ❑ Understand and identify a medical assistant's role
- ❑ Describe and evaluate other possible roles for medical office assistants
- ❑ Understand and perform different methods of examinations
- ❑ Obtain accurate weight and height measurements
- ❑ Understand and perform different patient positioning and draping procedures

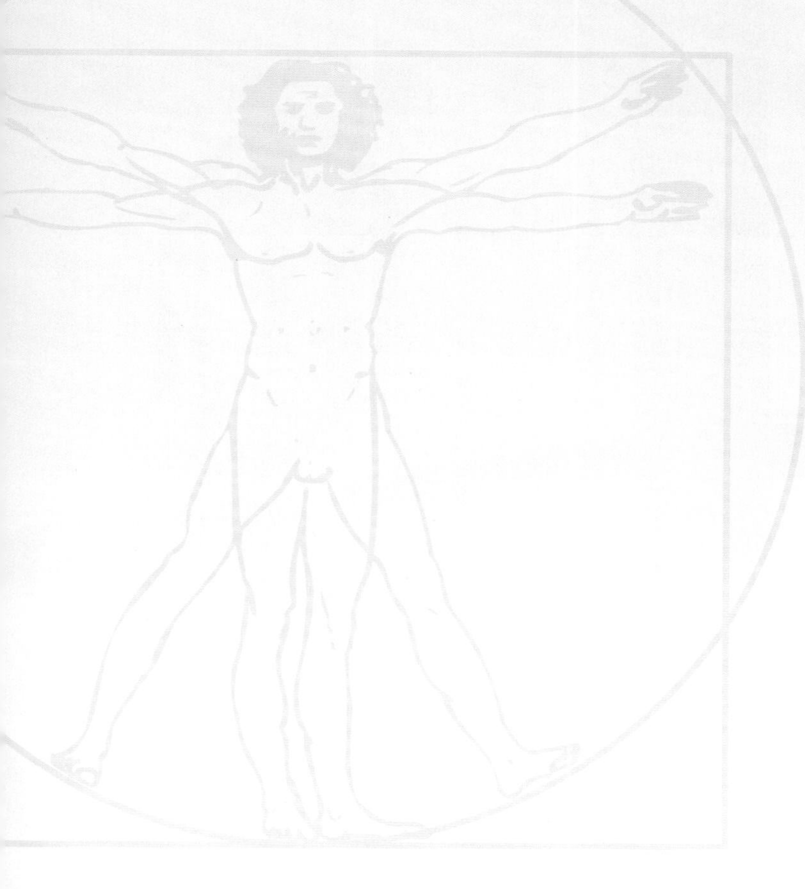

The purpose of a **physical examination is to** determine the overall state of wellbeing of the patient. During a physical exam, the physician will examine the appropriate organs and systems. The physician's interpretation forms an initial diagnosis, and he or she may order diagnostic testing to specify or confirm any diagnoses that arise. If a patient diagnosis is confirmed, the physician will prepare a treatment plan or refer them to a specialist.

Physical examination: *The process of evaluating overall state of wellbeing through observation of vital signs, palpation, percussion, mensuration, manipulation, and auscultation.*

A complete patient exam consists of three parts:

- Health history
- Physical exam of each body system
- Laboratory and diagnostic tests

Annual physical exams are important for detecting early signs of illnesses and preventing more serious health problems. The physician will approach the exam systematically, often starting from the head and work down towards the feet. This type of approach requires the least patient positioning. The medical assistant may have to adjust the patient, or help with draping and positioning if requested by the physician.

All findings must be written in the patient's medical file for paper-based patient records. In the case of electronic medical records, the physician may use free-text entry where there are drop-down lists and check boxes to record findings in the patient file. The EMR will generate a physical examination report so the physician does not have to dictate findings later.

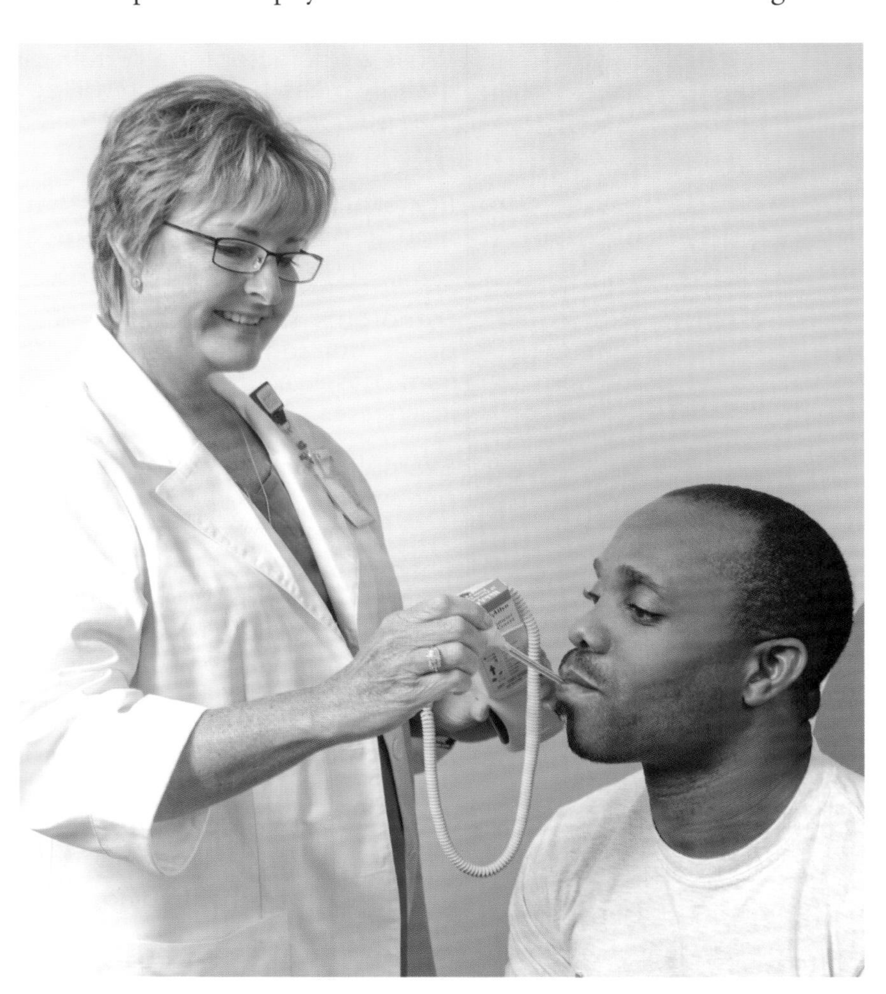

Definition of Terms Associated with Physical Examination	
Final diagnosis	Also known as diagnosis, this is the method of determining and identifying a patient's condition through a complete patient exam. A final diagnosis provides a logical basis for treatment and prognosis.
Clinical diagnosis	A diagnosis made on the basis of medical signs and patient-reported symptoms, rather that diagnostic tests.
Laboratory diagnosis	A diagnosis based signficantly on laboratory reports or test results, rather than the physical examination of the patient.
Differential diagnosis	The process of differentiating and distinguishing between two or more conditions that share similar signs or symptoms.
Prognosis	The probable course and outcome of a patient's condition and recovery prospects.
Risk factor	Physical or behavioural conditions that increase a person's chances of developing a particular condition. Risk factors include genetic factors, habits, environmental factors, and physiological conditions. While a risk factor for a certain disease does not necessarily mean the disease will develop, the chance of that person developing the disease is greater than a person without those factors. For example: An individual that lives in an area of high air pollution, may be at greater risk for developing lung diseases like asthma or emphysema.
Acute illness	Symptoms that have a rapid, severe, and intense onset, but subside after a relatively short period. In some cases, acute episodes may progress into chronic illnesses. Examples include colds, influenza, strep throat, and pneumonia.
Chronic illness	Characterized by symptoms that persist for longer than three months with little change or improvement. Depending on the illness, it may be a long-term disease that can be controlled or treated, but not cured.
Therapeutic procedure	Performed to treat a patient with the goal of eliminating the disease and/or promoting as much recovery as possible.
Laboratory testing	Analysis and study of specimens obtained from patients to assist in diagnosing and treating disease.
Diagnostic procedure	Performed to assist in diagnosing of a patient's condition.

The Medical Assistant's Role in an Exam

Medical assistants work together with physicians in medical offices and clinics, mainly in outpatient or ambulatory care facilities. According to census data reported by Service Canada, in 2006 almost all medical secretaries worked in the health sector (95%), primarily in hospitals (51%), but also in physician offices (29%) and local community service centres (7%). Cross-trained to perform administrative and clinical duties, a medical assistant's responsibilities may vary from office to office.

Medical assistants are also responsible for administrative duties—these duties include greeting patients, answering telephones, scheduling appointments, and updating and filing patient medical records. You may be asked to process insurance forms by coding and filling out the appropriate forms. Medical assistants also handle correspondence, billing, and bookkeeping. Additionally, as part of the medical team, this role involves arranging hospital admissions and laboratory services.

Medical assistants are not usually allowed any physical contact with the patient. However, some physicians choose to have their assistants attend and assist with the examination. Unless Canadian medical assistants have gone through the proper training and are supervised by their employer, assistants are not allowed to perform certain procedures. Clinical duties may include:

- Recording medical histories
- Preparing patients for examinations
- Taking vital signs
- Assisting physicians during exams
- Collecting and preparing laboratory specimens
- Performing basic laboratory tests
- Instructing and educating patients about medication and special diets
- Preparing and administering medication as directed by a physician
- Drawing blood
- Removing sutures and changing dressings
- Explaining treatment procedures to patients

Medical assistants act as a liaison between physicians and patients— in addition to explaining the physician's instructions, assistants help patients feel at ease. Medical assistants are essential for keeping a medical office running smoothly while providing optimal patient health care. It is necessary to have medical assistants as a part of a primary health care team as they help maintain an organized and clean working environment.

Possible Clinical Roles for Medical Office Assistants

There are many possible roles for a medical office assistant (MOA) and they vary between offices. In large practices, specialization may occur in particular areas under the supervision of department administrators. One of the primary roles includes making the patient feel relaxed and comfortable from the moment they enter the office. Listed below are possible roles for MOAs that might be encountered during their work:

	Examination room preparation
	Checking for cleanliness
	Emptying waste receptacles and replacing full biohazard containers.
	Ensuring that exam rooms are well-lit and clean.
	Cleaning and disinfecting examination tables, countertops, and faucets.
	Changing the examining table paper after each patient with a fresh sheet.
	Refilling supplies (syringes, vacutainers, tongue depressors, gloves, drapes, etc.)
	Making sure exam rooms are well stocked and restocking if supplies are getting low.
	Assembling any needed equipment or supplies and operating some equipment or instruments.
	Checking equipment and instruments regularly to confirm that they are in working condition to prevent using faulty equipment.
	Making sure the room is well-ventilated and installing air fresheners to eliminate odours.
	Maintaining comfortable room temperatures, especially for patients who need to disrobe for their appointment.
	Ensuring the exam room door is closed during the examination—patients have a right to privacy.

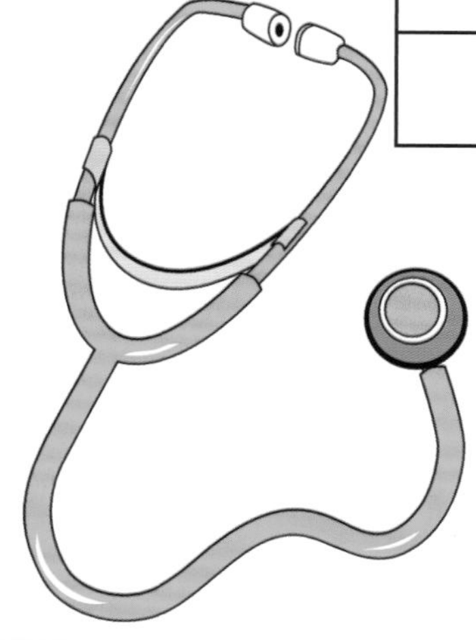

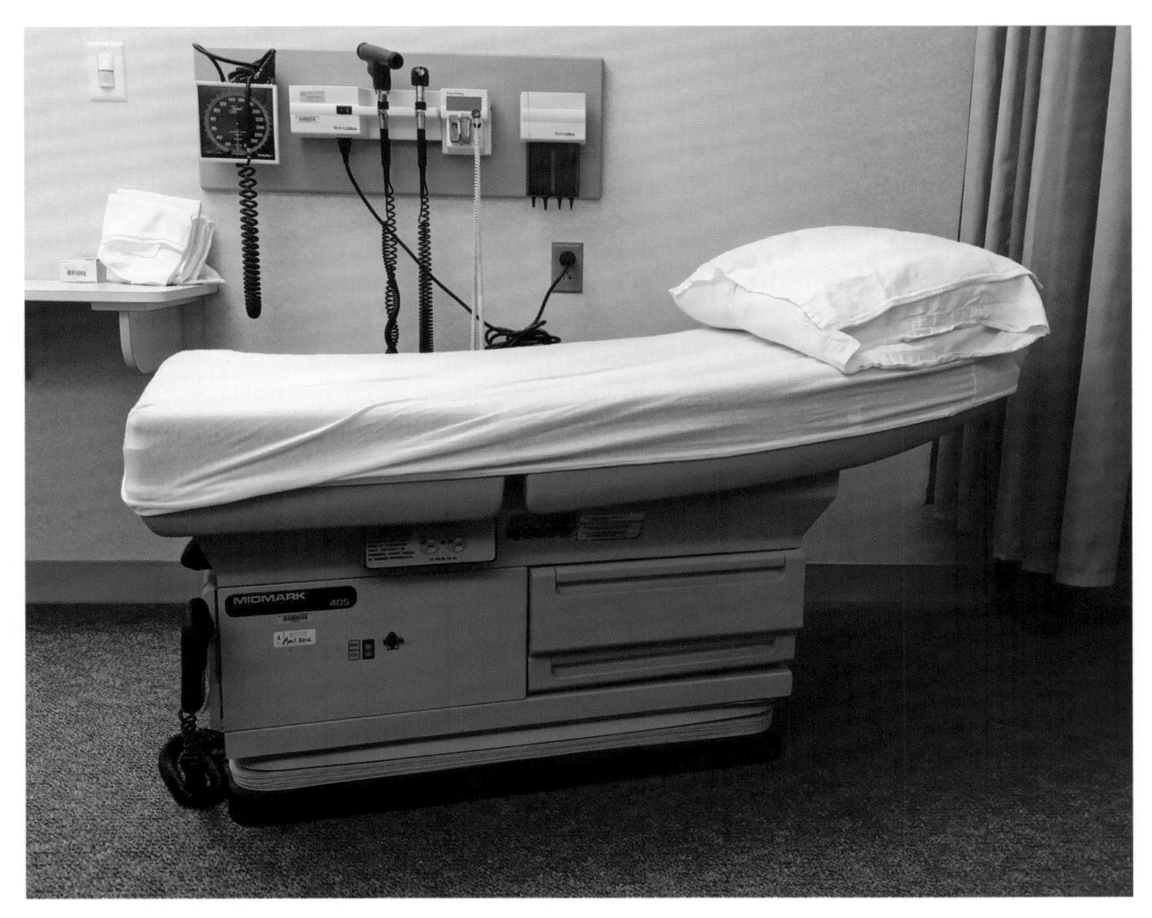

Patient Preparation

The medical office assistant prepares the patient for the physical exam. Prior to the appointment, check the medical record for completeness and make sure that the patient has signed any required consent forms. Verify the patient's health card and gather any additional patient information. Proper identification is essential to avoid mistaking one patient for another.

After greeting the patient upon check in, escort them to the exam room and identify the patient by asking for their full name and date of birth. Try to avoid asking a patient to confirm any information as they may mistakenly identify themselves as someone else if they are not paying attention or mishear you. Have them confirm information by asking detailed, non-leading questions. If the wrong medical procedure is performed on the patient by mistake, the physician or the entire practice may be held liable.

Maintain a friendly and professional composure after confirming the patient's identity. The medical office assistant should explain the purpose of the exam and offer to answer any questions. Ask the patient if they need to use the washroom before the exam—an empty bladder is more comfortable and a urine sample can be collected at this time if needed.

Try to anticipate a patient's needs by their demeanor in the exam room. If they appear cold or warm, ask if you can help by adjusting the thermostat. Patients may be uncomfortable from thirst, hunger, pain, stress, or fear. Keep these things in mind when working with the patient.

Depending on the assistant's responsibilities, preliminary evaluation of the patient may include measuring vital signs and recording the height and weight of the patient. Once these are noted in the patient's file, help the patient prepare for the exam by providing a gown. Explain which items of clothing can be removed and which can stay on during the exam. Disrobing instructions should be specific so the patient understands what items of clothing need to be removed and where to place their clothing.

The area where the patient disrobes should be comfortable and private. There should be an area where the patient can leave their clothes. If the patient is elderly and/or disabled and may have trouble disrobing, the assistant may offer assistance. After the patient has disrobed, instruct the patient where to sit and wait for the physician to arrive.

Paper-based patient charts and records should be placed so that identifiable information is not visible to the patient, but is available for review by the physician. The medical office should keep in-use records in a designated place that protects the privacy of the client's health information.

A patient's positioning for the examination depends on the purpose of the exam. For patient safety, the patient should be provided with help on and off the examination table at all times. See "Patient Positioning" later in this chapter for proper positions based on the type of exam. Answer any questions that the patient may have.

Assisting the Physician

As mentioned at the beginning of this section, part of a medical assistant's role is to work alongside the physician. Besides preparing the patient for the physical examination, being present for examinations such as gynecological appointments may fall under the responsibilities of an assistant. If necessary, helping the patient with positioning and draping will speed up the process of the examination by allowing the physician to access a particular part of the body.

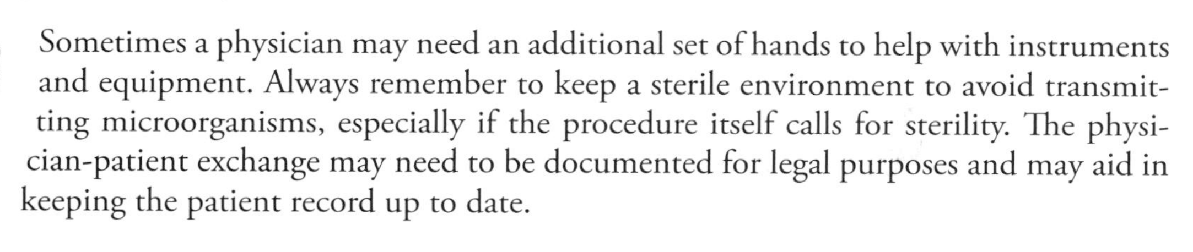

Sometimes a physician may need an additional set of hands to help with instruments and equipment. Always remember to keep a sterile environment to avoid transmitting microorganisms, especially if the procedure itself calls for sterility. The physician-patient exchange may need to be documented for legal purposes and may aid in keeping the patient record up to date.

Supplies and Equipment

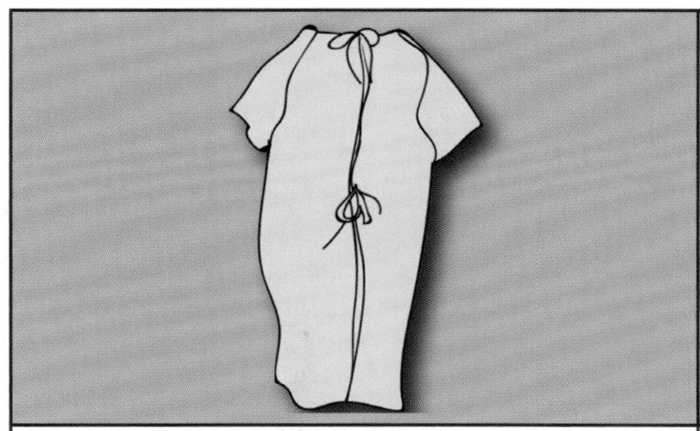	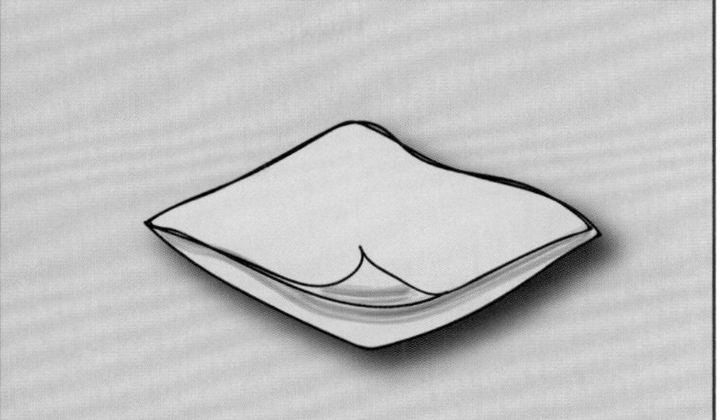
Patient examination gown: A gown made of cloth or disposable paper that provides patient modesty, comfort, and warmth.	**Drape:** A length of disposable paper or cloth to cover a patient or parts of a patient to provide comfort, warmth, and reduce exposure.
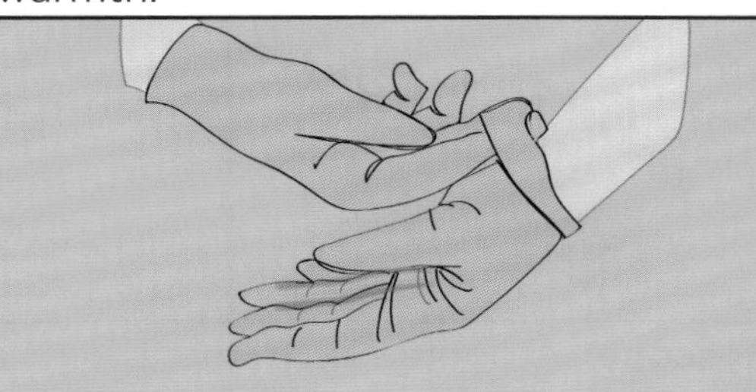	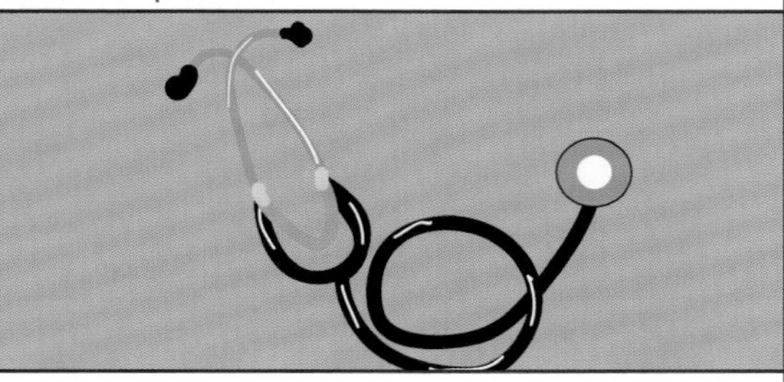
Gloves: Usually made of latex (although alternatives exist for those with a latex allergy), gloves are worn only once before being discarded to provide protection from bloodborne pathogens and other potentially infectious materials.	**Stethoscope:** An instrument used to auscultate body sounds, such as blood pressure, lung, and bowel sounds.
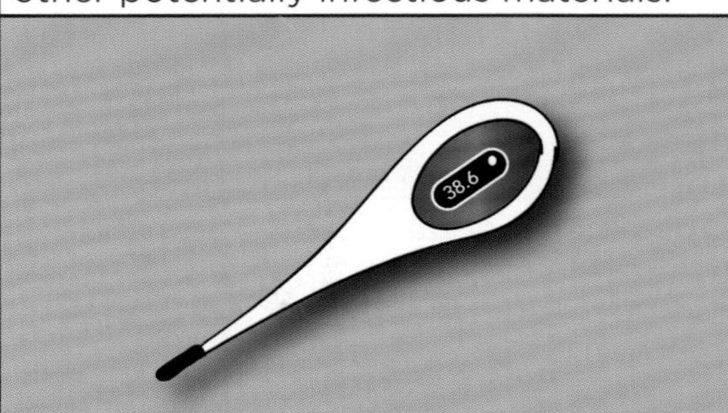	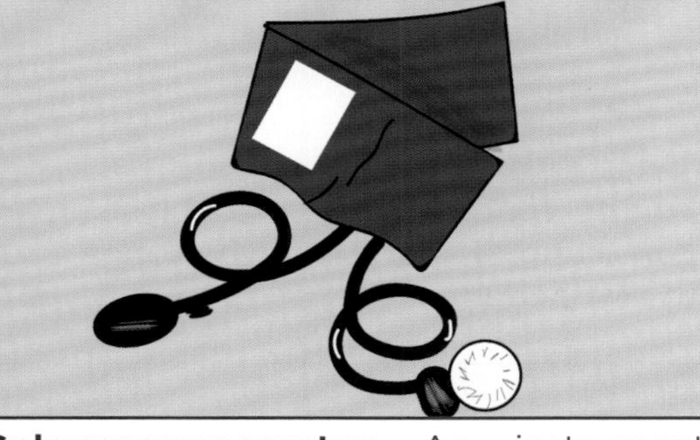
Thermometer: An instrument used to measure body temperature.	**Sphygmomanometer:** An instrument used to measure blood pressure (often called a blood pressure cuff).
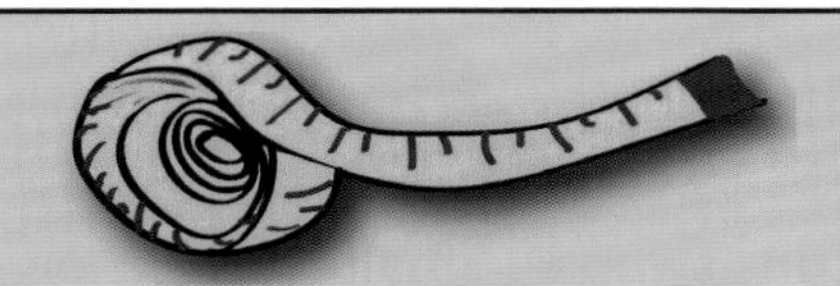	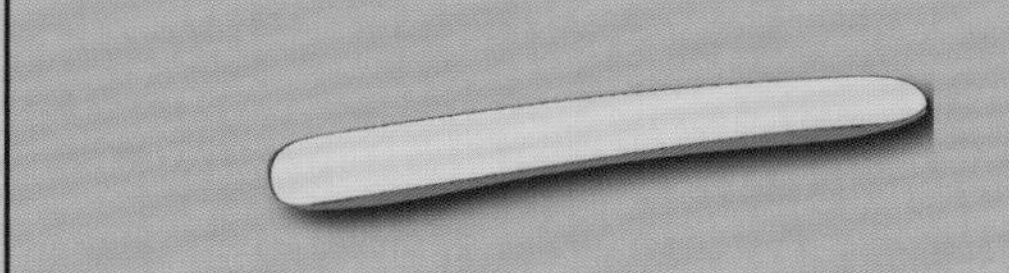
Tape measure: A flexible length of fabric or plastic, calibrated in inches and/or centimetres, used to measure patient dimensions (e.g., diameter of limb and head circumference).	**Tongue depressor:** A flat, thin, rounded, and smooth wooden blade used to depress a patient's tongue during examination of mouth and pharynx.

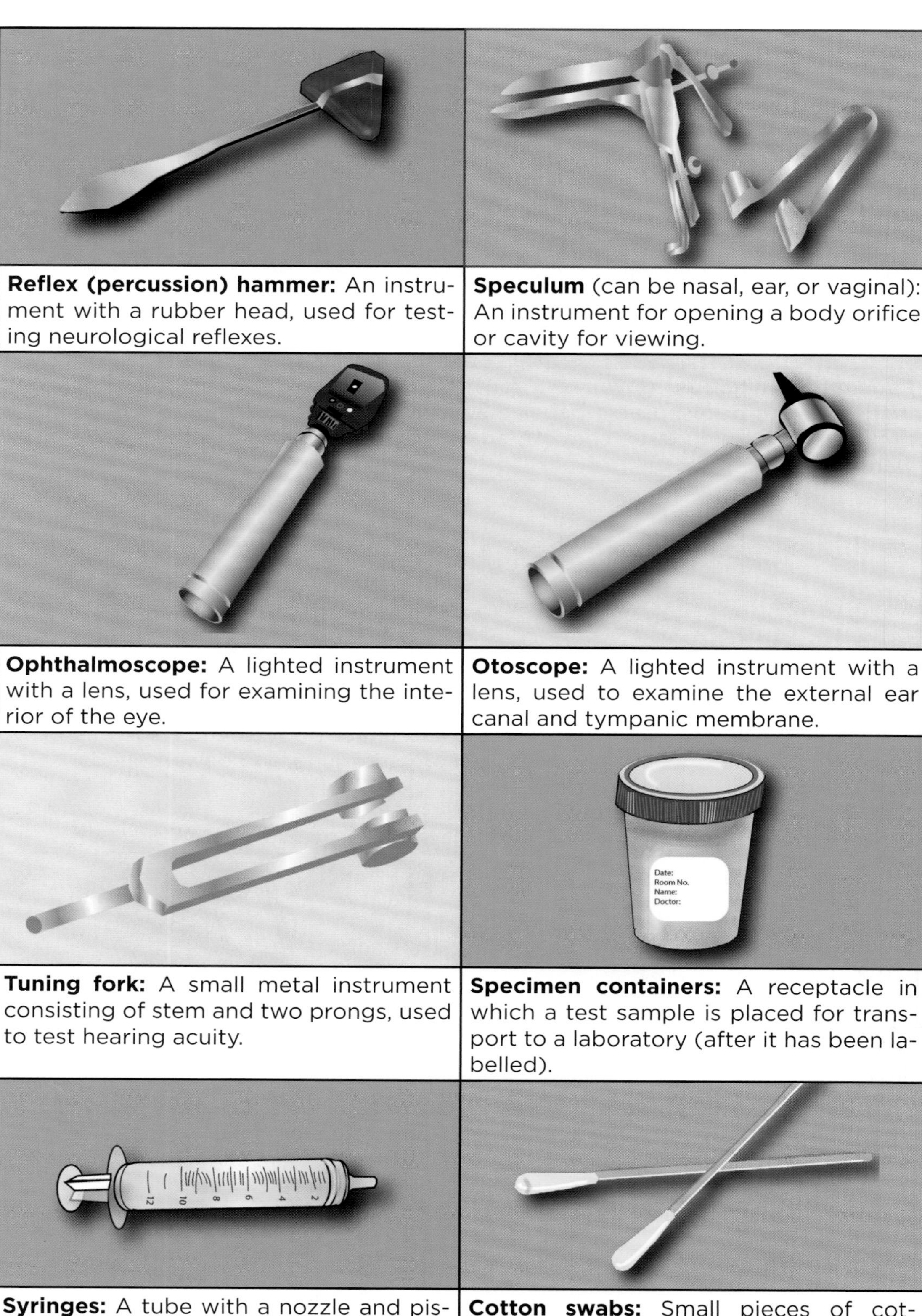

Reflex (percussion) hammer: An instrument with a rubber head, used for testing neurological reflexes.	**Speculum** (can be nasal, ear, or vaginal): An instrument for opening a body orifice or cavity for viewing.
Ophthalmoscope: A lighted instrument with a lens, used for examining the interior of the eye.	**Otoscope:** A lighted instrument with a lens, used to examine the external ear canal and tympanic membrane.
Tuning fork: A small metal instrument consisting of stem and two prongs, used to test hearing acuity.	**Specimen containers:** A receptacle in which a test sample is placed for transport to a laboratory (after it has been labelled).
Syringes: A tube with a nozzle and piston for drawing in and ejecting liquid in a thin stream. Used for cleaning wounds or body cavities. It can also be fitted with a hollow needle for injecting or withdrawing fluids.	**Cotton swabs:** Small pieces of cotton wrapped around the end of a slender wooden stick, used for cleaning of wounds and specimen collection from the body.

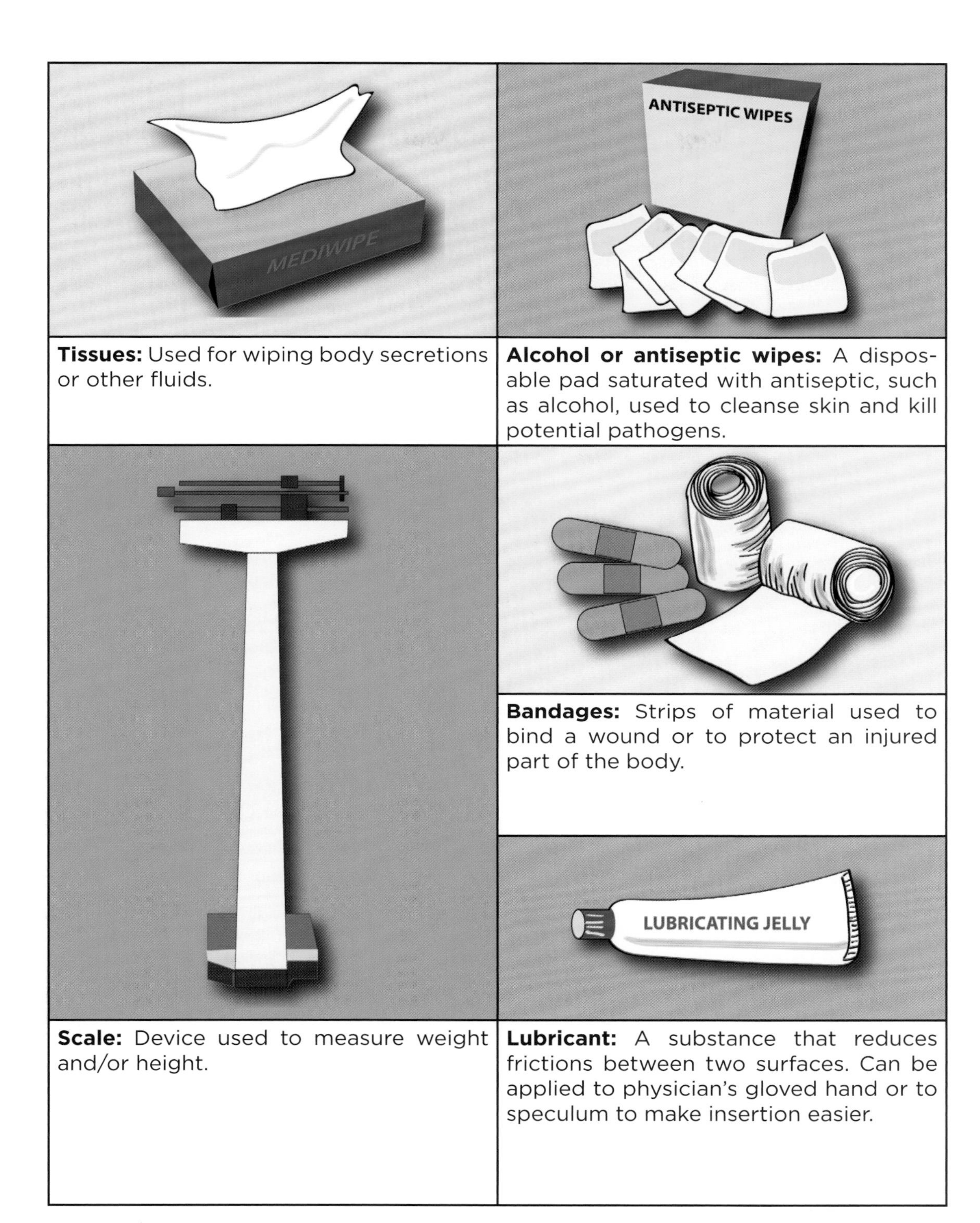

Tissues: Used for wiping body secretions or other fluids.

Alcohol or antiseptic wipes: A disposable pad saturated with antiseptic, such as alcohol, used to cleanse skin and kill potential pathogens.

Bandages: Strips of material used to bind a wound or to protect an injured part of the body.

Scale: Device used to measure weight and/or height.

Lubricant: A substance that reduces frictions between two surfaces. Can be applied to physician's gloved hand or to speculum to make insertion easier.

my notes

Patient Preparation Examples

Type of Examination	Patient Preparation

Physical – Adult; Major Prenatal	• Vitals (blood pressure), height, weight
	• Complete dipstick urinalysis and record results (keep specimen in case it needs to be sent to lab)
	• Ensure venipuncture (blood collection) supplies are available
	• Place adult physical form/Antenatal Record 1 in chart
	• Physician may require patient to be gowned —especially females due for a pap smear or breast exam, and men due for a prostate exam
	• If pap is required, also assemble pap supplies:
	  • Speculum
	  • Lube
	  • Specimen collection kit

Subsequent Prenatal Exam	• Weight, blood pressure • Complete dipstick urinalysis and record results (keep specimen until patient has left) • Ensure Doppler is available for heart sounds • Patients should be gowned and ready if in last four weeks of pregnancy • Ensure Antenatal Record 2 is in chart
Allergy shot	• Allergy serum and supplies prepped
Physical – Infant or Child	• Height or length, weight (infants should be undressed, no diaper), head circumference • Immunizations (card prepped and supplies assembled according to immunization schedule) • Ensure baby record/child physical form is in chart
Suspected Infection or Internal Complaint	• Temperature • UTI – dipstick urinalysis • Sore throat—Quick strep kit
All other adult visits	• Blood pressure • Ensure all supplies are refilled
All other elderly adult visits	• Height • Blood pressure
All other child (<16) visits	• Height and weight for medication dosage

Methods of Examination

Vital Signs

The four vital signs taken during a routine exam by a physician are: body temperature, pulse rate, respiration rate, and blood pressure. Vital signs are important for detecting or monitoring medical problems.

Body Temperature

The normal body temperature of a patient may vary depending on gender, recent activity, amount of food and fluid consumption, time of day, and the stage of menstrual cycle in women. For a healthy adult, the range of normal body temperature can be from 36.5 °C to 37.2 °C (97.8 °F to 99 °F). A patient's body temperature can be obtained in one of several ways:

- **Orally:** Temperature can be taken by mouth to measure the body temperature where the average normal is 37°C (98.6°F).
- **Rectally:** Temperatures taken rectally tend to be 0.3°C to 0.5 °C (0.5°F to 0.7 °F) higher than when taken by mouth.
- **Axillary:** Temperature taken under the arm tends to be 0.4°C to 0.6 °C (0.3°F to 0.4 °F) lower.
- **Tympanic:** A special thermometer is used to quickly measure the temperature of the eardrum, but tends to be 0.3°C to 0.6°C (0.5°F to 1.0°F) higher than an oral temperature.
- **By Skin:** This is the least invasive way to measure temperature and is most useful for monitoring a fever. A special thermometer is used to quickly measure the temperature of the skin on the forehead and tends to be 0.3°C to 0.6°C (0.5°F to 1.0°F) lower than an oral temperature.

If the patient has a fever (high temperature) or hypothermia (low temperature), the body temperature may be dangerously abnormal. According to The College of Family Physicians of Canada, a fever is present when the body temperature rises one degree or more over the normal temperature of 37.0 °C (98.6 °F). Hypothermia is classified as when the body temperature drops below 35.0 °C (95.0 °F).

Pulse Rate

Pulse rate (or heart rate) is the number of times the heart beats in a minute. The normal pulse for healthy adults can range anywhere from 60 to 100 beats per minute (BPM), though it may fluctuate and increase with exercise, illness, injury, or emotional state. Normal is relative, though. For example, athletes may have heart rates near 40 beats per minute and experience no problem as a result of cardiovascular conditioning. Also, females aged 12 and older tend to have faster heart rates than males.

There are multiple points of the body where the pulse can be found, such as on the side of the neck, on the inside of the elbow, or at the wrist. There are more locations that the pulse can be felt, but these three are the easiest to access in a typical clinical setting.

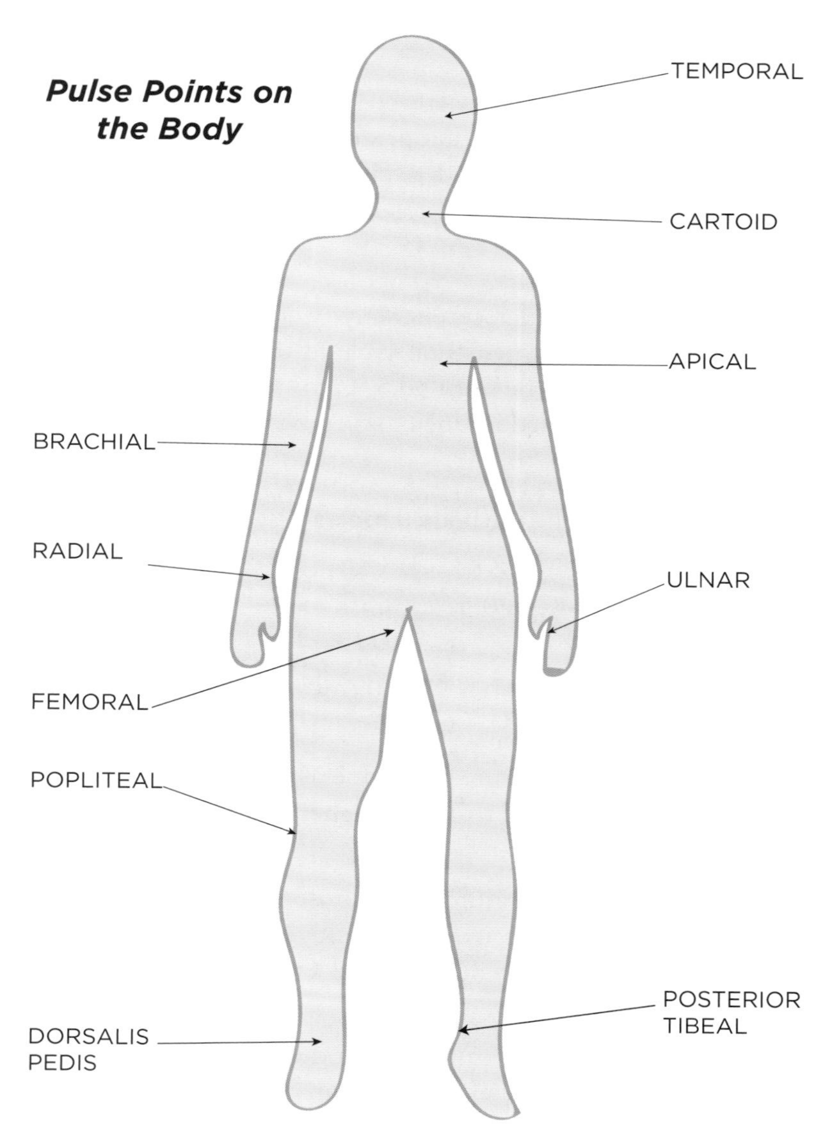

Pulse Points on the Body

The pulse can be felt throughout the body, wherever an artery is easily felt through soft tissues. When the heart forces blood through the arteries, you feel the beats by firmly pressing on the arteries located close to the surface of the skin. Never use your thumb when taking a pulse rate, as your thumb has its own pulse rate and can be confused with the patient's.

For most people, it is easiest to take the pulse at the wrist (radial pulse) by using the first and second fingertips to press firmly on the inside of the wrist and just below the thumb. Begin counting the pulse when the clock's second hand is on the 12. Count the pulse for 60 seconds or you can count for 30 seconds and multiply the number by two to calculate beats per minute. Alternatively, you can count for 10 seconds and multiply the number by six to calculate beats per minute. Concentrate on the beats of the pulse instead of focusing on the clock while counting. If the pulse is difficult to find, you can easily shift upwards to the inner elbow (brachial pulse). The brachial pulse is a good option for infants.

Taking pulse at the wrist

If you do decide to take the pulse on the side of the neck (carotid pulse), make sure you do not press too hard and never press on the pulses on both sides of the lower neck at the same time—this may block blood flow to the brain.

Start by placing your first and second fingertips on the neck to the side of the windpipe. When you feel a pulse, start counting the number of beats in 10 or 15 seconds. Ask another person to assist or count for you if you are ever unsure about the results you have calculated.

Respiration Rate

Respiration rate is the number of breaths a person takes per minute, and is usually measured when a person is at rest. Measure the number of breaths (counting how many times the chest rises) for 30 seconds and multiply this number by two. A normal respiration rate for an adult at rest may range from 12 to 16 breaths per minute. It is important to note whether or not a person has difficulty breathing. The respiration rate may increase with fever, illness, or other medical conditions.

Blood Pressure

Measured with a blood pressure cuff and stethoscope or an electronic sphygmomanometer, blood pressure is the force of blood pushing against the artery walls. Each time the heart beats, it pushes blood through the arteries—at this moment, blood pressure is at its highest. A nurse or a health care provider records two numbers when measuring blood pressure. The higher number (systolic pressure) refers to the pressure inside the artery when the heart contracts and pumps blood through the body.

The lower number (diastolic pressure) refers to the pressure inside the artery when the heart is at rest and is filling with blood. Both of these numbers are recorded using the pressure unit, mmHg (millimetres of mercury).

According to the National Heart, Lung, and Blood Institute of the National Institutes of Health, high blood pressure for adults is defined as 140 mmHg and greater systolic pressure or 90 mmHg and greater diastolic pressure. A new category was added called prehypertension and is defined as 120 mmHg to 139 mmHg systolic pressure or 80 mmHg to 89 mmHg diastolic pressure. Normal blood pressure is any measurements that are less than 120 mm Hg systolic pressure and any measures less than 80 mmHg diastolic pressure.

High blood pressure or hypertension directly increases the risk of coronary heart disease and stroke. With high blood pressure, the arteries may strengthen and increase resistance to the flow of blood, forcing the heart to work harder to pump blood throughout the body.

As with all measurements, keep in mind that these ranges may vary between patients, and a single elevated blood pressure is not necessarily an indication of a problem. A person who normally runs a lower-than-usual blood pressure may be considered hypertensive with lower blood pressure measurements than 140/90. In order to interpret the results, the physician may order multiple blood pressure measurements over a period of time (several days or weeks) before making a diagnosis and starting treatment.

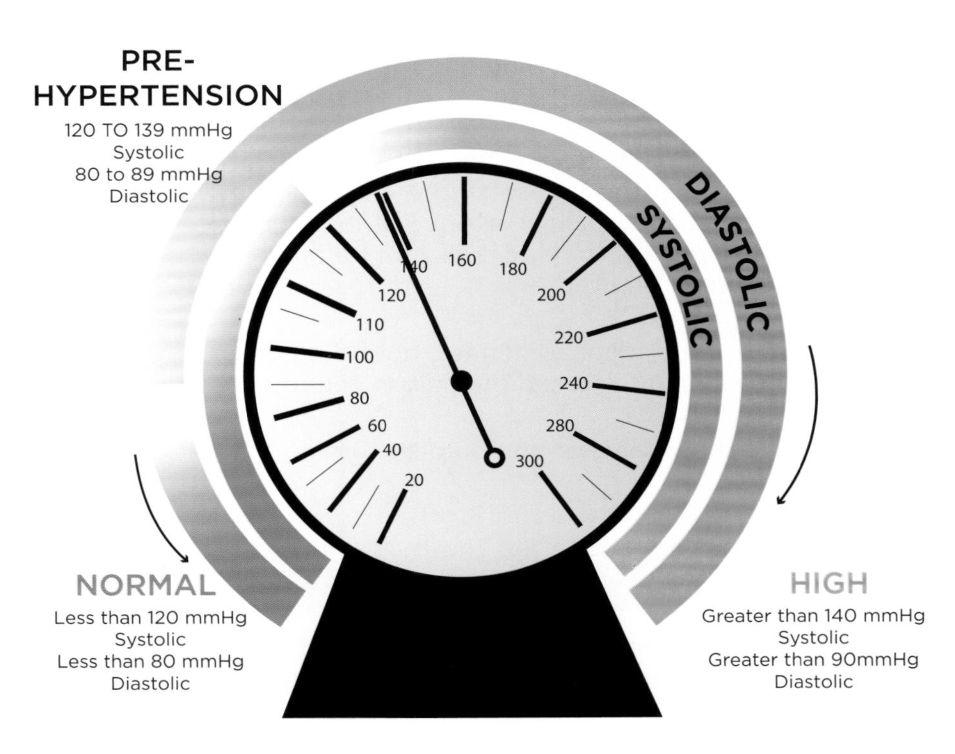

How to

MEASURING BLOOD PRESSURE

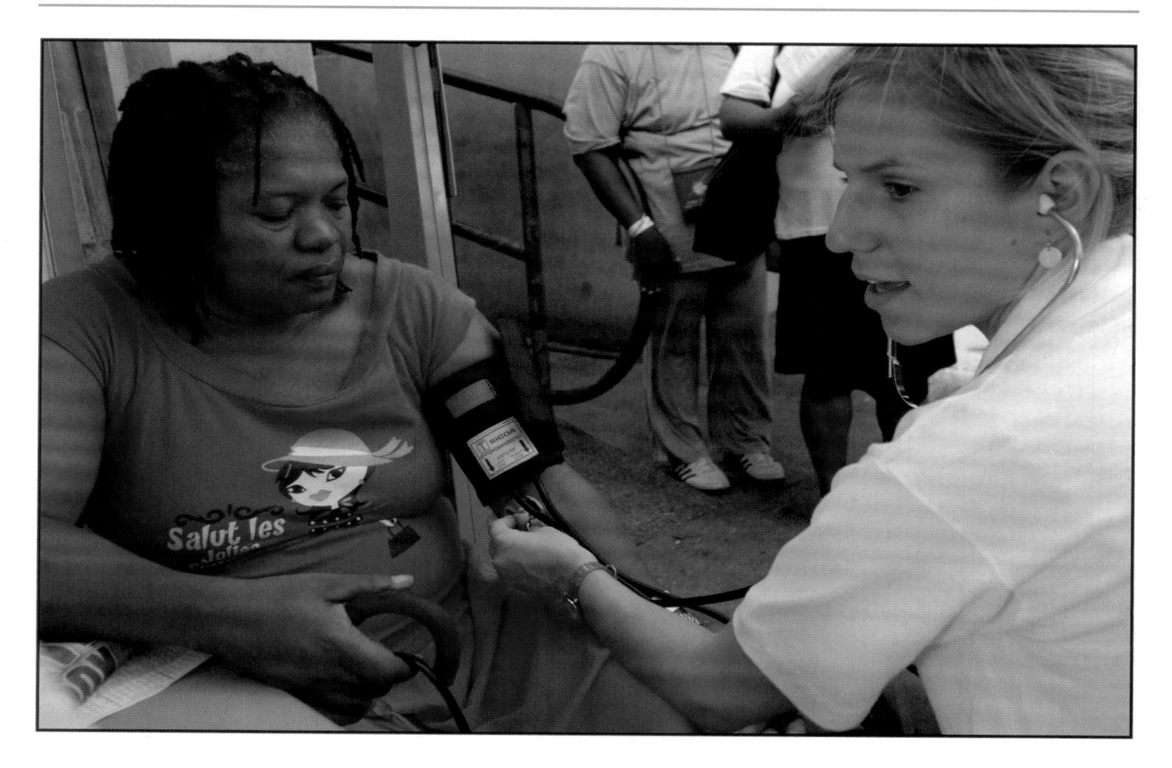

Before you measure blood pressure, it is a good idea to have the patient rest without talking for three to five minutes before taking a measurement. Have the patient sit in a comfortable chair with their back supported, with their legs and ankles uncrossed. With the arm raised to the same level as the heart, wrap the cuff smoothly and snugly around the upper part of the arm. The cuff should be sized to fit smoothly while still allowing enough room for one fingertip to slip under it.

1. Make sure that the bottom edge of the cuff is at least one inch above the crease of the elbow. Place the stethoscope at the brachial artery, just below the cuff. Instruct the patient to relax their arm before beginning to take their blood pressure.

2. If you are using a manual monitor, hold the pressure gauge in your left hand and the bulb in your right.

3. Close the airflow valve on the bulb by turning the screw clockwise.

4. Inflate the cuff by squeezing the bulb with your right hand—you may hear a pulse in the stethoscope.

5. Watch the gauge and keep inflating the cuff until the gauge reads about 30 points (mmHg) above the expected systolic pressure—around 180 mmHg. At this point, you should not hear a pulse in the stethoscope.

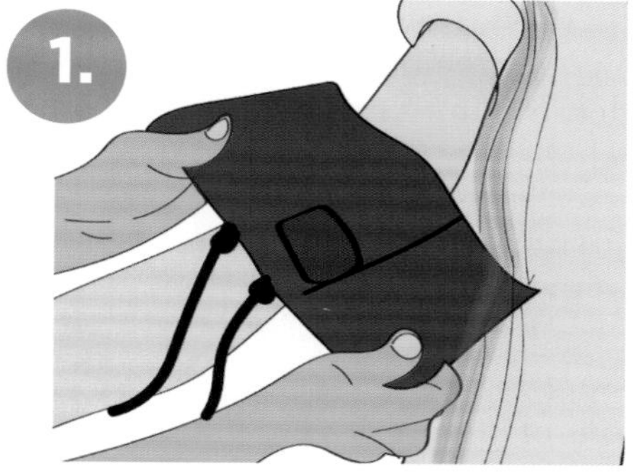

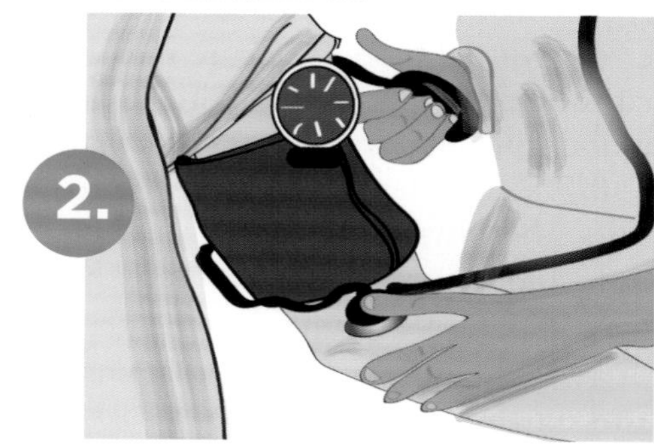

6. Slowly release the pressure in the cuff at a moderate rate of 3mm/sec by opening the airflow valve counter clockwise while keeping your eyes on the gauge. The gauge should fall only two to three points with each second.

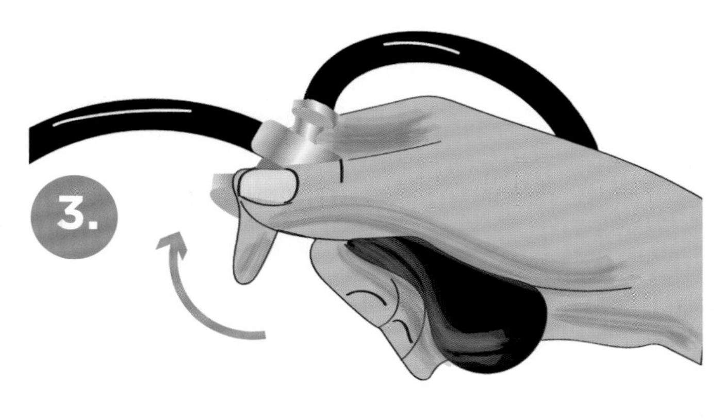

7. Listen carefully for a knocking sound (**Krotkoff sound**) and note the reading on the gauge. This measurement is the systolic pressure.

8. Continue to deflate the cuff slowly and listen until the sound disappears. As soon as you no longer hear the knock, note the reading on the gauge as this is the diastolic pressure.

9. Deflate the cuff completely and remove the cuff from the patient's arm. Note in the patient's chart the date and time their blood pressure was taken.

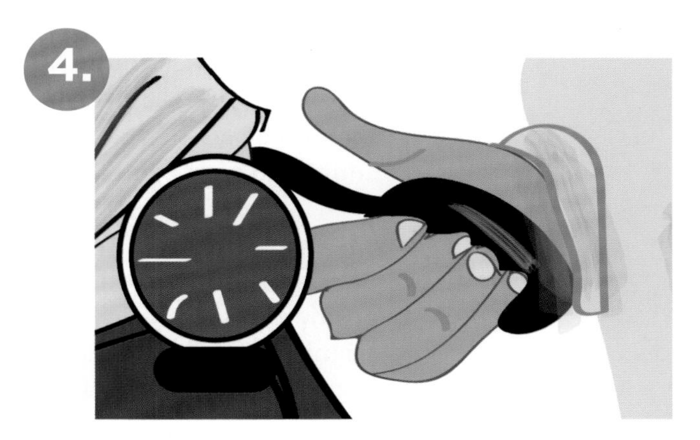

Note: Do not inflate the cuff right away again if you released the pressure too quickly or if you cannot hear a pulse. Wait one minute before trying to measure the blood pressure again. Start by reapplying the cuff and going through the same steps. If you still have trouble listening to the pulse, have additional medical personnel help you.

If the patient's pressure is elevated, measure blood pressure two additional times, waiting a few minutes between measurements.

Krotkoff sounds: *The knocking sounds you hear when taking blood pressure are called Krotkoff sounds. This is actually the sound of turbulent blood spurting through the artery! The sound disappears when the blood flow is restored.*

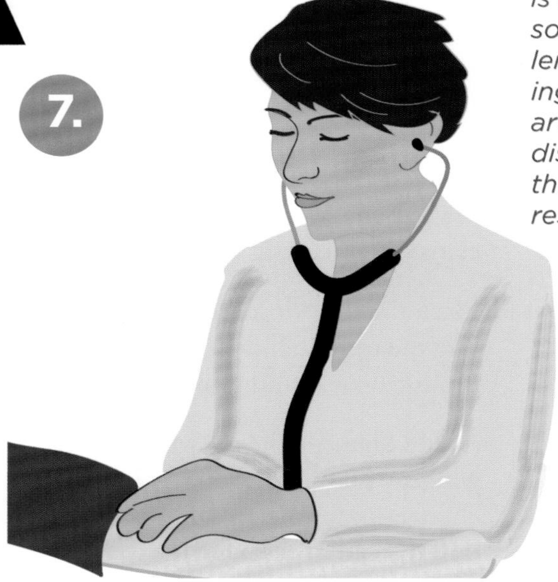

Height and Weight

In order to monitor and keep track of how well a patient is developing or growing, it is best to measure the height and weight of a patient. This is useful for children, a developing fetus, a pregnant woman, the elderly, and someone who has been recently placed on a medication or treatment. For detailed information on how to measure height and weight, read the mensuration section in this chapter.

Inspection

Observation of visual signs is part of the inspection method of examination, and is the one that is most frequently used. For effective observation, it is important to have a well-lit space to conduct the examination.

The patient's colour, speech, deformities, skin condition, body contours, and symmetry can all be assessed through inspection. The patient's body movement and anxiety level can also be inspected through detailed observation. Physicians and medical office assistants should pay attention to details and practice a high level of observational skills for this examination technique.

Palpation

Palpation uses the sense of touch to distinguish size, temperature, vibrations, form, and position to help verify data obtained by inspection. Palpation (along with many of these examination techniques) is not a procedure done by the medical office assistant, but it is important to know what it is to be able to explain the process to a patient.

The patient's facial and verbal communication (E.g. wincing, crying, tensing, and/or rocking) is also observed during palpation to assist the physician in detecting any abnormalities. Examining breasts and taking pulses are examples of palpation.

There are two types of palpation: light and deep. These are characterized by the amount of pressure applied to the examined area. Light palpation is used to determine areas of tenderness where fingertips are placed on the part of examination and is gently depressed approximately one half inch. Deep palpation is used to examine organ condition within the abdomen. One hand supports the body from below and the other presses over the area to be palpated—for example, when a physician is performing a bimanual pelvic exam.

Percussion

Percussion assesses the size, density, and location of the organs. Percussion involves tapping the patient with fingers and listening to the sound elicited or vibratory sensation. Physicians often use this technique when examining the lungs or abdomen.

Place the non-dominant hand with the fingers separated on the area needing assessment. Use the other hand to strike the joint of the non-dominant hand's middle finger. This will produce the sound vibration.

A dull sound is heard when the structures are dense, such as the liver, spleen, and heart whereas a hollow sound is heard from empty or air-filled structures, like the lungs. Any change in condition will result in an abnormal sound (e.g., fluid filled lungs will sound dull instead of resonant).

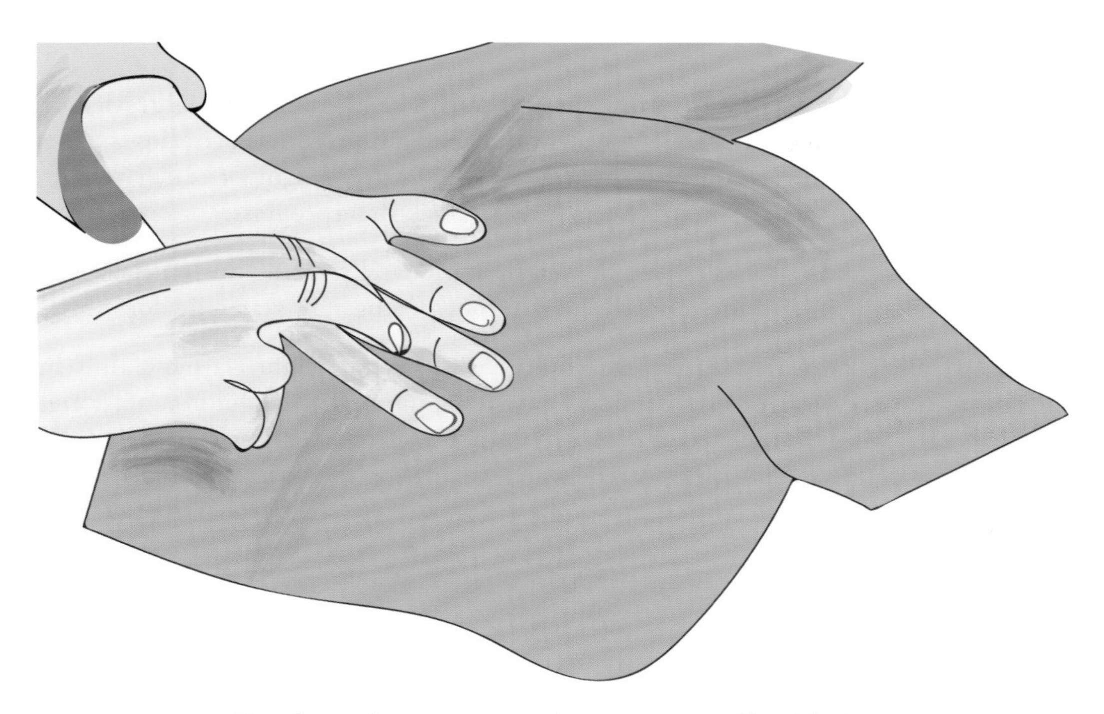

Performing percussion on a patient's lung

Auscultation

This examination technique involves a stethoscope to listen to sounds in the patient's body. Auscultation is used to listen to the heart and lungs and to distinguish between normal and abnormal sounds. The diaphragm of the stethoscope is used to assess high-pitched sounds, like lung and bowel sounds. The bell of the stethoscope chest piece is used to listen to low-pitched sounds, such as those produced by the heart and vascular system.

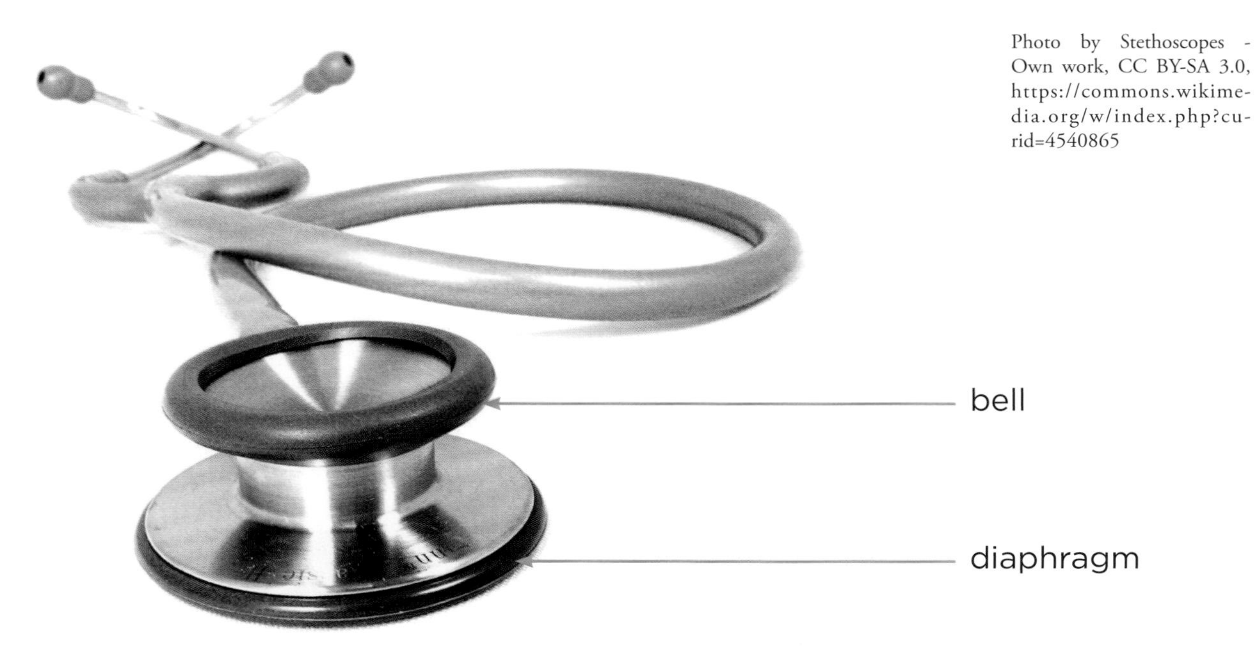

Mensuration

Mensuration is the process of measuring physical traits like height and weight. Measuring weight is important because a change in weight may be significant in diagnosing a patient's condition and prescribing a course of treatment. Weigh overweight or underweight patients following a diet therapy program regularly to track their progress.

Medical office assistants may take part in weighing prenatal patients during each visit to assess fetal development and the mother's health, but nursing staff generally does this.

An adult's weight is measured during each office visit, but the height is usually only measured during the first visit or at a complete physical examination. Children are weighed and their height will be measured during each office visit to keep track of their growth. Obtaining an accurate weight is important when calculating medication dosages.

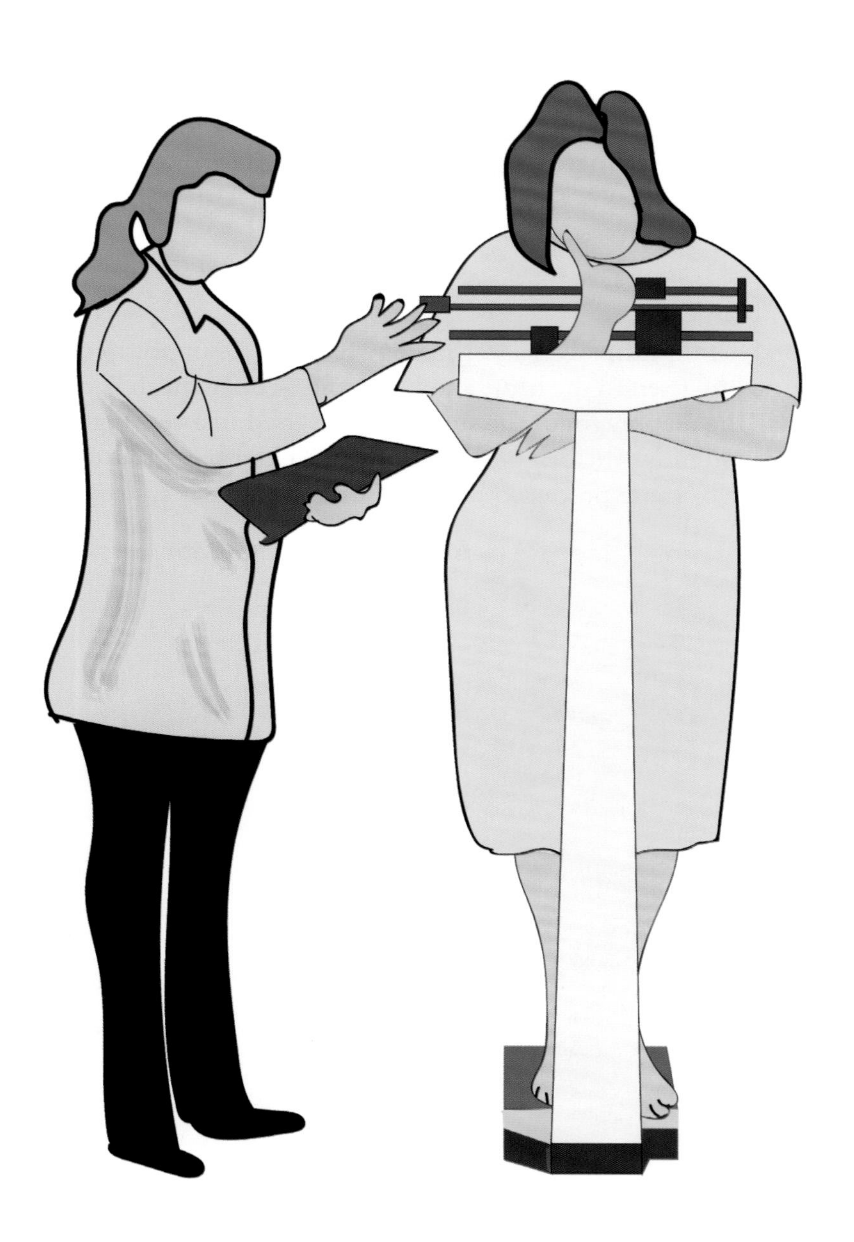

To Obtain an Accurate Weight Measurement

1. Make sure the scale is balanced before measuring the patient's weight by checking to see if upper and lower weights are on zero. The indicator should be in the centre of the balance area to avoid inaccurate readings.
2. Assist the patient onto the scale after asking the patient to remove their shoes and any heavy outer layers such as a coat or jacket.
3. To determine the patient's weight accurately, add the measurement on the lower scale to the upper scale measurement rounding to the nearest quarter pound.

- **Weight conversion:**
  Pounds (lbs) to Kilograms (kg): divide the number of pounds by 2.2
  E.g. 150 lbs ÷ 2.2 = 68.2 kg
  Kilograms (kg) to Pounds (lbs): multiply the number of kilograms by 2.2
  E.g. 60 kg x 2.2 = 132 lbs

Obtaining Accurate Height Measurements

1. With the use of an upright balance scale, slide the movable calibration rod upward until the measuring bar is above the patient's head. Open the measuring bar to its horizontal position.
2. Have the patient remove their shoes and step onto the scale with their back facing the scale and front towards you. Instruct the patient to stare straight ahead with a straight back posture.
3. Lower the measuring bar slowly until it gently rests on top of the patient's head with their hair compressed. There should be a 90-degree angle between the measuring bar with the calibration rod.
4. Keep the measuring bar in place and ask the patient to step down from the scale.
5. At the junction of the stationary calibration rod and movable calibration rod is the height measurement. Record this number in the patient's file.
6. Slide the movable calibration rod to its lower position after the measuring bar has returned to its resting position.
7. Record an accurate height measurement in feet and inches, along with the date and time when this measurement was taken. If you measured in inches, divide the measured number of inches by 12. For example, if a measure of 75 inches is obtained: 75 inches ÷ 12 = 6 feet, 3 inches.

- **Height conversion:**
  Inches to Centimetres: multiply the number of inches by 2.54
  E.g. 75 inches x 2.54 = 190.5 cm
  Centimetres to Inches:
  E.g. 180 cm ÷2.54 = 70.9 inches

Other categories that fall under mensuration include the length or diameter of a patient's extremities or the growth of the uterus during pregnancy. These measurements are important to record when patients come in for their office visit, as they will allow the physician to monitor the patient's progress. Knowing the conversion for weight and height is necessary when it comes to prescribing medication. Accurate mensuration goes hand-in-hand with patient health care and wellbeing.

Manipulation

Manipulation is the systemic moving of a patient's body parts. The physician will exert forceful, but passive movement of a joint to determine range of motion. It is only used in certain types of physical exams, such as a patient with joint difficulties.

my notes

PHYSICAL EXAMINATION

Jim Jones is complaining of abdominal pain with an unknown cause. What types of examination methods will the physician perform to assess Jim's condition?
Answer:

Draping

When you are draping the patient with an examination sheet, remember to explain to them exactly what to expect during the examination. Offer the bathroom or changing area and instruct the patient on how to properly disrobe and put on an exam gown. Once the patient is comfortable and ready, help the patient assume the needed exam position. Draping the patient with an exam sheet will provide privacy and keep the patient warm.

During the physical examination, one body part is exposed at a time and the drape is kept clear from the examination area. The provided drape at the medical office is usually made of paper, but may also be made of cloth. Discard the gown and drape in a waste container after use. Don't forget to sanitize your hands before and after any examination.

Patient Positioning for Physical Examination

Correct positioning helps facilitate the physician's examination. The type of position depends on the sort of examination or procedure to be performed. There is often more than one position to examine the same body part, and it is important to know the correct position for each examination or treatment. There are eight basic positions used in the medical office.

When guiding and assisting patients into different positions, keep in mind that you should follow natural body movements to avoid musculoskeletal injury from occurring. If a patient cannot move into position without pain, reconsider the positioning. The patient's endurance and degree of wellness should also be considered; weak or ill patients may not be able to assume a position. Sometimes special assistance is required for patients to attain the position.

Patient Position	Description	Purpose	How to Drape	Additional Notes
Supine	The patient is lying flat on their back, facing the ceiling.	Used for examination of the front of the body including head, heart, breasts, chest, and abdominal organs. Patient may be placed in this position for radiographs, upper gastrointestinal series, lower gastrointestinal series, intravenous urography, arthrogram, cardiovascular radiography, angiography, CAT scan, MRI, or ultrasound.	Place drape over patient's thigh and legs. Once patient is laying down with legs together, extend the drape lengthwise over the patient. Move drape accordingly to body parts being examined.	Gown should open in front.
Dorsal recumbent	The patient is on their back, with legs bent and rotated outward.	Used for examination of rectal, vaginal, and perineal areas, as well as during the insertion of a urinary catheter.	The drape should be positioned diagonally, with one corner over the patient's chest; the opposite corner falls between the patient's legs and completely covers the pubic area.	This position is more comfortable for patients with respiratory problems, back injury, or lower back pain. Once examination is done, have the patient assume the supine position, then into the sitting position, and finally down from the table.
Sitting	Standard patient position where the patient is in a semi-upright sitting position (80-90 degrees) with their knees bent or straight.	Used for examination of the head, neck, chest and upper extremities.	Place the drape over the patient's thighs and legs	The patient can be placed in this position for radiographs. This is also an effective position for measuring vital signs.

Lithotomy	The position is the same as the dorsal recumbent position except that the patient's feet are placed in stirrups.	Used primarily for vaginal examination that requires the use of a speculum and pap smears. Also used for pelvic and rectal examinations. This position provides maximal exposure to the genital area and facilitates insertion of a vaginal speculum.	Position the drape diagonally with one corner over the patient's chest and the opposite corner between the patient's feet. Reposition the drape as needed so one corner is over the patient's chest and the opposite falls between the patient's legs, completely covering the perineal area. When the genital area is ready to be examined by the physician, pull the centre corner of the drape and fold it back over the knees.	The patient may feel uncomfortable and embarrassed. They shouldn't be kept in these positions for any longer than necessary and not placed in this position until just before examination.
Fowler's	The head of the patient's bed is raised 30 to 90 degrees, with the knees sometimes also elevated.	Used for postsurgical exams, patients with difficulty breathing, and patients with head trauma. Used to examine the upper body of patients with cardiovascular and respiratory problems, including emphysema, congestive heart failure, and asthma. Use this position for patients who are likely to faint when they are having blood drawn.	Place drape over patient's thighs and legs then position the drape lengthwise over the patient. As the physician examines the patient, move the drape accordingly to the body parts being examined.	Patients find it easier to breathe in this position, rather than in a sitting or supine position, as the chest is open. Patient may be placed in this position during a cardiovascular radiography, or angiography.
Prone	The patient is lying on their stomach with head turned to the side. The arms can be straight or folded underneath the head.	Used for examination of the back, assessing extension of the hip joint and for postsurgical examination.	Place the drape over the patient's thighs and legs. Then, ask the patient to lie down and position the drape lengthwise over them.	Instruct the patient to turn onto their stomach by rolling towards you and adjust the drape to keep the patient covered. Do not have them roll away, as they may accidently roll off the table. The patient may be placed in this position for radiographs, upper gastrointestinal series, lower gastrointestinal series, arthrogram, or myelogram. The gown should open to the back.

Patient Position	Description	Purpose	How to Drape	Additional Notes
Sims' Left Lateral	The patient lies on their left side and stomach, with the left leg slightly bent. The right leg has a more severe bend and is pulled up. The positioning is designed to give room for the right leg to be bent and rotated outwards at the hip.	Used for rectal and some pelvic examinations, instillation of rectal medication and rectal thermometer readings. Used to perform flexible sigmoidoscopy, and to administer enema.	Position the drape lengthwise over the patient and ask them to turn onto their left side. The patient's left arm should be positioned behind the body and right arm forward with the elbow bent. Adjust the drape as needed. When the physician is ready for examination, a small portion of the drape is folded back to expose the anal area. After examination, assist the patient into a supine position and into a sitting position, and then down from the table.	Patient may be placed in this position for radiographs, an upper gastrointestinal series, or a lower gastrointestinal series.
Knee-chest	The patient rests on the knees and chest with head turned to one side, arms extended on the bed, and elbows flexed and resting so that they partially bear the patient's weight. The abdomen remains unsupported, though a small pillow may be placed under the chest.	Sometimes used for proctological, rectal, vaginal, and sigmoid examinations. This position provides complete access to the rectal area.	Position the drape diagonally over the patient to provide warmth and modesty with one corner over the patient's back and the opposite corner over the buttocks and falling between the patient's legs. When the physician is ready to examine the patient, a small portion of the drape is folded back to expose the anal area.	The position can be uncomfortable and embarrassing for the patient. Hence, they should not be kept in this position for longer than necessary and should not be placed into it until just before examination. Patients, especially elderly patients, may become dizzy after some time in this position—allow the patient to rest on the examination table before they get off. Assist the patient off the examination table to prevent falls.

Activity

CRITICAL THINKING

Determine the correct patient position and method of gowning/draping for the following:

Instillation of rectal suppository

Pap smear

Examination of the back

Patient with dyspnea

Breast examination

Patient with a head injury

Examination Sequence

What position would the patient be in for each of the steps in the physical exam?

Presenting or General Appearance

Skin

Head

Neck

Eyes

Ears

Nose and sinuses

Mouth and throat

Chest

Breast

Abdomen

Genitalia and Rectum

Extremities

Neurologic

Quiz

CHAPTER 8 QUIZ

1. What is the purpose of a physical examination, and what happens during this assessment? ____________________

____
____
____
____
____
____
____
____

2. What are the three parts that a patient exam consists of?

   a) Health history, physical exam, and laboratory or diagnostic tests

   b) Heart history, physical exam, and prescription

   c) Health history, physiological exam, and laboratory or diagnostic tests

   d) Heart history, physiological exam, and prescription

3. Fill in the blanks: A ____________________ diagnosis determines which disease is producing the patient's symptoms whereas a ________________ diagnosis provides logical basis for treatment and ________________.

4. True or false? A clinical diagnosis helps determine a final diagnosis. A final diagnosis is reached after the physician has analyzed the test results.

5. Colds, influenza, strep throat, and pneumonia are all examples of a(n) ________ illness?

   a) Acute

   b) Chronic

   c) Therapeutic

   d) Diagnostic

6. True or false? Upon check in, the medical office assistant should identify the patient by stating the patient's name and health card number.

7. The patient's colour, speech, deformities, skin condition, body contour, and symmetry can all be assessed through:
   a) Inspection
   b) Palpation
   c) Percussion
   d) Auscultation

8. Tapping the patient with fingers and listening to the sound elicited is which examination technique?
   a) Inspection
   b) Palpation
   c) Percussion
   d) Auscultation

9. Using touch and pressure to verify data obtained by inspection to detect any abnormalities is considered which of the following?
   a) Inspection
   b) Palpation
   c) Percussion
   d) Auscultation

10. Obtaining the height and weight of a patient is an example of: ____________________.

11. Patients with joint difficulties will undergo which type of examination by the physician?

12. True or false? The lithotomy position is used to examine the head, neck, chest, and extremities of patients who have difficulty maintaining the supine position.

13. True or false? The Fowler's position is used for examination of the head, neck, chest, and upper extremities when vital signs are taken.

14. True or false? The prone position is used for examination of the back, assessing extension of the hip joint, and for postsurgical examinations.

15. Which position should the patient be guided into when a urinary catheter is being inserted? ________________________________.

my notes